GASTROINTESTINAL RADIOLOGY

Performing and Interpreting Fluoroscopic Examinations

GASTROINTESTINAL RADIOLOGY

Performing and Interpreting
Fluoroscopic Examinations

David W. Gelfand, M.D.

Professor and Chief of
Gastrointestinal Radiology
Department of Radiology
Bowman Gray School of Medicine
Wake Forest University
Winston-Salem, North Carolina

CHURCHILL LIVINGSTONE
NEW YORK, EDINBURGH, LONDON, AND MELBOURNE   1984

Acquisitions editor: William R. Schmitt

Copy editor: Donna C. Balopole

Production editor: Karen Goldsmith Montanez

Production supervisor: Kerry Ann O'Rourke

Compositor: Progressive Typographers, Inc.

Printer/Binder: Halliday Lithograph

Distributed in the United Kingdom by Churchill Livingstone, Robert Stevenson House, 1-3 Baxter's Place, Leith Walk, Edinburgh EH1 3AF and by associated companies, branches and representatives throughout the world.

First published 1984

Printed in USA

ISBN 0-443-08096-8

9   8   7   6   5   4   3   2   1

Library of Congress Cataloging in Publication Data

Gelfand, David W.
  Gastrointestinal radiology.
  Includes bibliographies and index.
  1. Gastrointestinal system—Radiography. 2. Diagnosis, Fluoroscopic. I. Title. [DNLM: 1. Fluoroscopy.
2. Gastrointestinal System—radiography. WI 141 G316g]
RC804.F55G45 1984   616.3'307572   84-9497
ISBN 0-443-08096-8

Manufactured in the United States of America

To my loving wife, Eva, and to my daughters, Deborah and Miriam

Preface

The intention of this book is twofold. First, it attempts to provide a compact but reasonably thorough reference volume usable by the practicing radiologist. It is also intended as a guide to the resident physician training in gastrointestinal radiology or preparing for the certification examinations. The text limits itself to those studies employing barium sulfate as the contrast medium, which represent most of a typical day's fluoroscopic schedule.

The book is informally divided into two sections: one on performing the gastrointestinal examinations and one on interpreting those examinations. The first section devotes itself to fluoroscopic and radiographic methodology, with descriptions of the accepted techniques for performing the various examinations. The second section discusses the interpretation of these examinations, beginning with fundamental diagnostic principles and proceeding to the radiographic appearances of specific lesions. Included in this section are lists of differential diagnosis closely following the approach of Reeder and Felson in *Gamuts in Radiology.*

Every attempt has been made to keep this book compact. In this regard, I have been influenced by the author and philosopher Eric Hoffer who has said that when confronted with two books by the same author, one thick and one thin, he always chooses to read the thin book first. Hoffer's observation has been that the thin book usually presents what the author knows, while the thick book represents what he does not know.

David W. Gelfand, M.D.

Acknowledgments

The benevolent influence and kind help of many individuals were required to bring this book into being.

My deepest debt is to Dr. Benjamin Felson, under whom I trained, and who managed to convey to me a very small part of his love of radiology and an appreciation of the value of scholarship. His unwavering support through the years has been typical of the generosity of this remarkable man. While a resident at the University of Cincinnati, I was introduced to gastrointestinal radiology by Dr. Jerome F. Wiot, whose skills as a radiologist are formidable and whose training has served me well.

A particular debt is owed to Dr. Herbert L. Abrams, with whom I trained for a year at Stanford University. From Dr. Abrams one learned the necessity for meticulous work in both clinical and investigative pursuits.

While at Stanford, I met Dr. Gerald W. Friedland who many years later, as Chief of Diagnostic Radiology at Bowman Gray, asked me to join him and to assume responsibility for gastrointestinal radiology. For this opportunity, and for his friendship over the years, I hold an immense gratitude. I hold in similar regard Dr. Isadore Meschan and Dr. C. Douglas Maynard, the successive Chairmen of the Bowman Gray Radiology Department, for providing that rare atmosphere in which academic endeavors are supported and encouraged.

I also wish to express my good fortune in having as my very capable associate Dr. David J. Ott, who performed many of the studies illustrated in this book and who unselfishly made available much of the photographic material incorporated in the text. Finally, I thank Mrs. Carolyn Shaver and Mrs. Carolyn Ezzell for their efforts in preparing this manuscript.

Contents

1

Characteristics of Barium Sulfate Suspensions

Barium sulfate is unique among contrast media by virtue of being a suspension rather than a solution. Its inert nature and insolubility in water have made it for over fifty years the contrast medium of choice for examining the gastrointestinal tract. Although the barium sulfate in all suspensions intended for diagnostic purposes is chemically identical, to a large extent the differing physical characteristics of the commercially available suspensions determine the possibilities and limitations of the gastrointestinal examination.

SUSPENSION STABILITY

The great differences in stability among the barium sulfate preparations are illustrated in Figure 1-1. This illustration demonstrates that within ½ hour after mixing, certain commercial barium sulfate suspensions intended for the single-contrast barium enema will have completely settled. When this happens in a patient, most of the column of barium suspension will be almost totally water, and those lesions surrounded by the portion devoid of

barium will not be visible radiographically. Because a poor quality suspension may jeopardize the ability to make a diagnosis, and because excellent suspensions are available, there is no reason for using a poorly suspended material.

For practical purposes, commercially available barium suspensions fall into two groups based on suspension stability. The first group is comprised of poorly suspended preparations of low viscosity, which can be prepared by manually shaking or stirring the powdered barium sulfate with water, and which include several very popular preparations. Most of these materials stay in uniform suspension for only a few minutes, and signs of flocculation or settling are visible during various examinations.

The second group is more effectively suspended, with considerable adjuvant material added to maintain the suspension for long intervals. Generally, these adjuvants are large, complex organic molecules that raise viscosity, physically slowing the settling of the barium sulfate particles. In certain of these preparations, the barium sulfate particles may be held in suspension almost indefinitely. Virtually all suspensions in this second

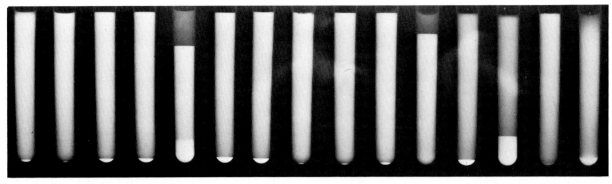

Fig. 1-1 In vitro settling test of fifteen commercially available barium suspensions as used for the full column barium enema at 15 percent weight per volume. The considerable differences in suspension stability are immediately apparent on this film taken 30 minutes after original agitation of the suspensions. All of the suspensions showing virtually complete stability at this low density were suspended in pectin and were of submicron average particle size (Gelfand DW, Ott DJ: Barium sulfate suspensions. An evaluation of available products. AJR 138:935, 1982. © 1982 Am Roentgen Ray Soc.).

group require high-speed mechanical mixing. Increasingly, these suspensions are prepared by the manufacturer and sold as ready-to-use liquids.

Certain fallacies regarding barium sulfate particle size should be mentioned. First, there are no truly colloidal barium sulfate suspensions for purposes of diagnostic radiology. Although colloidal suspensions can be produced, the required particle size is extremely small (0.1 μm or less) and the maximum density of the resulting suspension is so low as to preclude practical application. A second

fallacy is that small particle size per se is a guarantee of a high quality barium sulfate suspension. In reality, the adjuvants in a suspension are more important than particle size in determining clinical usefulness.

COATING ABILITY

Good coating ability, as assessed on radiographs, is a combination of two qualities. First, the barium

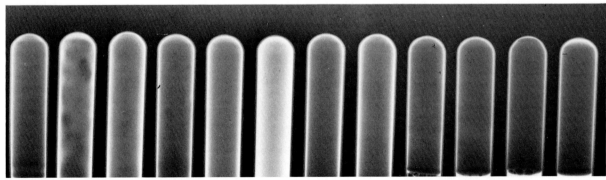

Fig. 1-2 Film of an inverted rack of test tubes half filled with barium suspension showing differences in coating opacity and uniformity of twelve commercially available products. Those showing greatest opacity were viscous materials specifically intended for the double-contrast barium enema. Several low viscosity suspensions of the manually mixed variety (on the right) are of significantly lower opacity (Gelfand DW, Ott DJ: Barium sulfate suspensions: An evaluation of available products. AJR 138:935, 1982. © 1982 Am Roentgen Ray Soc.).

sulfate suspension coating the mucosa must have sufficient radiographic opacity so as to be clearly visible (Fig. 1-2). Second, the film of liquid covering the mucosal surface should be uniformly distributed, and it should maintain that uniformity long enough for radiographs to be obtained.

The apparent radiographic density of a film of barium sulfate suspension is the result of its density and the thickness of the film of liquid deposited on the mucosal surface. Adjustment of density is an easy matter, but production of a thick, uniform coating is more difficult. In general, viscous barium sulfate suspensions produce a thicker film of barium sulfate on the mucosa than do suspensions of watery consistency. Thus, barium sulfate suspensions intended for double-contrast examinations are usually very dense, very viscous, or both.

The coating ability of a barium suspension also depends on its interaction with the physiologic characteristics of the organ being examined. The esophagus may be difficult to coat because of the stripping acting of peristalsis, but it neither excretes nor absorbs fluids to any great extent. The stomach is a secretory organ whose volume of acid secretions may be sufficient to wash the barium suspension off of its mucosal surface and may flocculate the barium sulfate particles if the suspension is not acid resistant. On the other hand, the colon absorbs water and may dry out a barium sulfate suspension deposited on its mucosal surface, re-

Table 1-1. Adjuvants Commonly Employed in Commercially Available Barium Sulfate Suspensions

Suspending Agents	**Defoaming Agents**
Alginic acid	Dimethyl polysiloxane (simethicone)
Avicel°	Ethyl polysilicate
Carbopols	
Carboxymethylcellulose	
Carboxymethyldextran	**Humectants**
Gelatin	Glycerin
Gum arabic (acacia)	Sodium chloride
Gum ghatti	Sorbitol
Gum karaya	
Gum tragacanth	
Kaolin	**Acidifiers and Antacids**
Methylcellulose	Aluminum hydroxide
Mucilaginous gels	Citric acid
Pectin	Magnesium aluminum silicate
Polyvinyl pyrolidone	Magnesium trisilicate
Sodium alginate	Sodium bicarbonate
Sodium carboxymethylcellulose	Sodium carbonate
Sodium cellulose acetate sulfate	Tartaric acid
Sodium hydroxyethylcellulose	
Sodium montmorillonite (bentonite, Veegum°)	
Sorbitol	**Preservatives**
Starch	Methyl paraben
	Potassium sorbate
Dispersing Agents	Propyl paraben
Alkalinated polysaccharide—sulfuric acid esters	
Carageenan	
Sodium carboxymethylcellulose	**Flavoring Agents**
Sodium citrate	Chocolate
Sodium dextran sulfate	Dextrose
	Ethyl vanillin
Wetting Agents	Levulose
Dioctyl sodium sulfosuccinate	Maltose
Lecithin	Palatone°
Mono-oleate of sorbitan polyethylene glycol	Sodium cyclamate
Myrj 45°	Sodium saccharin
Polyoxyethylenes	Sucrose
Sodium lauryl sulfate	Sugar
Tween 80°	Vanillin

°Brand name.

sulting in an uneven or flake-like appearance of the coating during double-contrast studies.

COMMONLY USED ADJUVANTS

Virtually all barium suspensions contain adjuvant materials designed to enhance suspension or coating. These may be divided into the several groups summarized in Table 1-1. A detailed description of these materials and their use in barium sulfate suspensions is beyond the scope of this text. The best resumé of this subject appears in *Radiographic Contrast Agents*, edited by Miller and Skucas.

PROPER PREPARATION AND STORAGE

Proper preparation of a barium sulfate suspension is complicated by the fact that barium sulfate powder cannot be accurately measured by volume. Barium sulfate powder from the top of a large container may be appreciably less dense per unit volume than that finally taken from the bottom of the same container. As a result, the practice of simply adding a certain number of cups of barium sulfate powder to a given volume of water is guaranteed to result in barium suspensions of inconsistent density.

The more accurate method is to weigh the barium sulfate powder on a small dietary scale, available at restaurant supply shops, and add it to a known volume of water, mixing it either manually or by machine as required. A chart of the amounts of barium sulfate powder and water required to produce approximately 500 ml or 2 cups (16 oz) of barium suspensions of various densities is given in Table 1-2. Increasingly, however, radiologists are using unit-dose barium powders weighed and packaged in plastic cups or disposable enema bags, or they are using barium suspensions prepared and bottled by the manufacturer.

The refrigeration of stored barium sulfate suspensions should be stressed. Suspensions made on site from powders will contain bacteria and may be capable of supporting bacterial growth. They must therefore be refrigerated for long-term storage. Generally speaking, factory-prepared liquid bariums contain preservatives that prevent bacterial growth, and refrigeration is less critical.

Certain further precautions should be observed. All mixers and storage vessels should be cleaned with hot water after each fluoroscopy session. Also, disposable bags and tips should be used for barium enemas, since pressures within the colon can propel barium from the colon into an enema can several feet above the table. Cultures of non-disposable enema tips, tubing, and cans invariably show contamination by fecal organisms, raising the possibility of iatrogenic contagion.

Table 1-2. Preparation of Barium Sulfate Suspension°

%wt/vol†	%wt/wt‡	Specific Gravity	H₂O oz	H₂O ml	BaSO₄ oz	BaSO₄ g
15	13	1.12	16.3	483	2.8	79
20	17	1.17	16.2	478	3.7	105
30	24	1.25	15.8	467	5.6	158
45	32	1.37	15.2	450	8.4	237
60	40	1.50	14.6	433	11.1	318
75	46	1.62	14.1	417	13.9	395
100	55	1.82	13.1	382	18.5	526

° This table shows the preparation of 500 ml of barium sulfate suspension from powder containing 95% barium sulfate. Densities are listed as percent weight per volume, percent weight per weight, and specific gravity. Final density may vary slightly due to the differing amounts of adjuvant material, usually 3 to 9% by weight, in commercial preparations. For example, to prepare a 75 % wt/vol suspension, add 14-oz barium sulfate powder to 14-oz water. Rounding off quantities for convenience has little practical effect.
† % wt/vol = weight of BaSO₄ per volume of suspension × 100.
‡ % wt/wt = weight of BaSO₄ per weight of suspension × 100.

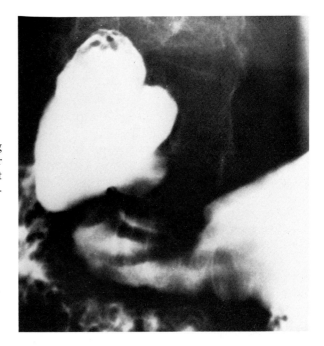

Fig. 1-3 Compression film of the distal stomach showing the deformity and converging folds of a gastric ulcer scar. The easy compressibility of the 72 percent weight per volume suspension employed during this conventional upper gastrointestinal series is illustrated.

DESIRABLE CHARACTERISTICS FOR INDIVIDUAL EXAMINATIONS

The Standard Upper Gastrointestinal Series

Barium suspensions used for the standard upper gastrointestinal series usually fall between 60 and 100 percent weight per volume. In this range, it is relatively easy to see pathologic lesions through the column of barium sulfate when compression is applied (Fig. 1-3). Also, the barium is easily seen fluoroscopically and double-contrast films are usually of adequate quality.

In general, the barium used for the full column upper gastrointestinal series should be as well sus-

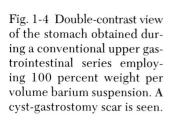

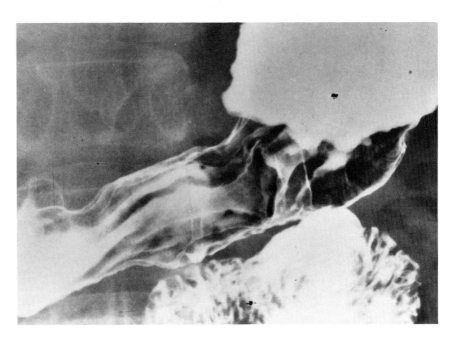

Fig. 1-4 Double-contrast view of the stomach obtained during a conventional upper gastrointestinal series employing 100 percent weight per volume barium suspension. A cyst-gastrostomy scar is seen.

pended as possible. The same barium is commonly used for any subsequent small bowel examination and it must therefore possess the suspension stability needed for the small bowel examination. Good coating ability is also required, since the conventional upper gastrointestinal examination usually includes double-contrast films of various areas of the stomach and of the duodenal bulb (Fig. 1-4). Overall, a moderately viscous preparation is usually best for achieving the desired combination of suspension stability and good coating.

The Double-Contrast Upper Gastrointestinal Series

In the double-contrast upper gastrointestinal series, superior coating ability is the primary quality desired of the barium sulfate suspension (Fig. 1-5). Radiologists performing these examinations have been employing high density barium sulfate suspensions ranging up to 250 percent weight per volume. To date, all of the barium suspensions recommended for this examination have been formulated specifically for this purpose, and they are not appropriate for other examinations.

Most suspensions marketed for the double-contrast upper gastrointestinal examination are sold in conjunction with a specific gas-producing agent. These tablets or powders usually contain sodium bicarbonate, a weak acid, and an antifoaming agent. Best results are usually achieved using a particular manufacturer's barium suspension and gas producer together.

Because of its extreme density, a minimal volume of high density barium suspension should be used if a small bowel series is to follow. A small bowel series can be performed with these high density, poorly suspended materials, but it will be suboptimal, particularly when there is malabsorption. In general, it is best to switch to a lower density, more stable suspension suitable for the small bowel examination after double-contrast films of the esophagus, stomach, and duodenal bulb have been obtained.

The Small Bowel Examination

Barium intended for the peroral examination of the small bowel should be as well suspended as possible (Fig. 1-6A). Unabsorbed food products

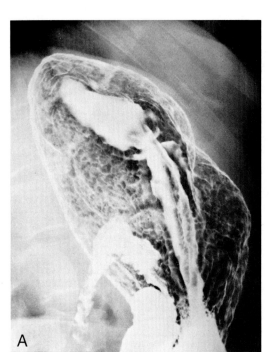

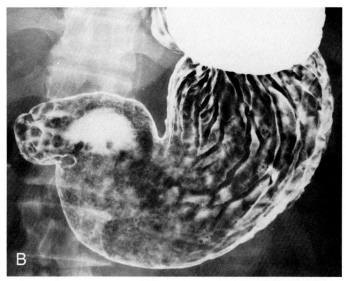

Fig. 1-5 Double-contrast views of the stomach employing 250 percent weight per volume barium suspension of low viscosity to show maximum surface detail. (A) Prominent areae gastricae in the proximal stomach. (B) Erosive antral gastritis.

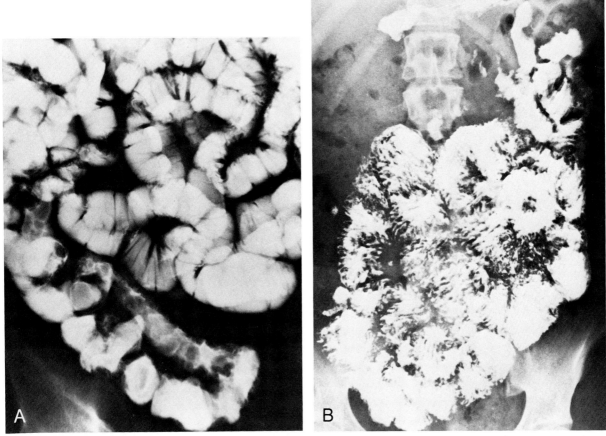

Fig. 1-6 Examples of well-suspended and poorly suspended barium suspensions during small bowel examinations. (A) A very well-suspended preparation employed at 18 percent weight per volume during an enteroclysis examination showing Crohn's disease of the distal ileum. (B) Severe sedimentation of a poorly suspended barium preparation in a patient with nontropical sprue.

and mucous encountered during the examination of the abnormal small bowel tend to force barium sulfate particles out of suspension, a process often termed *flocculation* or *sedimentation* (Fig. 1-6B). It is preferable that the barium remain well suspended so as to demonstrate the structural abnormalities of the small bowel, since this allows differentiation of the specific condition causing malabsorption. In general, the more viscous barium suspensions are most likely to remain suspended in the face of malabsorption.

The appropriate density for barium for the peroral small bowel examination is in the range of 50 to 75 percent weight per volume. At lower densi-

ties, radiographic contrast may be insufficient and structural detail is lost, particularly with large patients. At higher densities, it becomes impossible to see through superimposed small bowel loops.

A special case exists for the enteroclysis examination, or small bowel enema. This examination may be performed satisfactorily with any well-suspended barium sulfate preparation, using a density of 15 to 30 percent weight per volume.

The Full Column Barium Enema

Barium sulfate suspensions intended for the full column enema must excel in their ability to stay

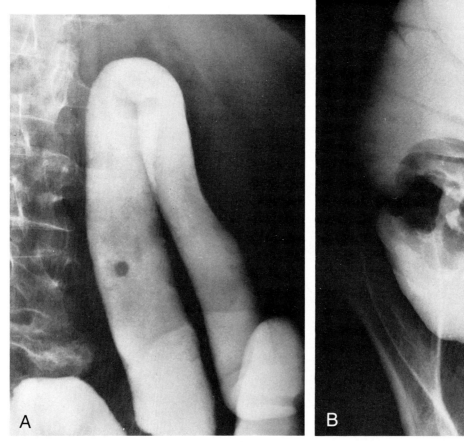

Fig. 1-7 Full column barium enema films employing 18 percent weight per volume barium suspension, 100 to 110 kVp, and compression. (A) A 6-mm polyp at the splenic flexure. (B) A circumferential carcinoma of the ileocecal valve region.

well suspended at low densities. Because the standard barium enema is basically a "see through" technique, barium density is usually held to 15 to 25 percent weight per volume (Fig. 1-7). Keeping barium sulfate particles well suspended at these low densities is difficult, since there is considerable dilution of the suspending agents.

Other characteristics desired for the standard barium enema are the ability to produce good postevacuation films and a reasonable air-contrast examination following the full column study if required (Fig. 1-8). In general, the ability to produce good postevacuation and air-contrast films is related to both the density of barium sulfate and the viscosity of the suspension. Increasing the barium

sulfate density to about 25 percent weight per volume is helpful, but decreases the ability to see filling defects, such as polyps, through the column of barium.

The Double-Contrast Barium Enema

The most effective preparations for the double-contrast barium enema have been designed specifically for this purpose. They range from 60 to 125 percent weight per volume density, and tend to be quite viscous so as to produce a thick, easily visible coating (Fig. 1-9). Most contain wetting agents and humectants to achieve uniform coating and pre-

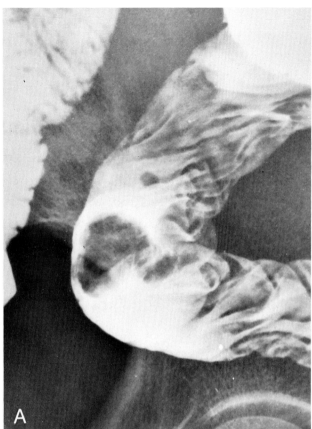

Fig. 1-8 (A) Postevacuation spot film showing a large peduculated polyp of the sigmoid colon and a second smaller adjacent polyp. A 24 percent weight per volume viscous barium suspension was employed using 80 kVp to enhance contrast. (B) Postevacuation film taken in conjunction with a biphasic (single-contrast and double-contrast phases) barium enema employing 24 percent weight per volume viscous barium suspension. The postevacuation film clearly shows the diffuse abnormality of the mucosa in this patient with Crohn's disease. The double-contrast phase of this examination was normal.

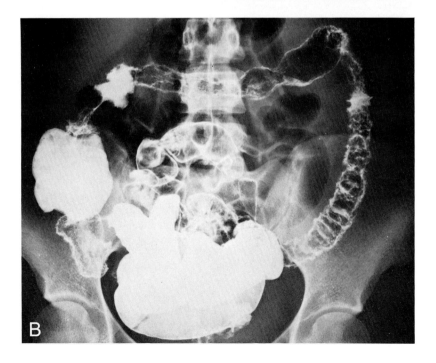

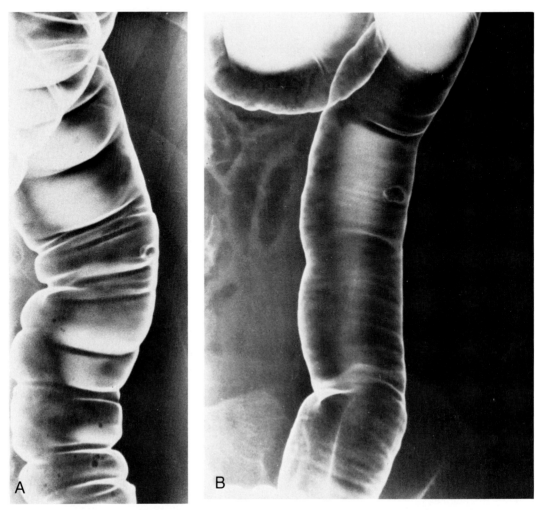

Fig. 1-9 Examples of small polyps shown on double-contrast barium enema employing the two most popular preparations used in the United States for this examination. (A) An 85 percent weight per volume factory-prepared suspension of extreme viscosity. (B) A 100 percent weight per volume factory-prepared suspension of moderately high viscosity.

vent drying of barium on the wall of the colon. Their viscosity dictates that a large diameter enema tube (0.5 inch) and tip be employed to administer the necessary amount of suspension quickly.

SUGGESTED READINGS

Gelfand DW: High density, low viscosity barium for fine mucosal detail on double-contrast examinations. **AJR** 130:831, 1978.

Gelfand DW, Ott DJ: Barium sulfate suspensions: An evaluation of available products. AJR 138:935, 1982.

Leininger V: The concentration of enema materials. In: Detection of Colon Lesions—First Standardization Conference—1969. Chicago, American College of Radiology, 1973, pp 10–17.

Miller RE: Barium sulfate suspensions. Radiology 84:241, 1965.

Miller RE, Skucas J: Radiographic Contrast Agents. Baltimore, University Park Press, 1977, pp 3–167.

Virkkunen P, Retulainen W: Visualization of the areae gastricae in double-contrast examination. Gastrointest Radiol 5:325, 1980.

2

Fluoroscopic Apparatus

Types of Apparatus

Three general types of fluoroscopic apparatus intended for gastrointestinal studies are commercially available. Differences in their basic design and radiographic capabilities are considerable and greatly influence the manner in which the individual examinations are performed.

Conventional Radiographic-Fluoroscopic Table

The most widely employed fluoroscopic apparatus is the conventional radiographic-fluoroscopic table (Fig. 2-1). This device typically consists of a tilting table containing both an under-table x-ray tube and a film holder with Bucky apparatus. A spot-film device with an image intensifier is cantilevered over the table and scans the table in coordination with the under-table tube. An additional overhead tube is mounted on an independent tube crane and is used in conjunction with the table Bucky apparatus at the conclusion of a study to obtain overall views of the organs being examined.

Since the gastrointestinal organs are located anteriorly in the abdomen, most fluoroscopy on a conventional fluoroscope is best performed with the patient's back against the table and his anterior abdominal wall against the spot-film device. This allows the fluoroscopist access to the gastrointestinal organs for palpation and compression. It also keeps the anteriorly located gastrointestinal organs close to the spot-film device, maintaining maximum radiographic sharpness. An experienced fluoroscopist will always keep the spot-film device pressed against the patient to achieve optimally sharp fluoroscopic and radiographic images.

The major advantage of the conventional radiographic-fluoroscopic table is that the examiner remains adjacent to the patient. This allows the radiologist to turn the patient directly and perform manual palpation of the abdomen. The disadvantages are exposure of radiologist and technician to radiation during fluoroscopy, and the short source-image distance of the spot-film device, which often results in films of poor definition.

The Remote Control Radiographic-Fluoroscopic Table

The remote control radiographic-fluoroscopic table (Fig. 2-2) is the second type of apparatus in general use, and represents a more recent ap-

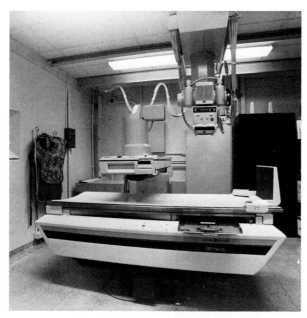

Fig. 2-1 Conventional radiographic-fluoroscopic apparatus of modern vintage designed for gastrointestinal fluoroscopy. The spot film device, cantilevered over the table, supports a large image intensifier and moves in coordination with an under-table tube, which cannot be seen in this photograph. The overhead tube operates in conjunction with the Bucky device, shown with its film tray extended.

proach that became possible with the advent of the image intensifier coupled to television. The usual remote control machine consists of a tilting table containing a spot-film device capable of handling 14- × 17-inch films backed up by an image intensifier equipped with a television camera. An overhead tube is integrated with the table and moves in conjunction with the spot-film device and image intensifier. Generally, the table also provides tomographic capabilities and the ability to angle the tube during fluoroscopy. Movements of the table, spot-film device, and overhead tube are remotely controlled by an operator behind a radiation barrier.

The advantages of the remote control fluoroscope include virtually complete radiation protection, flouroscopic control of all filming, a uniformly long source-image distance, and the ability to angle the beam during fluoroscopy. The long source-image distance produces uniformly sharp films and makes patient positioning considerably less critical than with the conventional fluoroscope. The ability to angle the tube allows unobstructed visualization of redundant or angulated portions of the gut not possible with the conventional fluoroscope (Fig. 2-3). Disadvantages include loss of direct contact with the patient, inability to perform manual palpation of the abdomen, and inconvenience in performing those studies requiring injection of contrast materials or manipulation of instruments under fluoroscopy. In my opinion, the balance of advantages versus disadvantages tends to favor the remote control apparatus over the conventional fluoroscope.

The Rotating Cradle-Type Fluoroscopic Table

A third type of fluoroscopic device mounts the patient on a rotating cradle with the tube and spot-film device also having the ability to rotate around the patient. The advantage of this arrangement is that one can obtain both vertical and horizontal beam films under direct fluoroscopic control, desirable when performing double-contrast examinations. Several such devices are available, but to date thay have met with limited acceptance. Because of their rarity, no attempt is made in this text to describe examinations performed on these machines.

IMAGE RECORDING METHODS

Conventional Film-Screen Combination

The image recording method employed for most gastrointestinal examinations is the conventional film-screen combination in individual cassettes, this technique having the advantages of maximum definition and life-size viewing. Resolution ranges from 4.0 to 7.0 line pairs per mm, depending on the film-screen combination employed. Most fluoroscopic spot-film devices have the ability to record one large image or several small images on a single cassette.

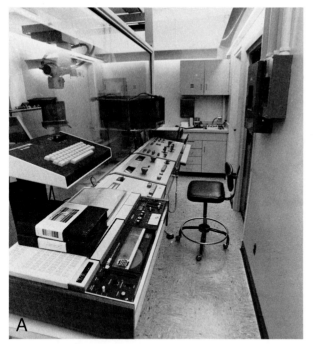
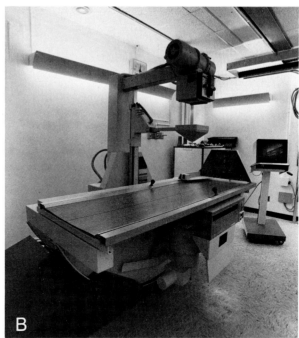

Fig. 2-2 (A) Control area showing the remote control console, generator controls, and videotape recorder. The large glass radiation barrier, which is open on both ends, and a suitably placed microphone allow good communication between the fluoroscopist and the patient. (B) Remote control table with x-ray tube mounted above the table and the spot-film device and image intensifier mounted below the table. Using the coordinated movement of the overhead tube and table top, the entire patient can be scanned fluoroscopically. The long source-image distance maximizes radiographic resolution.

Several general statements may be made concerning the choice of films and cassettes for gastrointestinal procedures. First, standard contrast films are usually more satisfactory than so-called latitude or low contrast films, the latter having a deliberately restricted gray scale. Second, most radiologists will prefer to use screens faster than par speed in an attempt to reduce radiation exposure and obtain short exposure times. Rare earth screens may be employed for maximum speed, but often produce lower definition than the best conventional screens. A very important recent advance is the curved-back cassette, which retains excellent screen-film contact even after years of rough handling.

Spot-Film Cameras

Spot-film cameras are an alternate method of recording images during fluoroscopy and offer distinct advantages and disadvantages. These record the image produced by the image intensifier onto roll film or small cut films contained within the camera. Advantages include lower patient radiation per exposure, short exposure times, rapid sequence filming, and the ability to record many images without changing cassettes. Disadvantages include high initial cost, lower resolution, restricted gray scale, inability (on certain machines) to control spot film kilovoltage, and having to complete fluoroscopy before the films can be developed. Generally speaking, the lower resolution of the typical spot-film camera (Fig. 2-4) renders it somewhat less satisfactory, in my opinion, than use of individual cassettes, and any saving on film costs never compensates for the high initial cost of the device. However, spot-film cameras are appropriate in high volume situations where rapidity of the fluoroscopic examination is of importance and where the radiologist is willing to make a slight sacrifice in image quality.

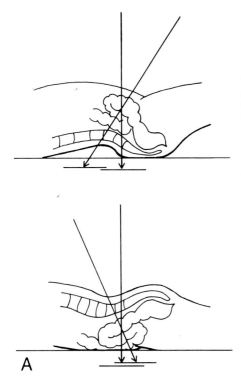

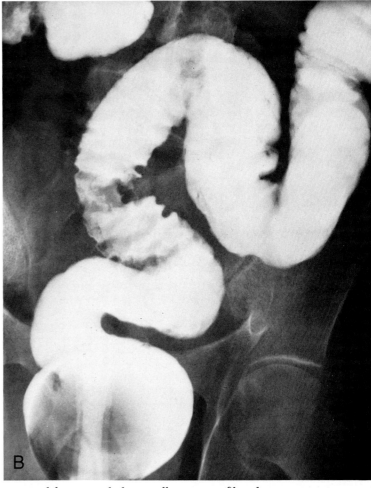

Fig. 2-3 (A) Diagrammatic illustration of the ability of tube angulation to prevent foreshortening and overlap of sigmoid colon loops during barium enema. Fluoroscopically controlled tube angulation is a routine aspect of remote control fluoroscopy. (B) Supine view of the sigmoid colon during barium enema with the central beam angled cranially, as spot-filmed on a remote control apparatus. Significant overlap of the sigmoid loops has been prevented by this means.

Cineradiography

Cineradiography was the first widely used method for recording motion during fluoroscopy, with most cameras used for gastrointestinal radiology being of the 16 millimeter size. Cineradiography is useful in examining the pharynx and the esophagus, where motion and peristalsis is rapid, and it produces an easily stored permanent record. Cineradiography was initially popular after the advent of the image amplifier, but the technique has been almost completely supplanted on newer installations by television recorders.

Videotape Recording

Videotape recording has increasingly become the method of choice for motion recording during gastrointestinal fluoroscopy, the recorder being simply wired into the television circuit. Events occurring during fluoroscopy may be recorded and reviewed without processing. Videotape recorders are of considerable use for recording the rapidly occurring events in the pharynx and esophagus during swallowing. While the cost of the tapes precludes permanent storage, recordings may be retained several days for consultation and review, all that is generally necessary.

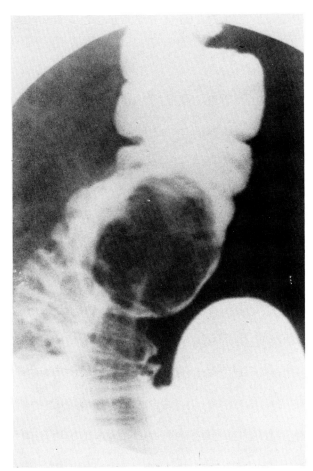

Fig. 2-4 Pedunculated colonic polyp as recorded with a 90-mm spot-film camera. The slightly lower radiographic definition of these devices is apparent on this film.

IMAGE INTENSIFIERS

The advent of the x-ray image intensifier was one of the major advances in gastrointestinal radiology. Image intensification allows the radiologist to perform fluoroscopy in a lighted room and, more importantly, provides a fluoroscopic image of considerable clarity. An equally important benefit has been the reduction of the amount of radiation necessary to produce an acceptable fluoroscopic image.

Modern image intensifiers range in size from 6 to 14 inches in diameter (Fig. 2-5). In general, the smaller image intensifiers are least costly and of high resolution, but their restricted field of view

can be an inconvenience. The largest image intensifiers are expensive and often of lower definition, but they allow viewing of large areas of the abdomen and thus speed fluoroscopy. Generally, 9- and 10-inch image intensifiers are most often installed when possible, representing a reasonable compromise between cost, size, definition, and convenience.

Considerable variation in performance characteristics of image intensifiers can be expected. Useable resolution, as measured at the input phosphor, varies from 3.5 to 5.0 line pairs per mm.

The image recording and viewing method chosen for a fluoroscope determines the degree of excellence required from an image intensifier. If

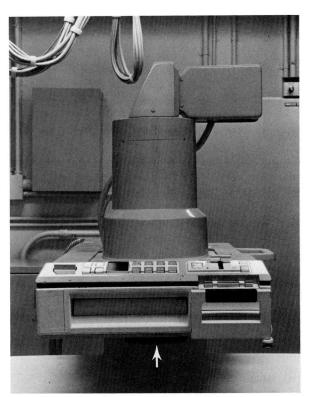

Fig. 2-5 Typical image intensifier with attached television camera mounted on a large front-loading spot-film device. The use of the modern spot-film device has rendered it difficult to perform manual palpation of the patient during fluoroscopy. The compression cone (arrow) projecting from the bottom of the spot-film mechanism is now often used as a substitute for the palpating hand.

the output of the image intensifier is to be recorded by a spot-film camera, obtaining an image intensifier of the highest possible resolution is of considerable importance. If the image intensifier is coupled only to a television camera, the resolution of the television system tends to be the limiting factor and an image intensifier of extremely high resolution, often a costly option, is generally not necessary.

RADIOGRAPHIC CONSIDERATIONS

Specifications of the X-Ray Tube

The specifications of the x-ray tube employed in a particular apparatus to a large extent determine the overall radiographic capabilities of the machine. Virtually all quality fluoroscopes now employ tubes with 4-inch anodes and large focal spots of 1.0 to 1.5 mm dimension. Choice of a 1.0-mm focal spot allows greatest possible sharpness consistent with reasonably short exposure times under most circumstances, and a 1.0-mm focal spot is often employed for spot-filming in the under-table tubes of conventional fluoroscopes. Larger focal spots of 1.2 to 1.5 mm are generally used in overhead tubes and remote control units, the longer source-image distance minimizing focal spot blur but requiring greater applications of power to the tube to achieve short exposures.

Generator Power

Several generalities can be made concerning the relationship of generator power to x-ray tube capacity. First, the typical 1.2 to 1.5 mm large focal spot used in the overhead tubes of many machines is incapable of absorbing the full power of a 100-kW, 1,000-MA generator for much more than one-tenth of a second. As a result, most manufacturers restrict generator power at the higher kilovoltages employed for gastrointestinal radiology, often limiting current to 600 MA or 700 MA at the 100 to 120 kVp often used for gastrointestinal radiography. For 1.0-mm focal spots, the maximum current allowed may be as low as 400 MA. Thus, the typical radiographic-fluoroscopic unit equipped with a 600- to 1,000-MA generator is usually "tube limited."

Grid Ratio

The grid ratio of the grids in the spot-film device and Bucky apparatus should be adequate to suppress most scattered radiation. A rough rule in abdominal radiography is that the grid ratio should equal or exceed kilovoltage ÷ 10. Since kilovoltages of 120 or more must occasionally be employed during gastrointestinal radiology, both the spot-film device and the Bucky apparatus of a fluoroscope should be equipped with 12:1 grids if possible.

Phototiming

A final, desirable radiographic feature of a good fluoroscope is that all of its radiographic functions should be phototimed. The importance of phototiming all exposures during a gastrointestinal examination cannot be overemphasized. As will be discussed later, the accuracy of gastrointestinal examinations decreases radically if exposures are poorly controlled, and it is impossible for most technologists to duplicate the consistency of a phototimer.

SUGGESTED READINGS°

Hamelin L, Hurtebise M: Remote control technique in double-contrast study of the colon. Am J Roentgenol 119:382, 1973.

Hayt DB, Simon DF, Collica CJ: Grid choice in high-kilovoltage 70 mm radiographic spot filming. Radiology 93:135, 1969.

°Only a minimal list of suggested readings can be provided for this chapter, since there are few journal publications or texts providing the practical information needed to properly select and use the fluoroscope employed for gastrointestinal examinations. The specifications of the individual fluoroscopic tables, generators, tubes, image amplifiers, etc. change constantly, and the pertinent information can only be obtained from the manufacturers.

Hendee WR, Rossi RP: Performance specifications for diagnostic x-ray equipment. Radiology 120:409, 1976.

Hynes DM, Edmonds EW, Krametz KR, Baranowski D: Radiographic, photofluoroscopic and television imaging systems: An evaluation. Radiology 133:751, 1979.

Janower ML, Urie M: Routine fluoroscopy using mini-spot cameras. Radiology 133: 527, 1979.

Jutras A, Duckett G: Roentgen diagnosis by remote control tele-fluoroscopy and cineradiography. Medica Mundi 4:77, 1958.

Lee D, Sourkes AM, Holloway AF, Reed MH: Performance evaluation of image-intensifier tubes. Radiology 138:455, 1981.

Maglinte DDT, Dolan PA, Miller RE: Angled radiography in upper gastrointestinal examinations. AJR 137:1082, 1981.

Rossi RP, Niemkeiwicz JM, Mulvaney JA, Hendee WR: X-ray equipment performance: A 3.5 year case history. AJR 136:1199, 1981.

Templeton FE: X-ray Examination of the Stomach. Chicago, University of Chicago Press, 1964, pp 7–21.

3

Capabilities and Limitations of Barium Examinations

Two basic methods are available for examining the gastrointestinal tract with barium sulphate suspensions. *Single-contrast* techniques rely on filling the organ examined with barium suspension, the mass of barium taking the contours of the organ and delineating any abnormal structure. *Double-contrast* techniques depend on coating the mucosal surface of the organ with a film of barium suspension, while filling most of the lumen with air or carbon dioxide. The film of barium then coats the mucosa and outlines both normal and abnormal structures.

SINGLE-CONTRAST TECHNIQUES

Information about the mucosal surface of an organ filled with barium is obtained in two ways with single-contrast techniques. The most obvious visual information is the outline of the barium-filled organ. Large abnormalities of structure, such as those caused by a bulky, circumferential tumor or large ulcer disturb this outline and are readily apparent (Fig. 3-1). Smaller or more localized abnormalities of the mucosa, such as small sessile polyps or a small ulcer, will also be visible in outline, but only if the lesion happens to be on the limited, marginal portion of the organ being struck tangentially by the x-ray beam (Fig. 3-2).

A second, more complex and productive type of information is derived from the demonstration of lesions en face, rather than as abnormalities of outline. Lesions seen by this means form their image either as a radiolucency caused by a mass lesion displacing barium within the lumen (Fig. 3-3) or as a radio-opacity caused by barium in an ulcer, diverticulum, or fistula extending beyond the normal confines of the organ (Fig. 3-4). The major challenge when performing single-contrast examinations is in arranging all factors so that small abnormalities of the mucosal surface can always be seen en face through the overlying barium.

The ability of the single-contrast technique to consistently visualize abnormalities of the mucosal surfaces en face depends in great measure on the interaction of three factors controlled by the radiologist: organ thickness, barium density, and kilovoltage. Other factors, such as grid ratios and film gamma (contrast) also play a part but are generally not varied during the examination.

19

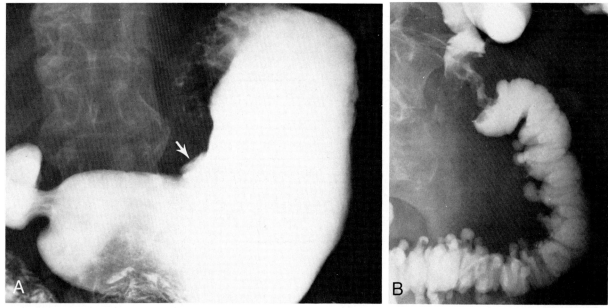

Fig. 3-1 Single-contrast barium-filled films with large lesions visible as contour defects. (**A**) Large lesser curvature ulcer at the angularis (arrow). (**B**) Circumferential adenocarcinoma of the descending colon.

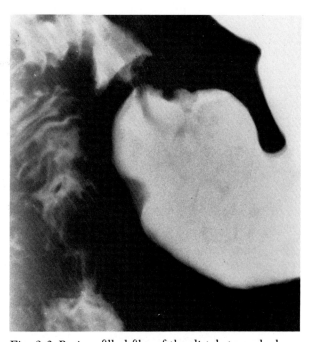

Fig. 3-2 Barium-filled film of the distal stomach showing indentation of the barium column by ectopic pancreatic tissue located on the greater curvature. A mass lesion of similar size located on the anterior or posterior wall would almost certainly be rendered invisible by the overlying barium.

Organ Thickness

Organ thickness is the major determinant of the effectiveness of single-contrast radiography. As a rule, large organs such as the stomach and colon are difficult to penetrate radiographically when filled with barium suspension, even when the suspension is rather dilute. However, this difficulty can be ameliorated by compressing the organ so that it presents a greatly lessened thickness of barium to be penetrated.

The clarity with which a lesion is visible through a barium column depends on the fraction of the barium column displaced by the lesion if it projects into the lumen, or added by barium lying beyond the lumen as in an ulcer. Thus, a polypoid neoplasm displacing virtually all of the barium column in the lumen of a stomach that has been thinned out by compression will appear as a striking radiolucency (Fig. 3-3). On the other hand, the same lesion in a stomach distended by barium and not compressed might be barely visible, since it would not displace enough of the barium to be clearly seen as a radiolucency. Total invisibility occurs if the mass of barium in front of a lesion is too dense to be penetrable, or if the lesion displaces such a

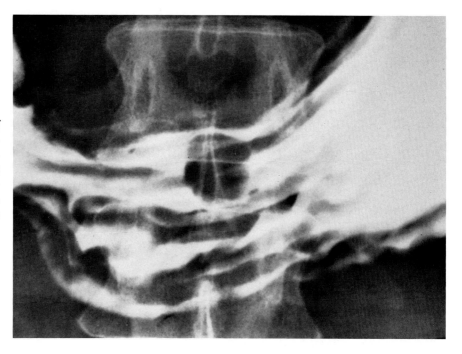

Fig. 3-3 Polypoid lesion of the distal stomach demonstrated en face by compression filming. The lesion is clearly outlined by displacement of the barium column. Bone detail is visible through the barium.

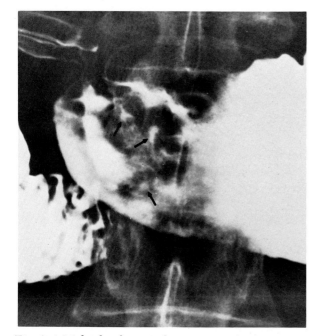

Fig. 3-4 Multiple ulcers and erosions in the gastric antrum (arrows) demonstrated by compression filming. The lesions and their surrounding mounds of edema are demonstrated en face.

small fraction of the overlying barium that contrast between it and surrounding areas cannot be detected by the radiographic-fluoroscopic system or by the eye.

As a result of the above, compression is almost always desirable during single-contrast examinations. Compression thins out the mass of barium in the lumen of an organ and thus increases the relative amount of abnormally displaced or protruding barium. This results in a more visible lesion. (Figs. 3-3 and 3-4).

Barium Density

Barium density is the second controllable factor. In general, the larger the organ to be examined, the more dilute the barium suspension must be to allow adequate penetration of the barium in its lumen. On the other hand, a small diameter segment of bowel, such as the duodenum, may be successfully examined with a more dense barium suspension, since any mass lesion or ulcer present is likely to displace or add a considerable fraction of the barium in the lumen and will thus be easily visible. Other factors considered in the choice of barium density for a single-contrast examination include the need to obtain double-contrast films during upper gastrointestinal single-contrast examinations and the desirability of postevacuation films after barium enemas. The choice of barium density for the various single-contrast studies is described in Chapter 1, but may be summarized as follows in light of the above discussion:

1. The single-contrast upper gastrointestinal series usually employs barium densities of 60 to 100 percent weight per volume. This allows radiographic penetration of the barium column in the esophagus and duodenum, but presupposes compression of the stomach (Figs. 3-3 and 3-4) and duodenal bulb as well as a double-contrast examination of the duodenal bulb and limited areas of the stomach.

2. The oral small bowel examination is best performed with barium densities of 50 to 75 percent weight per volume. The small bowel is sufficiently small in diameter that both normal folds and abnormal structural changes will usually be visible through the barium column. However, because of the barium density, overlapping loops may not be fully penetrated by the x-ray beam and the small bowel loops must be separated by compression. (Fig. 3–5). For enteroclysis, barium density is usually 15 to 30 percent weight per volume to allow penetration of the distended small bowel and of overlapping loops (Fig. 3–6).

3. Single-contrast barium enemas generally employ barium densities of 15 to 25 percent weight per volume. The colon is a large organ, not all of which can be adequately compressed, and a rather thin barium suspension is used to allow radiographic penetration (Fig. 3–7). If routine postevacuation or double-contrast films of the colon are obtained following the barium-filled examination, a barium density of approximately 25 percent

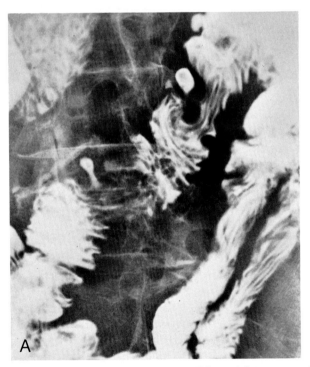 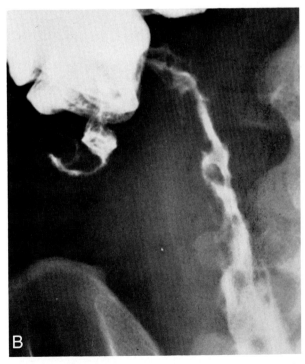

Fig. 3-5 Normal and abnormal small bowel features easily visible on films taken with mild compression, using 72 percent weight per volume barium suspension. Since the peroral small bowel examination does not greatly distend the lumen, barium suspensions of moderate density may be used and will show considerable detail. (A) Multiple jejunal diverticula. (B) Crohn's disease of the distal ileum, cecum, and appendix.

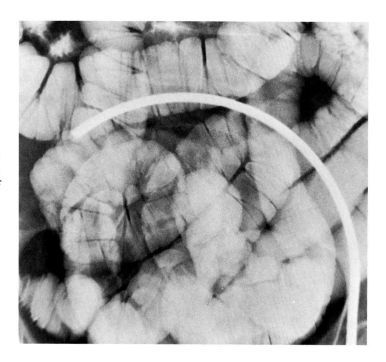

Fig. 3-6 Small bowel enema employing 18 percent weight per volume barium suspension to allow radiographic penetration of distended small bowel loops.

is desirable. If such films are not to be obtained, barium densities of 15 to 20 percent will allow more consistent radiographic penetration.

Kilovoltage

Kilovoltage is the third variable influencing the visibility of lesions during single-contrast examinations. Kilovoltage interacts with organ size and barium density in determining both the size and density of an organ that can be penetrated, and the apparent contrast of a lesion as seen radiographically. In general, kilovoltages much below 90 kVp are to be avoided during single-contrast filming, since in many instances the barium may not be radiographically penetrated. On the other hand, high kilovoltages greater than approximately 110 kVp cause a loss of intrinsic radiographic contrast between the barium and the lesion it surrounds, as well as a further loss of radiographic contrast due to increased scattered radiation. When using modern three-phase equipment, the best compromise between adequate penetration of the barium column, short exposure times, and minimizing scattered radiation occurs in the range of 90 to 110

kVp. Higher kilovoltages should be used only to achieve short exposures when examining very large patients.

Practical Limitations

Practical limitations exist concerning the size and shape of lesions routinely detectable with single-contrast examinations. Most lesions demonstrated during single-contrast examinations must be visualized through varying amounts of overlying barium suspension. Where the amount of barium overlying a lesion is considerable, very small ulcers or neoplasms may be impossible to detect. Thus, these lesions are frequently missed on single-contrast examinations consisting primarily of barium distended views. On the other hand, small ulcers or neoplasms will usually be visible during single-contrast examinations when the examination is accompanied by careful compression filming (Figs. 3-4 and 3-7). Supplementation with double-contrast and mucosal relief films taken as part of the single-contrast examination also aids in the detection of small, subtle lesions.

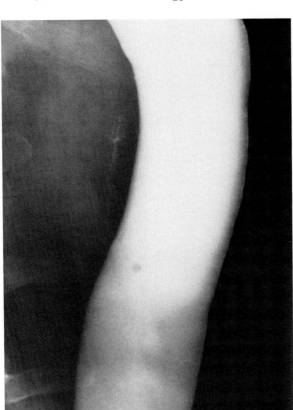

Fig. 3-7 Single-contrast barium enema film using 18 percent weight per volume barium suspension and employing compression. A 3-mm polyp is clearly demonstrated.

Quality Control

Quality control during single-contrast studies is necessary to ensure that the barium is always adequately penetrated for an en face detection of lesions, since the outline of an opaque, barium-filled organ provides limited information. A valuable test of adequate penetration is whether skeletal shadows are consistently visible through the barium column (Figs. 3-3, 3-4, and 3-7). If, for example, the vertebrae are visible through the barium during compression filming of the gastric antrum or duodenal bulb, a polyp displacing several millimeters of barium or a gastric ulcer superimposing several additional millimeters of barium should be easily discernible (Figs. 3-3 and 3-4). An

additional quality control for the single-contrast barium enema is the ability to see through two loops of bowel that are superimposed on each other. This is helpful during single-contrast barium enemas because it is often impossible to position the patient or angle the x-ray beam in a manner demonstrating all portions of the colon without superimposition of loops, particularly in the sigmoid region.

DOUBLE-CONTRAST TECHNIQUES

Double-contrast examinations, as stated earlier, depend on outlining abnormalities of the mucosal surface with a film or shallow pool of barium, the lumen of the organ being inflated by air or carbon dioxide. The kilovoltage-barium density-organ size relationship in double-contrast work is far less critical than during single-contrast studies for several reasons. First, the x-ray beam need only penetrate two thin layers of barium during double-contrast studies, and the challenge of producing adequate penetration of a large barium column under widely varying conditions is not present. Second, since the organ is not filled with barium, the size of its lumen is relatively unimportant. Third, barium density is generally not varied for organ size. Fourth, kilovoltage is usually kept in the region of 100 kVp, to minimize the amount of scattered radiation, with higher kilovoltages being used only to achieve short exposure times when examining large patients. Finally, there is considerably more latitude of exposure allowable, as compared to single-contrast examinations.

Radiographic Capability

The radiographic capability of double-contrast studies to delineate small alterations of the mucosal surface is considerable. Because the film of barium covering the mucosal surface is quite thin, very small protrusions or excavations of the mucosal surface are easily detectable. Thus, the areae gastricae, which are normally 1 to 2 mm in diameter and protrude into the lumen approximately 0.5 mm, and gastric erosions with similar dimensions, are readily demonstrated (Fig. 3-8).

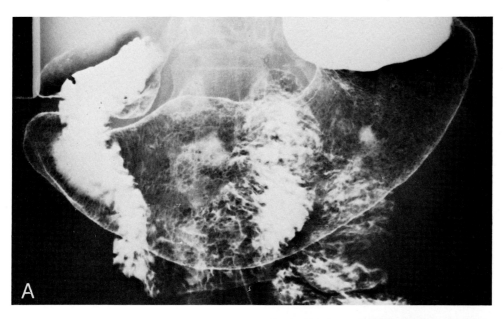

Fig. 3-8 Illustration of the considerable detail visible on double-contrast films of the stomach. (A) Slightly disorganized areae gastricae in a patient with atrophic gastritis. (B) Multiple gastric erosions in the distal stomach.

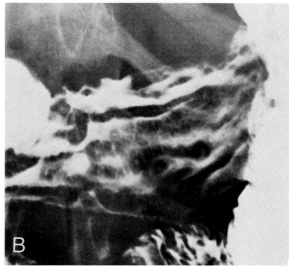

Limitations

The limitations of double-contrast examinations lie elsewhere, and revolve around two related problems inherent to the double-contrast method.

The first problem is created by the tendency of barium to drain by gravity from the nondependent areas of an organ onto its dependent wall, forming shallow pools on the dependent wall. Very small abnormalities are easily seen on the dependent wall, since a lesion or normal structure that is basically a protrusion, such as a polyp or rugal fold, will displace the shallow barium pool and will be very clearly visible (Figs. 3-9, and 3-10). On the other hand, both lesions and normal structures on the more superiorly located walls of the organ will be covered with merely a thin coating of barium and can only be seen in outline and, moreover, can only be seen when and where their sides are sufficiently steep that the beam strikes the coating of

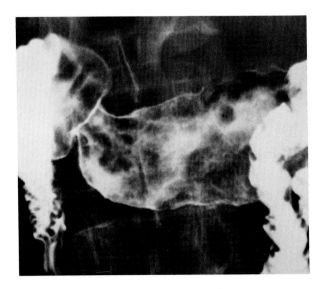

Fig. 3-9 Polypoid swellings of the gastric mucosa in a patient with antral gastritis, visible by displacement of barium suspension in the shallow pool on the posterior wall.

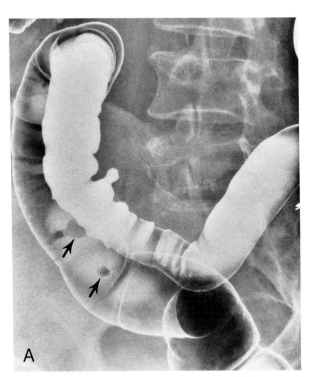

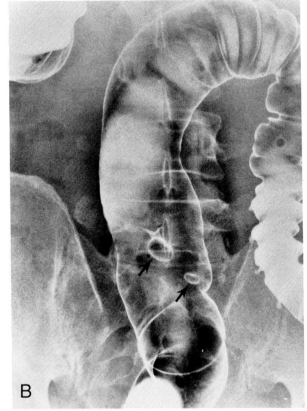

Fig. 3-10 Colonic polyps (arrows) detected during a double-contrast barium enema. (A) Prone film showing the polyps displacing the barium pool on the dependent anterior wall. (B) Supine film demonstrating the polyps as ring shadows.

barium suspension tangentially (Fig. 3-10). Detection of superiorly located lesions may therefore be quite difficult.

The second limitation of the double-contrast technique is related to the shape of any lesions that do not lie on the dependent wall and are thus potentially visible only in outline. To produce this outline, as noted above, the x-ray beam must tangentially strike the barium suspension covering the lesion. The classic example of this is the polyp on the anterior gastric or colonic wall, which is seen as a ring shadow (Fig. 3-10). However, many ulcers and plaque-like neoplasms of the anterior wall of the stomach do not possess steep enough margins to produce a contour that can be tangentially impinged upon by the x-ray beam. Such lesions are totally invisible during double-contrast examinations unless films can be taken in several projections so that the lesion is certain to be seen partially or completely in profile, or unless the examination includes compression or mucosal relief films designed to show abnormalities on the nondependent wall (Fig. 3-11). Thus, a thorough double-contrast examination of the colon will include double-contrast films of each area in several positions, so as to minimize dependent versus superior wall prob-

lems. Moreover, a thorough "double-contrast" upper gastrointestinal study must include compression films, mucosal relief films, or both as a means of demonstrating lesions on the anterior wall of the stomach and duodenum.

Quality Control

Quality control during double-contrast filming consists mainly of insuring that all portions of the organ being examined are in fact thoroughly coated and properly radiographed in double-contrast. Areas not thoroughly coated or optimally positioned are in fact "invisible" during double-contrast studies, and these areas may represent most of the organ being studied.

Thorough and uniform coating of the mucosa is best insured by two measures: (1) use of adequate amounts of an appropriate barium suspension and (2) constant turning of the patient so that each portion being examined is freshly washed by barium suspension prior to filming. To insure proper radiography, the organ being examined must be moderately distended by gas or air, but a reasonable amount of barium suspension must also be

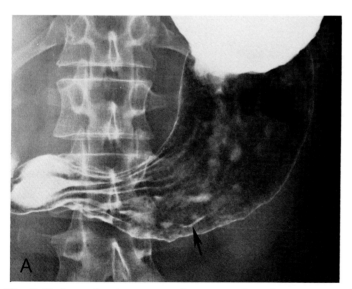
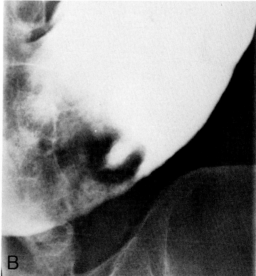

Fig. 3-11 Large benign gastric ulcer situated on the anterior wall of the stomach near the greater curvature. **(A)** Supine double-contrast film of the region shows only one edge of the ulcer; it appears as a somewhat inconspicuous white line (arrow), which could easily be missed during interpretation of the study. **(B)** Compression film clearly showing the ulcer and its surrounding mound of edema.

present to maintain a generous coating over the entire mucosal surface. Attempts to perform double-contrast studies with minimal amounts of barium suspension often result in poor or incomplete coating of the region being examined.

SUGGESTED READINGS

Amaral NM: The value of the compressive technique associated with pharmacological hypotonia in the diagnosis of erosive gastritis. Gastrointest Radiol 3:161, 1978.

Figiel SJ, Figiel LS, Rush DK: Study of the colon by use of high-kilovoltage spot-compression technique. JAMA 166:1269, 1958.

Gelfand DW, Ott DJ: Single- vs double-contrast gastrointestinal studies: Critical analysis of reported statistics. AJR 137:523, 1981.

Gelfand DW, Ott DJ, Tritico R: Causes of error in gastrointestinal radiology: I. Upper gastrointestinal examination. Gastrointest Radiol 5:91, 1980.

Gianturco C, Miller G: Routine search for colonic polyps by high voltage radiography. Radiology 60:496, 1953.

Horikoshi H: Characteristics of x-ray examination of the stomach. In Murakami T, ed: Early Gastric Cancer. GANN Monograph on Cancer Research 11. Tokyo, University of Tokyo Press, 1971, pp 93–103.

Kawai K, Tanaka H: Differential Diagnosis of Gastric Diseases. Chicago, Yearbook Medical Publishers, 1974, pp 11–53.

Kressel HY, Laufer I: Principles of double contrast diagnosis. In: Double Contrast Gastrointestinal Radiology. Philadelphia, WB Saunders, 1979, pp 21–44.

Leininger V: The concentration of enema materials. In: Detection of Colon Lesions. First Standardization Conference—1969. Chicago, American College of Radiology, 1973, pp 10–17.

Miller RE: The clinical aspects of barium concentration. In: Detection of Colon Lesions. First Standardization Conference—1969. Chicago, American College of Radiology, 1973, pp 18–22.

Miller RE: Examination of the colon. Curr Prob Radiol 2:1, 1975.

Ott DJ, Gelfand DW, Ramquist NA: Causes of error in gastrointestinal radiology: II. The barium enema. Gastrointest Radiol 5:99, 1980.

Ott DJ, Gelfand DW, Wu WC, Kerr RM: Sensitivity of the double-contrast barium enema: Emphasis on polyp detection. AJR 135:327, 1980.

Schatzki R: You still have to work for it: Analysis of the impact of screen intensification. Radiology 87:759, 1966.

Sellink JL: Radiological atlas of common diseases of the small bowel. Leiden, HE Stenfert Kroese BV, 1976, pp 43–52.

Stein GN, Martin RD, Roy RH, Finkelstein AK: Evaluation of conventional roentgenographic techniques for demonstration of duodenal ulcer craters. AM J Roentgenol 91:801, 1964.

Templeton FE: X-ray Examination of the Stomach. Chicago, University of Chicago Press, 1964, pp 36–50.

Welin S: Results of the Malmö technique of colon examination. JAMA 199:369, 1967.

4

A Description of the Upper Gastrointestinal Examinations

This chapter presents three methods for examining the upper gastrointestinal tract. Historically, the first of these to be developed was the *fluoroscopic examination*, usually supplemented by several films obtained after fluoroscopy. With the advent of the filming fluoroscope, or spot-film device, the *conventional upper gastrointestinal examination* came into being, the study most frequently performed today. More recently, Japanese physicians perfected the "double-contrast" examination, which as performed in Japan and as described in this text is in actuality a *multiphasic upper gastrointestinal series*.

The versions of these examinations to be described are more elaborate than performed in most institutions. First, it is thought best to present a thorough examination rather than one that is sketchy and might possibly yield poor results. Second, by presenting an extensive examination, most of the views and techniques employed by the majority of radiologists performing these studies will be included. Certain specialized techniques not described in this chapter are presented in subsequent chapters devoted to more detailed descriptions of the examination of the individual organs of the gastrointestinal tract.

In the descriptions of examinations which follow, *patient positions are listed in respect to the table.* This differs somewhat from the conventional practice of relating position to the portion of the body closest to the film. However, because the text describes examinations as performed with both conventional and remote control machines, it is least confusing to consistently list positions in relation to the x-ray table. For example, if a position is noted as right anterior oblique (RAO) with the table horizontal, it designates that the patient is lying with the right anterior aspect of his body closest to the table. This is regardless of whether the spot-film device is above the patient, as with conventional fluoroscopy, or within the table, as with remote control apparatus. As another example, the anteroposterior (AP) position with table erect designates that the patient is standing on the footboard with his back square against the surface of the table, whether the spot-film device is suspended in front of him or is within the table. A pictorial summary of the positional nomenclature and abbreviations used throughout the text is presented in Figure 4-1.

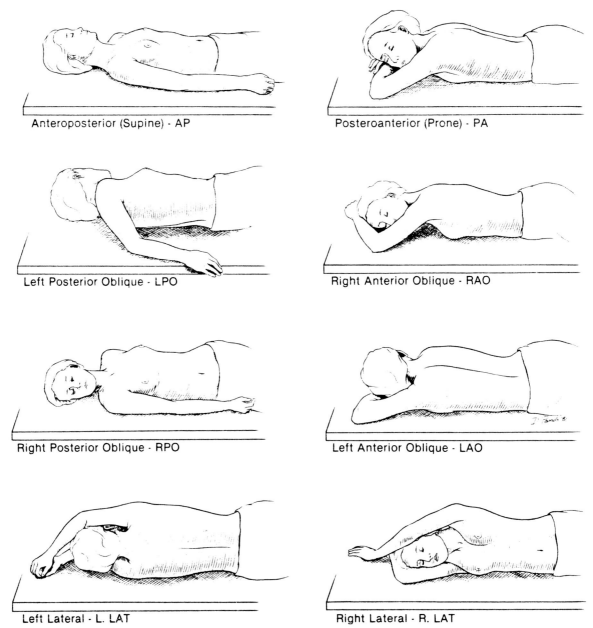

Anteroposterior (Supine) - AP

Posteroanterior (Prone) - PA

Left Posterior Oblique - LPO

Right Anterior Oblique - RAO

Right Posterior Oblique - RPO

Left Anterior Oblique - LAO

Left Lateral - L. LAT

Right Lateral - R. LAT

Fig. 4–1 Pictorial summary of the positional nomenclature and abbreviations used in this text. Patient positions are listed as the part of the body closest to the table.

THE PRIMARILY FLUOROSCOPIC EXAMINATION

Historically, the fluoroscopic examination was the first radiologic examination of the upper gastrointestinal tract. Subsequently it became apparent that the accuracy of the examination was improved by supplementing fluoroscopy with films of the esophagus, stomach, and duodenum, usually obtained after fluoroscopy was completed. This examination has the advantages of simplicity, speed, low cost, and minimum use of film. In skilled hands, it can be very accurate, with the fluoroscopic skills of the examiner being the determining factor. In situations where funds are limited or where large numbers of patients must be examined quickly with limited facilities, it may be the examination of choice. Most importantly, however, the fluoroscopic skills upon which this examination depends remain an integral and vital part of any skillfully performed examination of the upper gastrointestinal tract. It is primarily for this latter reason that the examination is described in some detail.

The fluoroscopic examination of the esophagus, stomach, and duodenum may be divided into the following five phases:

Phase 1: Erect Anteroposterior Position without Barium

The chest and abdomen are briefly fluoroscoped for any pathology visible without contrast material.

Phase 2: Erect Anteroposterior Position with Barium

As 2 to 4 mouthfuls of barium suspension (60 to 100 percent weight per volume) pass down the esophagus, visual search for strictures, neoplasms, diverticuli, and other abnormalities is performed (Fig. 4-2A). When the barium reaches the stomach, the stomach is carefully palpated and compressed. The gloved hand and/or compression cone is used to wipe the barium suspension into the spaces between the rugal folds. Any collection of barium in an ulcer niche or any filling defect is noted (Fig. 4-2B). By palpation and compression, any rigid areas of the stomach also are detected. The patient is then rotated slightly to his left, and a similar examination of the duodenal bulb is performed (Fig. 4-2C). If necessary, the gloved hand may be used to milk the barium into the duodenal bulb. During this phase, the stomach and bulb must be compressed sufficiently so that any lesion on the anterior or posterior wall may be seen en face through the overlying layer of barium. The patient is also rotated in both directions so that an

abnormality of contour of any portion of the stomach or duodenal bulb may be observed.

The patient then swallows more barium, and the esophagus is again observed from several angles. The additional volume of barium now in the stomach allows detection of areas of decreased gastric distensibility and also spreads the rugae apart. With palpation and/or compression, small ulcers or other small lesions between the rugae may now be observed. If the duodenal bulb did not fill following the initial swallows of barium, it is likely to do so at this time, and the palpation-compression examination of the duodenal bulb is performed. Both the stomach and duodenum are again observed in several obliquities for abnormalities of contour.

Phase 3: Supine (AP) Position

With the table now horizontal, the examiner again palpates or compresses the stomach in a manner similar to that described above. Because of the effects of gravity, and the limited double-contrast effect, this position is particularly apt to demonstrate lesions on the posterior wall of the distal half of the stomach. (Fig. 4-2D). With the patient turned to the left posterior oblique (LPO) position, the duodenal bulb may be observed first with a moderate amount of barium (Hampton's view) and then with an air-barium double-contrast technique after the bulb has filled with air (Fig. 4-2E).

Phase 4: Right Anterior Oblique and Prone (PA) Positions

The patient is now turned into the RAO and prone (PA) positions and filling of the duodenal bulb, which is now dependent, takes place. Abnormalities of contour of the gastric antrum or duodenum caused by ulcers, scarring, or neoplasm may be observed (Fig. 4-2F). Use of a compression device such as a padded or inflatable paddle or bolster beneath the distal stomach and duodenal bulb will help render most lesions visible en face through the barium.

With the patient still recumbent and in the RAO position, additional barium is administered through a straw. The esophagus is observed in both

(Text continues on page 34.)

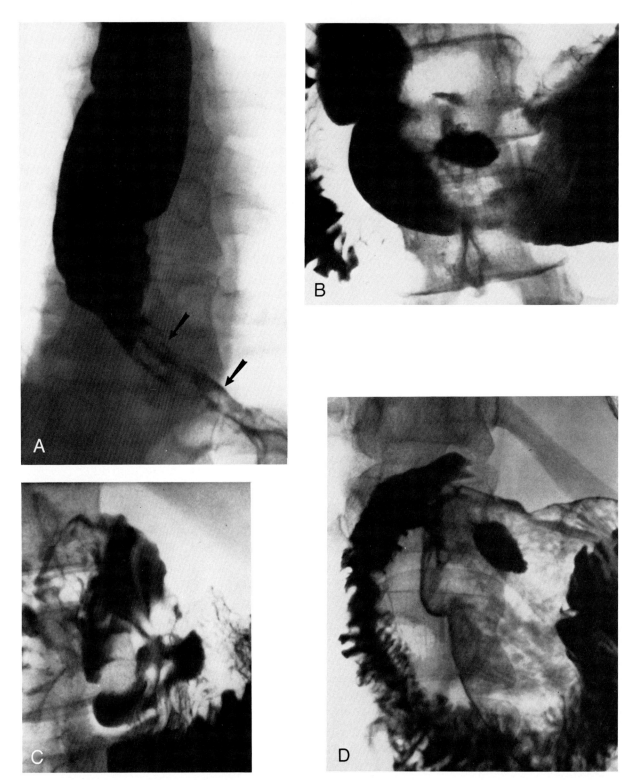

Fig. 4-2 Representation of the several phases of an upper gastrointestinal fluoroscopy as seen on the fluoroscope. The illustrations are spot-films printed as negatives to simulate fluoroscopic images. (A) Upright examination of the distal esophagus with an esophagogastric carcinoma visible as thickened, nodular folds (arrows). (B) Erect compression examination of the distal stomach showing a large benign antral ulcer. (C) Erect compression examination of the duodenal bulb showing an active ulcer surrounded by converging folds and a mound of edema. (D) Supine examination of the distal stomach in a double-contrast view demonstrating a large benign gastric ulcer.

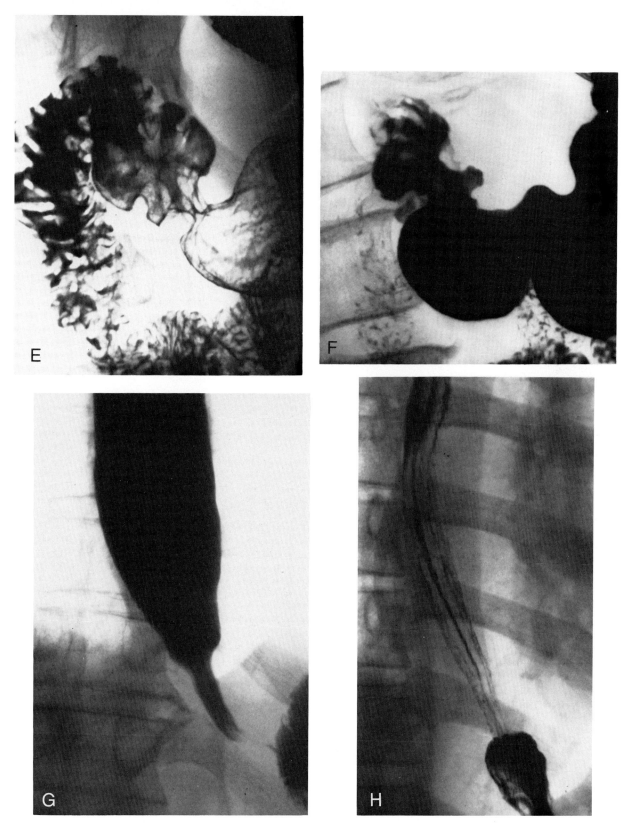

Fig. 4-2 *(continued)* (E) Double-contrast view of the distal gastric antrum and duodenal bulb in the LPO position in a patient with chronic duodenal ulcer disease. (F) Barium-filled view of the distal stomach and pyloric region obtained in a steep RAO position and showing a pyloric channel ulcer. (G) Prone barium-filled view of the distal esophagus in a patient with carcinoma of the esophagogastric junction simulating achalasia. (H) Mucosal relief view of the distal esophagus employing a very dense barium for maximum coating, and showing thick, irregular folds due to reflux esophagitis.

the distended and collapsed (mucosal relief) state (Figs. 4-2G and H). With the esophagus distended and the patient performing a deep Valsalva maneuver, hiatus hernias may be optimally detected. For thoroughness, this sequence for examining the esophagus should be repeated in the left anterior oblique (LAO) position. The mucosal relief study of the esophagus may be enhanced by using a very dense barium suspension or paste, in which case it is best performed at the very end of the examination, after the Bucky films, to avoid simulation of ulcers on the Bucky films by collections of the dense barium.

Phase 5: Obtaining Bucky Films

Bucky films are customarily taken by the technologist following fluoroscopy. Films obtained typically are as follows, although individual routines vary considerably.

1. Prone (PA) film of the stomach and duodenum (see Fig. 4-4A).
2. Right anterior oblique film of the stomach and duodenum (see Fig. 4-4B).
3. Right lateral (R Lat) of the stomach and duodenum (see Fig. 4-4C).
4. Supine (AP) film of the stomach and duodenum (see Fig. 4-4D).
5. Left posterior oblique film of the stomach and duodenum (see Fig. 4-4E).
6. Right anterior oblique film of the entire esophagus with patient drinking (see Fig. 4-4F).

The above and other similar fluoroscopic routines originated when the nonintensified fluoroscopic screen was in general use. Close proximity of the fluoroscopist to the patient was possible and manual palpation of the abdomen was easily performed. In recent years, the presence of an image amplifier atop a bulky spot-film device has unfortunately rendered it more difficult to perform the palpation maneuvers described. However, a reasonable substitute for the palpating hand is the careful use of the compression cone on the underside of the spot-film device as an extension of the examiner's hands; this has the advantage of sparing the hands from the radiation of the primary beam.

THE CONVENTIONAL UPPER GASTROINTESTINAL EXAMINATION

The conventional, mainly single-contrast upper gastrointestinal series evolved from the fluoroscopic examination when the filming fluoroscope, or spot-film device, came into general use approximately 40 years ago. With the spot-film device available, it became apparent that increased accuracy could be obtained by a combination of thorough fluoroscopy, strategically obtained spot-films, and an adequate number of Bucky films taken after fluoroscopy. This remains the most commonly performed barium examination of the upper gastrointestinal tract.

The description of the conventional upper gastrointestinal series may be divided into the following phases.

Phase 1: Erect Anteroposterior Position without Barium

The chest and abdomen are briefly fluoroscoped before barium is administered.

Phase 2: Erect Anteroposterior Position with Barium

With 2 to 4 swallows of barium, the esophagus is observed for lesions, but no film is routinely taken. Careful palpation and compression of the stomach is then performed, either manually or with the compression cone. During the upright examination of the stomach, compression spot films are taken (Fig. 4-3A), usually employing four exposures on a single film. Similarly, when the duodenal bulb has filled, a palpation examination is performed and compression spot films of the duodenal bulb are obtained (Fig. 4-3B).

Phase 3: Supine (AP) Position

With the stomach still containing a small amount of barium, the distal stomach and duodenal bulb are again palpated and compressed. A large spot film of the entire stomach and duodenum is ob-

(Text continues on page 38.)

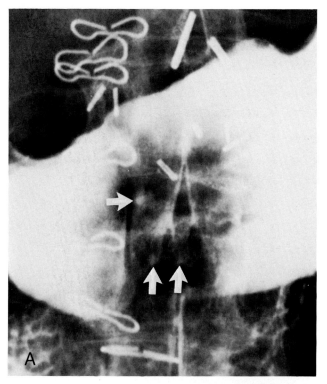

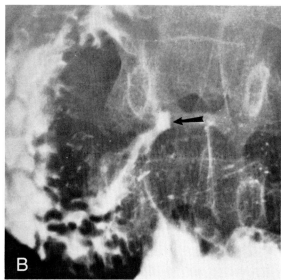

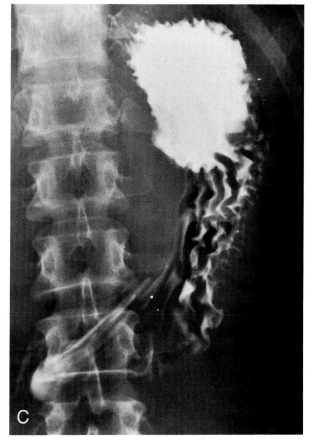

Fig. 4-3 Representative spot-films as obtained during
fluoroscopy in the performance of a conventional upper
gastrointestinal series. (A) Upright compression film of
the distal stomach showing gastric erosions (arrows) surrounded by edema. (B) Erect compression spot-film
showing an active duodenal ulcer (arrow). The barium in
the remainder of the duodenal bulb has been displaced
by the compression, with barium remaining only in the
ulcer crater. (C) Supine mucosal relief spot-film, which
shows to advantage structures on the posterior wall of
the distal stomach; in this instance normal folds are seen.

(Figure continues on next page.)

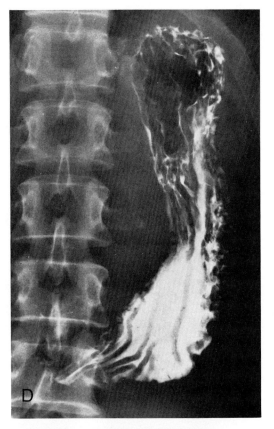

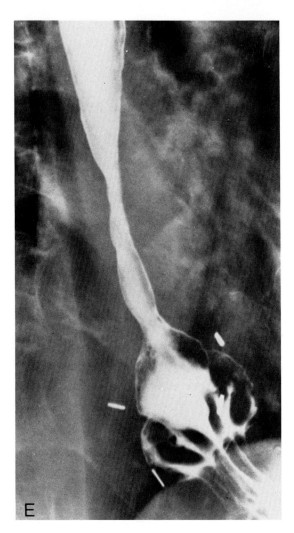

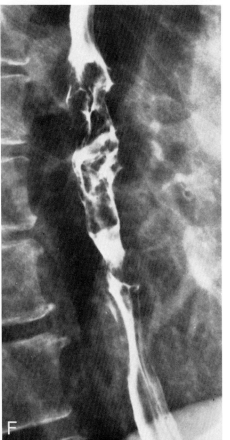

Fig. 4-3 (continued) (D) Prone mucosal relief spot-film of a normal stomach. This view shows to advantage structures on the distal anterior wall. (E) Spot-film with the distal esophagus taken in the RAO position showing a hiatal hernia and a distal esophageal stricture due to reflux esophagitis. (F) Mucosal relief film showing a large carcinoma of the midesophagus.

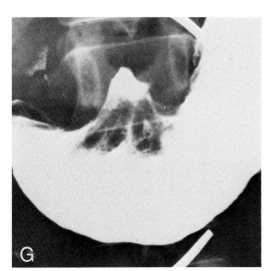

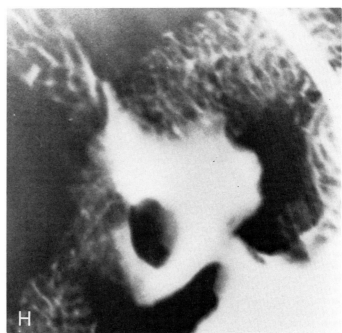

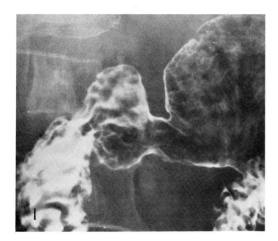

Fig. 4-3 *(continued)* (G) Prone compression spot-film using an inflatable paddle beneath the patient's abdomen. A large, benign, lesser curvature gastric ulcer is demonstrated. (H) Compression spot film of the barium-filled duodenal bulb obtained in the RAO position and showing an adenoma of the duodenal bulb. (I) Double-contrast view of the gastric antrum and duodenal bulb obtained in the LPO position showing deformity of the distal antrum and pyloric canal due to chronic peptic ulcer disease.

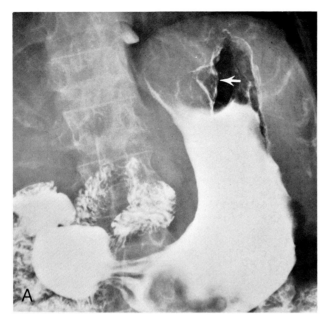

Fig. 4-4 Examples of Bucky films commonly taken at the conclusion of a conventional upper gastrointestinal series. (A) Prone (PA) film of the stomach demonstrating a large carcinoma of the fundus (arrow). (B) Right anterior oblique view of the stomach demonstrating elevation of gastric antrum by a large lymphomatous mass in the region of the pancreas. (C) Right lateral view of the stomach demonstrating shortening and narrowing of the gastric antrum due to gastric syphilis (Courtesy of Harry L. Stein, M. D., Manhasset, N.Y.).

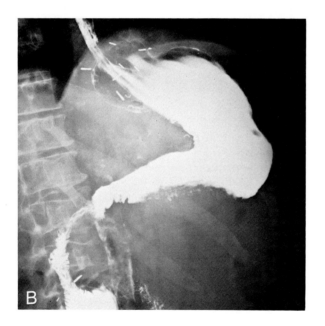

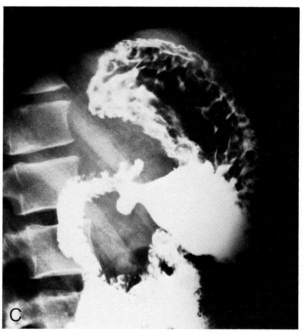

tained in the supine (AP) position (Fig. 4-3C). The patient is then turned to the prone (PA) position, and a second large spot film of the stomach and duodenal bulb is obtained (Fig. 4-3D). These prone (PA) and supine (AP) views are known as "mucosal relief" films.

Phase 4: Horizontal, Starting in the Prone (PA) Position

The patient now swallows additional barium rapidly via a straw. Spot films of the esophagus are taken when it is fully distended by the barium (Fig.

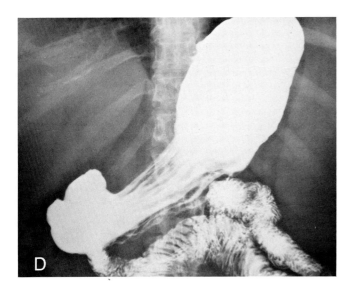

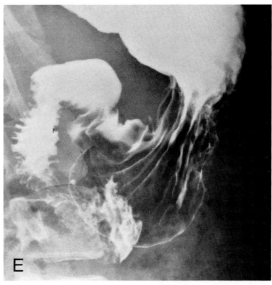

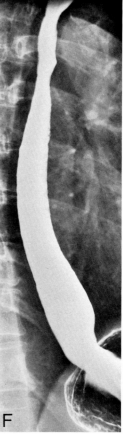

Fig. 4-4 *(continued)* (D) Supine (**AP**) view of the stomach with medial displacement of the proximal stomach by a greatly enlarged spleen. (**E**) Left posterior oblique view of a normal stomach demonstrating the double-contrast effect which can be obtained. (**F**) Full length view of the barium-filled esophagus obtained in the **RAO** position.

4-3E). The patient is asked to perform a deep Valsalva maneuver to help demonstrate any hiatus hernia that is present. Single swallows of barium are also employed to assess esophageal mobility. When peristalsis has stripped most of the barium from the esophagus, a mucosal relief film is taken with the patient in the RAO position to rotate the esophageal image clear of the spine (Fig. 4-3F). In this phase, with the patient in the RAO position, the duodenal bulb is allowed to fill with barium. The gastric antrum and duodenal bulb are then compressed from beneath with a compression paddle and spot filmed (Fig. 4-3G and H).

The patient is then turned onto his back to the LPO position. In this position, the gastric antrum and duodenal bulb will usually fill with air, giving an air-barium double-contrast view that is spot filmed (Fig. 4-3I).

Usually, at this point the fluoroscopy ceases and the patient is given over to the technologist for Bucky films of the esophagus, stomach, and duodenum.

Phase 5: Obtaining Bucky Films

A typical sequence of Bucky films of the esophagus, stomach, and duodenum is as follows.

1. Prone (PA) film of the stomach and duodenum (Fig. 4-4A).
2. Right anterior oblique film of the stomach and duodenum (Fig. 4-4B).
3. Right lateral film of the stomach and duodenum (Fig. 4-4C).
4. Supine (AP) film of the stomach and duodenum (Fig. 4-4D).
5. Left posterior oblique film of the stomach and duodenum (Fig. 4-4E).
6. Right anterior oblique film of the entire esophagus with patient drinking barium suspension (Fig. 4-4F).

With remote control machines, the above Bucky films are taken under fluoroscopic control at appropriate points in the course of the fluoroscopic examination. Table 4-1 presents a summary of the materials, positions, and films of the conventional upper gastrointestinal series.

Table 4-1. Summary of the Materials, Positions, and Films of the Conventional Upper Gastrointestinal Series

Materials
  60–100% wt/vol barium suspension, 6–8 oz

Fluoroscopic and Spot-Filming Sequence
  With patient upright
    Stomach AP—compression films
    Duodenal bulb LPO—compression films
  With table horizontal
    Stomach AP—mucosal relief film
    Stomach PA—mucosal relief film
    Esophagus PA and RAO—distended and mucosal relief
    Stomach and duodenal bulb PA and RAO—distended with barium and compressed.
    Gastric antrum and duodenal bulb LPO—double contrast films

Bucky films
  PA of stomach and duodenum
  RAO of stomach and duodenum
  R Lat of stomach and duodenum
  AP of stomach and duodenum
  LPO of stomach and duodenum
  RAO of esophagus with patient drinking

With remote control machines, the above Bucky films are taken under fluoroscopic control at appropriate points in the course of the fluoroscopic examination.

THE MULTIPHASIC OR "DOUBLE-CONTRAST" UPPER GASTROINTESTINAL EXAMINATION

Although in skilled hands the conventional, primarily single-contrast upper gastrointestinal series is very accurate, certain lesions causing minimal alterations of the mucosal surface of the esophagus, stomach, and duodenum may be difficult to detect, particularly early carcinomas, erosions, and scars. An upper gastrointestinal series incorporating double-contrast techniques allows more reliable detection of the lesions mentioned above. However, barium-filled and mucosal relief films of the esophagus and compression films of the stomach and duodenum are also required to reap maximum accuracy, and they are therefore included in the examination. As a result, the examination may most accurately be described as a multiphasic study. Due to the incorporation of double-contrast technique, the examination is performed in a somewhat different manner than the conventional upper gastrointestinal series, and may be divided into several phases as follows.

Phase 1: Table Erect

The patient is prepared for the examination with an intravenous injection of 0.1 to 0.25 mg of glucagon. In the upright or semiupright position, after 1 to 2 swallows of dense (200 to 250 percent weight per volume) barium, compression films of the distal two-thirds of the stomach are obtained (Fig. 4-5A and B).

Gas-producing granules or tablets sufficient to produce 300 to 500 cc of carbon dioxide are then administered with 10 to 15 ml of water, and the patient is provided with a cup with approximately 4 to 5 oz (120 to 150 ml) of the dense barium suspension. With the table upright and in the LPO position, the patient drinks the barium as rapidly as possible. Air swallowed with the barium and eructated from the stomach distends the esophagus, which is coated with the swallowed barium. When the esophagus is well distended and completely coated, double-contrast spot films of the esophagus are obtained (Fig. 4-5C).

Phase 2: Table Horizontal

The table is lowered to the horizontal position and the patient is rolled 360° three times. When the patient has finally been returned to the supine (AP) position, the gas-producing substance has dissolved and produced carbon dioxide, and the barium suspension has coated the stomach. The following representative series of films of the stomach are then taken under fluoroscopic control: supine (AP) (Fig. 4-5D), LPO (Fig. 4-5E), R Lat (Fig. 4-5F), RPO (Fig. 4-5G), and prone (PA) (remote control machines only) (Fig. 4-5H).

The entire stomach and duodenum are included on the films when possible. If the available spot films cannot encompass the entire stomach and duodenum, filming should be concentrated on those areas shown to advantage in double contrast.

Phase 3: Table Horizontal

The patient is placed in the RAO position and additional dense barium is given via a straw. Films are taken of the esophagus distended with barium (Fig. 4-5I) and in mucosal relief after peristalsis has passed (Fig. 4-5J). A Valsalva maneuver is performed to help demonstrate hiatus hernia. Single swallows of barium are also given to assess esophageal motility. With the patient recumbent, the following films of the duodenal bulb are also taken: RAO of the filled duodenum (Fig. 4-5K) and LPO of the duodenal bulb in double-contrast (Fig. 4-5L).

Phase 4: Table Elevated

The table is now elevated 45 to 90° and semierect or fully upright compression spot films of the duodenal bulb are obtained (Fig. 4-5M).

Phase 5: Bucky Film (Optional)

If the examination has been performed on a conventional fluoroscopic machine, the technologist now obtains a final prone (PA) Bucky film of the stomach and duodenum (Fig. 4-5F). This is not

Table 4-2. Summary of the Materials, Fluoroscopic Positions, and Films Employed During a Multiphasic Upper Gastrointestinal Series

Materials
  Glucagon, 0.1–0.25 mg IV
  Gas-producing granules
  Water, 10–15 ml
  High density barium suspension (200–250% wt/vol), 6–8 oz

Fluoroscopic and Spot-Filming Sequence
  With table upright and semierect
    Stomach AP—compression films
    Esophagus LPO—double-contrast films
  With table horizontal
    Stomach AP—double-contrast film
    Stomach LPO—double-contrast film
    Stomach R Lat—double-contrast film
    Stomach RPO—double-contrast film
    Stomach PA (Remote control only—barium-filled and
      double-contrast view)
    Esophagus PA and RAO—distended and mucosal relief
      films
    Duodenum RAO—barium-filled films
    Duodenum LPO—double-contrast films
  With table erect or semierect
    Duodenum AP or LPO—compression films

Bucky Film (Conventional Machines Only)
  Stomach and Duodenum PA—barium-filled film

(Text continues on page 46.)

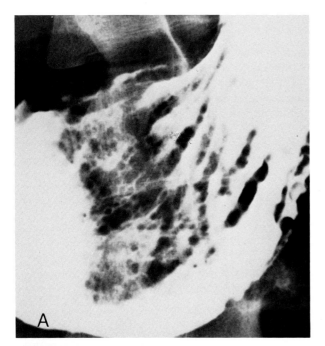

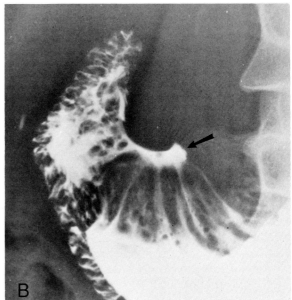

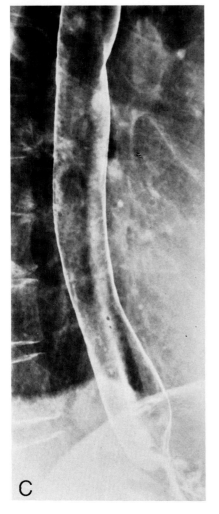

Fig. 4-5 Examples of films obtained during the course of multiphasic examination of the upper gastrointestinal tract. (A) Semierect compression film of the stomach showing multiple hyperplastic polyps. (B) Erect compression view of the distal stomach showing an active lesser curvature antral ulcer (arrow). (C) Erect double-contrast film of the esophagus showing slight mucosal irregularity due to mild esophagitis.

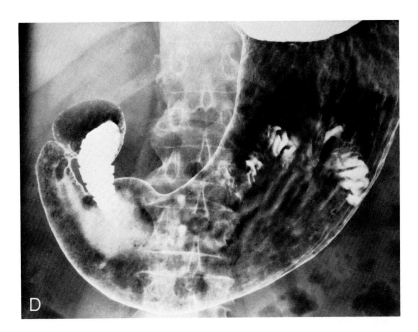

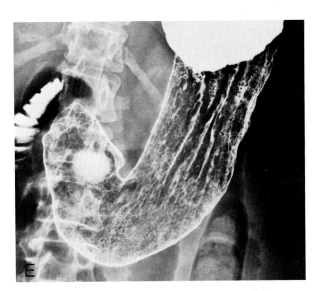

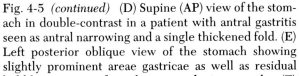

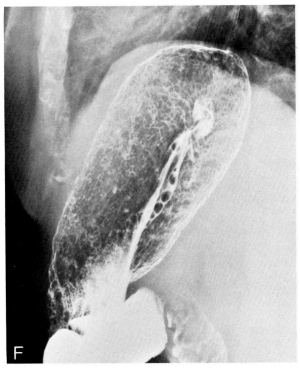

Fig. 4-5 *(continued)* (D) Supine (AP) view of the stomach in double-contrast in a patient with antral gastritis seen as antral narrowing and a single thickened fold. (E) Left posterior oblique view of the stomach showing slightly prominent areae gastricae as well as residual bubbles remaining from the gas-producing granules. (F) Right lateral (R Lat) view of the proximal stomach showing prominent areae gastricae and residual bubbles.

(Figure continues on next page)

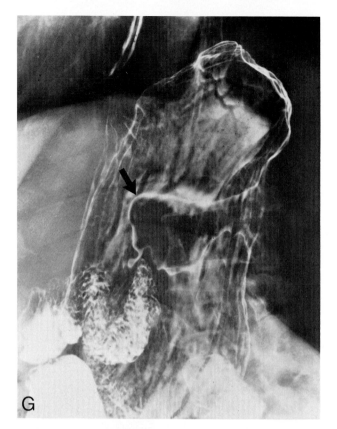

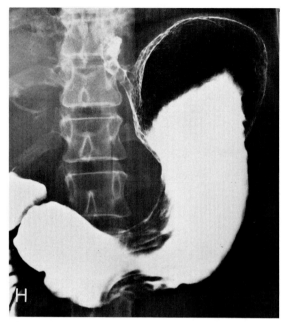

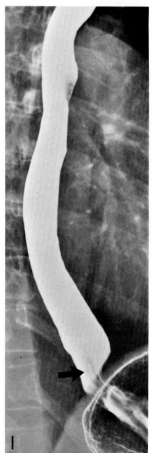
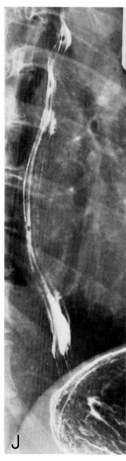

Fig. 4-5 *(continued)*   (G) Right posterior oblique view of the proximal stomach showing a tumor-like artifact (arrow) due to apposition of the anterior and posterior walls of the stomach. (H) Prone (PA) view of the stomach, which is normal except for a small hiatal hernia. (I) Recumbent RAO view of the esophagus with the patient drinking barium, showing a linear ulceration of the distal stomach surrounded by a halo of edema. (J) Mucosal relief view of the esophagus demonstrating thickened folds due to esophagitis.

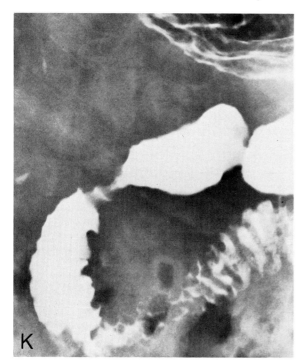

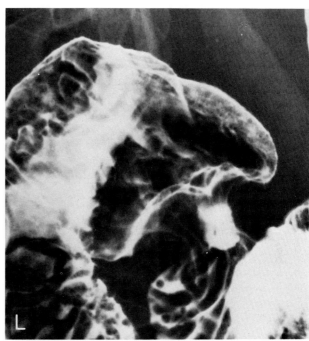

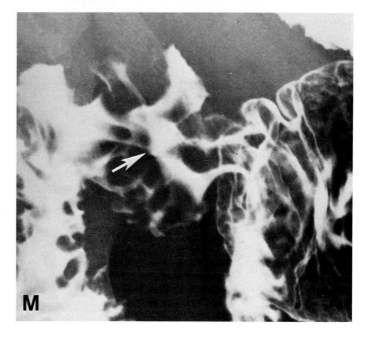

Fig. 4-5 *(continued)* (**K**) Right anterior oblique view of the barium-filled duodenum showing constriction of the postbulbar duodenum due to a postbulbar ulcer. (**L**) Left posterior oblique spot-film of the duodenal bulb and pyloric canal in double-contrast showing a large pyloric channel ulcer. (**M**) Semierect compression spot-film of the duodenal bulb showing an active ulcer (arrow) in the center of converging, edematous folds.

necessary with remote control fluoroscopy since a prone film taken with optimum geometry has already been obtained in the course of the examination.

Summary and Conclusions

Table 4-2 summarizes the materials, fluoroscopic positions, and films employed during the multiphasic upper gastrointestinal series.

In the above multiphasic examination, compression films are obtained at the onset using the same dense 200 to 250 percent weight per volume barium employed for the subsequent double-contrast phases of the study. The dense barium is used throughout the study, since it provides maximum mucosal detail on compression and mucosal relief films, as well as on the double-contrast films. The procedure for obtaining compression films with dense barium is detailed in Chapter 6, which explains in much greater detail the several techniques available for examining the stomach.

It should also be noted, however, that many radiologists prefer to obtain compression films toward the end of the study and to use a thin (30 to 40 percent weight per volume) barium suspension to dilute the dense barium given initially. They feel that the more dilute barium is more easily compressed. However, there are severe disadvantages to this technique including (1) the large volume of barium to be compressed, (2) interference by barium that has entered the small bowel, (3) destruction of the coating power of the barium suspension so that further double-contrast films are compromised, (4) difficulty in showing small lesions on the compression films, and (5) the unnecessary complexity of preparing two barium suspensions.

Although the use of dense barium suspension during compression filming requires a certain degree of skill, it provides greater radiographic detail and an unobstructed view of the stomach. It thereby maximizes the yield from the compression phase of the study without compromising the double-contrast films.

SUGGESTED READINGS

Gelfand DW: The Japanese-style double-contrast examination of the stomach. Gastrointest Radiol 1:7, 1976.

Gelfand DW, Ott DJ: Single- vs. double-contrast gastrointestinal studies; critical analysis of reported statistics. AJR 137:523, 1981.

Kawai K, Tanaka H: Differential diagnosis of gastric diseases. Chicago, Year Book Medical Publishers, 1974, pp. 11–54.

Laufer I: Double-Contrast Gastrointestinal Radiology. Philadelphia, WB Saunders, 1979, pp 59–77.

Op den Orth JO: The Standard Biphasic-Contrast Examination of the Stomach and Duodenum. The Hague, Martinus Nijhoff, 1979.

Ott DJ, Gelfand DW, Wu WC: Detection of gastric ulcer: Comparison of single- and double-contrast examination. AJR 139:93, 1982.

Storch CB: Fundamentals of Clinical Fluoroscopy. New York, Grune and Stratton, 1957, pp 111–115, 125–164.

Templeton FE: X-ray Examination of the Stomach. Chicago, University of Chicago Press, 1964, pp 36–78.

5

Techniques for Examining the Hypopharynx and Esophagus

Four examination modalities are commonly employed for the radiographic study of the hypopharynx and esophagus: barium-filled, double-contrast, mucosal relief, and motion-recording. Furthermore, there are four anatomic regions, each demanding a specific form of examination for optimal results: the hypopharynx, the cervical esophagus, the thoracic esophagus, and the esophagogastric junction. The modalities of examination most suitable for each of these areas are determined by the structure and function of each region, as well as the disease entities most frequently encountered. Examination techniques for the hypopharynx and esophagus are therefore described on a regional basis.

THE HYPOPHARYNX

The hypopharynx is that portion of the pharynx extending from the epiglottis to the esophageal inlet. Since dysphagia in the cervical region is a common complaint leading to the performance of esophagography, and since neoplasms or neuromuscular dysfunctions affecting the hypopharynx

are not uncommon, an ability to examine this area carefully is of considerable clinical importance.

The most satisfactory methods for performing a detailed radiographic examination of the hypopharynx are via double-contrast and motion-recording techniques. Although the hypopharynx is not often routinely examined, it is one of the simplest of all gastrointestinal examinations.

To accomplish the double-contrast examination of the hypopharynx, the patient is placed with his back against the upright fluoroscopic table, and is given a cup of high density barium suspension. The patient takes a mouthful of barium suspension, but refrains from swallowing it until asked to do so. The patient is told to elevate his chin and look straight ahead and is then asked to swallow. The swallow is viewed fluoroscopically, and its passage may be recorded by one of the motion-recording methods described below (Fig. 5-1). The patient is asked to refrain from swallowing again or clearing his throat. The swallow will have deposited a coating of barium on the walls of the hypopharynx producing a double-contrast effect that is easily seen and radiographed (Fig. 5-2). When a satisfactory frontal examination of the hypopharynx has

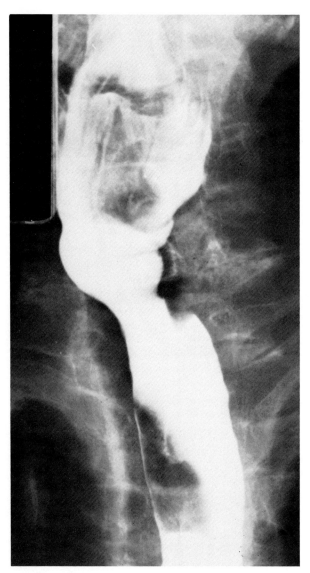

Fig. 5-1 Barium-distended view of the hypopharynx and cervical esophagus obtained with a rapid sequence spot-film device. Distortion of the pharyngoesophageal junction is caused by postsurgical scarring.

the patient tends to aspirate barium, the larynx proper and the proximal portion of the trachea are often delineated. Viewing and recording of the passage of the bolus through the hypopharynx (and cervical esophagus) allows assessment of any areas of nondistensibility or of displacement or diversion of the barium stream due to neoplasms or webs. Neuromuscular disorders affecting swallowing functions will also be appreciated.

THE CERVICAL ESOPHAGUS

Because of the normally rapid passage of a bolus through the cervical esophagus, in the absence of a motion-recording device it may be a challenge to obtain films of the barium as it traverses this region. A variety of "tricks" have been devised to accomplish this using ordinary spot films. The most common method is to place one's finger on the patient's thyroid cartilage, drawing it away and taking a film as the thyroid cartilage begins to rise during deglutition. Unfortunately, several films are usually required before a view of the cervical esophagus in a suitable state of distension can be obtained (Fig. 5-1). A second method can be described as the "counting" method. The patient is asked to swallow a bolus of barium, and the radiologist counts until he sees the bolus passing through the cervical esophagus. To then take a film of the barium-distended cervical esophagus, the patient is asked to swallow and the fluoroscopist begins counting, exposing the film at the appropriate count. As before, several films may be expended before a view with adequate distension is obtained.

An alternative method of filming the cervical esophagus, albeit not in distension, is to use a very dense barium suspension or paste, filming the mucosal relief pattern in the cervical esophagus after passage of the bolus (Fig. 5-3). The more dense and viscous the barium employed, the more certain the success of the method. Very small mucosal abnormalities can be demonstrated by this technique, but it must be supplemented by viewing and/or motion recording of the distended cervical esophagus during passage of the bolus to rule out constricting lesions.

Motion-recording techniques are perhaps the most reliable and simplest methods of recording

been obtained, the patient is turned 90° to his right, facing the examiner, and the sequence is repeated, providing lateral views of the same area (Fig. 5-2).

The above method produces double-contrast views of the posterior wall of the pharynx, the piriform sinuses, the epiglottis and valleculae, and the top of the arytenoid cartilages. In addition, if

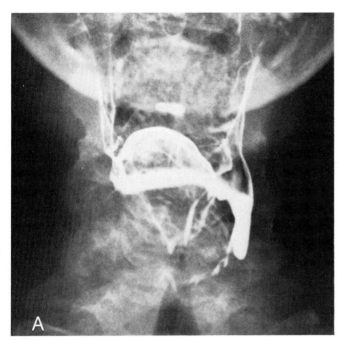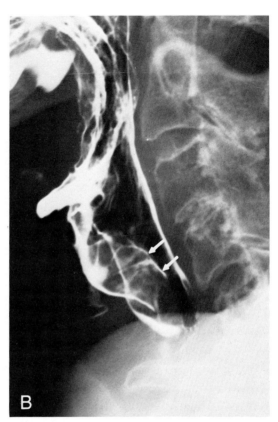

Fig. 5-2 Frontal and lateral double-contrast views of the hypopharynx obtained after a swallow of high density barium. (A) Frontal view showing a large carcinoma obliterating the right piriform sinus. (B) Lateral view showing enlargement of the arytenoid cartilages (arrows) due to spread of carcinoma of the larynx.

both the structure and peristalsis of the cervical esophagus. Motion-recording techniques that can be employed include videotape recording, cine radiography, and rapid sequence recording on standard x-ray film using a high speed spot-film device capable of sequential filming. Since motility disorders are relatively uncommon in the cervical esophagus, one is mainly looking for lack of distensibility or contour defects due to intrinsic neoplasm, extrinsic mass, web, stricture, or diverticulum.

THE THORACIC ESOPHAGUS

By definition, the thoracic esophagus extends from the thoracic inlet to the esophagogastric junction. It is the most frequent esophageal site of both malignant neoplasms and serious inflammatory disease. Its proximity to the mediastinal lymph nodes and heart often cause it to be invaded and/or displaced by masses or enlargement of these adjacent structures. Also, it is the usual site of esophageal dysmotility. As a result, the thoracic esophagus should be thoroughly examined using most or all of the available radiographic modalities both during esophagography as a separate examination and during the performance of an upper gastrointestinal series.

The most common and reliable method of examining the thoracic esophagus is by observing and radiographing it while it is distended with barium. This is the most basic form of examination and provides considerable information about the three most common and serious entities affecting the thoracic esophagus: cancer of the esophagus, se-

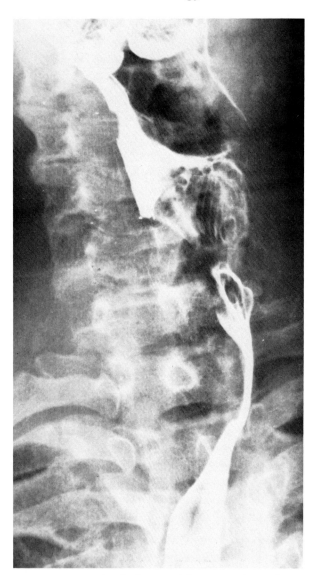

Fig. 5-3 Mucosal relief view of the cervical esophagus taken immediately after the patient had swallowed a bolus of very dense barium suspension. The esophagus is deviated to the left by a large metastatic carcinoma present in the right cervical region.

vere reflux esophagitis, and significant motility disorders. To produce a satisfactory barium-distended study of the thoracic esophagus, the patient is placed in the RAO position on the horizontal table and is asked to drink several swallows of barium suspension without hesitation. The barium usually distends the entire thoracic esophagus, and a film is then taken (Fig. 5-4). To evaluate esophageal motility, single swallows of barium are used, since multiple swallows reflexly suppress esophageal peristalsis. For thoroughness, a second view may be employed, usually the LAO position, allowing inspection of the esophagus in two views at 90° variance from each other.

Mucosal relief technique is the second method available for examining the thoracic esophagus, and is usually applied in conjuction with the distension films described above. After the distended views are obtained, the esophagus is allowed to empty, leaving a coating of barium on the collapsed mucosa, the so-called mucosal relief. The best mucosal relief films are obtained using dense barium suspension or paste (Fig. 5-5). The purpose of the mucosal relief films is to demonstrate structural abnormalities of small dimension that might be hidden by the mass of barium present in the esophagus during full distension. These include reflux esophagitis, candidiasis, herpes esophagitis, small ulcers, and early carcinomas that are of insufficient size to cause a significant filling or contour defect on barium-distended views.

Mucosal relief films are also the best modality for the detection and evaluation of esophageal varices. For maximal detection of varices, the examination should be preceded by administration of an anticholinergic agent capable of relaxing the esophageal musculature. This lowers intraluminal pressure and encourages filling of the varices (Fig. 5-5C).

Double-contrast esophagography may be employed in conjunction with the single-contrast films described above, and is useful for detecting esophagitis and small esophageal neoplasms. To obtain double-contrast films of the esophagus, the patient stands in front of the upright fluoroscopic table in the LPO position. Gas-producing granules or tablets are administered with 10 to 15 ml of water. The patient is then instructed to drink barium suspension as rapidly as possible. Usually, the patient ingests sufficient air with the barium to fill the lumen of the esophagus with air while barium running down the sides of the esophagus coats its mucosal surface, producing the double-contrast effect (Fig. 5-6). Often, the gas evolving in the

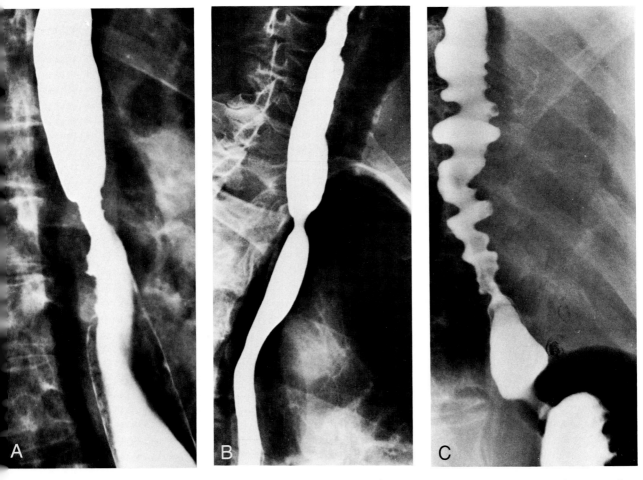

Fig. 5-4 Barium-distended views of the thoracic esophagus as employed to demonstrate constricting lesions and motility disorders. **(A)** Circumferential carcinoma of the midesophagus. **(B)** Constriction at the squamocolumnar junction in a patient with Barrett's esophagus. **(C)** Severe tertiary contractions (curling) in an elderly patient with dysphagia.

stomach will bubble up into the esophagus, increasing the degree of distension and providing a double-contrast view of the distal third of the esophagus.

An alternate method of examining the distal esophagus in double-contrast is with the patient prone and drinking as rapidly as possible. Considerable air will usually be ingested, producing a double-contrast effect in the distal esophagus (Fig. 5-7). Ingested air tends to collect in the distal esophagus because of the normal, posteriorly convex curve of the distal esophagus.

Motion-recording devices (videotape, cineradiography, spot-film camera, or rapid sequence spot-film device as described in Ch. 2) can be employed to record peristalsis and detect abnormal motility in the thoracic esophagus. The most precise procedure involves having the patient take a single swallow of barium, and then recording the primary peristaltic wave as it progresses distally in the esophagus. This accurately evaluates the patient's primary wave, which should move smoothly from the proximal esophagus to the esophagogastric junction. The act of deglutition may also stimu-

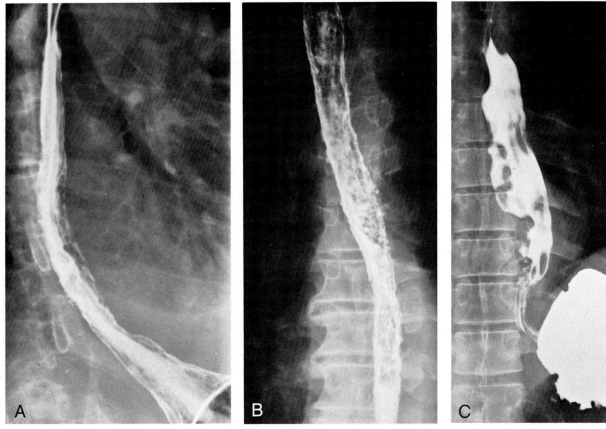

Fig. 5-5 Examples of pathology easily demonstrated with mucosal relief technique. (A) Reflux esophagitis with irregular thickening of distal esophageal folds, as well as a patulous esophagogastric junction. (B) Esophageal candidiasis demonstrating the irregular, coarsely granular, ulcerated appearance of this disease. (C) Esophageal varices with irregular, serpiginous swelling of distal esophageal folds.

late abnormal secondary and tertiary peristalsis, which should similarly be recorded. Quickly repeated swallows should be avoided, since they tend to reflexly inhibit propagation of the normal primary wave. The considerable variety of motility disorders that present in the thoracic esophagus are described in Chapter 13, Abnormalities of the Esophagus and Esophagogastric Junction.

THE ESOPHAGOGASTRIC JUNCTION

The frequency of hiatus hernia and reflux esophagitis as causes of upper gastrointestinal symptoms requires that particular attention be paid to the examination of the esophagogastric junction.

Single-contrast technique has been the dominant means of examining the esophagogastric junction, since it provides the reliable distension of the region necessary to show both hiatus hernia and any loss of distensibility or stricture due to reflux esophagitis. Also, both esophageal and gastric carcinomas occur with reasonable frequency in the region, and most are easily demonstrable by this means.

Reliable distension of the esophagogastric junction during the single-contrast examination may be achieved with the following procedure. The pa-

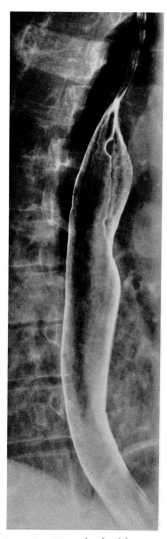

Fig. 5-6 Upright double-contrast film of the thoracic esophagus showing a small intramural neoplasm in the proximal thoracic esophagus.

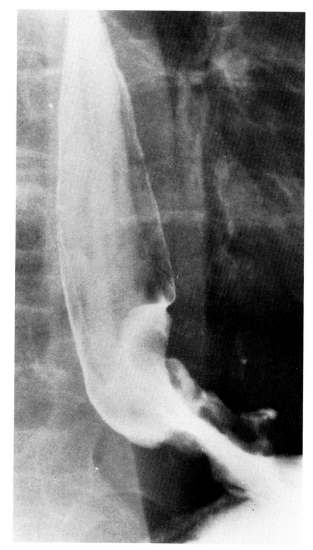

Fig. 5-7 Prone double-contrast view of the distal thoracic esophagus outlining the proximal extent of an esophagogastric adenocarcinoma (Ott DJ, Gelfand DW, Wu WC, Kerr RM: Secondary achalasia in esophagogastric carcinoma: Re-emphasis of a difficult differential problem. Rev Interam Radiol 4:135, 1979.)

tient is placed in the RAO position and drinks barium as rapidly as possible. When the esophagus is fully distended with barium, the patient is asked to perform a deep Valsalva maneuver. The pinchcock effect of the diaphragmatic crura occurring with the Valsalva maneuver causes the barium in the esophagus to accumulate in the esophagogas-tric region and distend it maximally (Fig. 5-8). The downward displacement of the diaphragm during the Valsalva maneuver also allows a more unobstructed view of the esophagogastric junction and of any hiatal hernia that is present. For thoroughness, this examination sequence can be repeated in the LAO position.

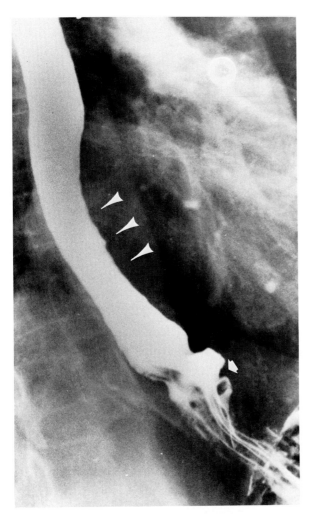

Fig. 5-8 Barium-distended view of the distal esophagus and esophagogastric junction with the patient performing a Valsalva maneuver to ensure maximum distention. The presence of hiatal hernia is indicated by visibility of the muscular A ring and a notch at the location of the B ring (lower arrow). Severe reflux esophagitis is present as manifested by restricted distensibility and marginal irregularity (upper arrows).

In addition to the barium-distended views described above, mucosal relief and/or double-contrast films of the esophagogastric region should be obtained. Mucosal relief films will usually show the earliest radiographic signs of reflux esophagitis, consisting of thickening and irregularity of the distal folds (Fig. 5-5A), and may occasionally show a hernial sac not clearly apparent on distended views. Films of the esophagogastric junction in double-contrast may also demonstrate signs of reflux esophagitis, such as mucosal granularity and erosions, and may occasionally show hiatus hernia in the form of areae gastricae extending above the diaphragmatic crura into the hernia. Also, mucosal relief and/or double-contrast films may be required to demonstrate an occasional early carcinoma of the esophagogastric region, which can be hidden by the mass of barium present on barium-distended views.

SUGGESTED READINGS

Cockerill EM, Miller RE, Chernish SM, et al: Optimal visualization of esophageal varices. Am J Roentgenol 126:512, 1976.

Dodds WJ: Current concepts of esophageal motor function: Clinical implications for cardiology. Am J Roentgenol 128:549, 1977.

Donner MW, Siegel CI: The evaluation of pharyngeal neuromuscular disorders by cinefluorography. Am J Roentgenol 94:299, 1965.

Friedland GW: Historical review of the changing concepts of lower esophageal anatomy: 430 BC–1977. AJR 131:373, 1978.

Gelfand OW, Ott DJ: Anatomy and technique in evaluating the esophagus. Semin Roentgenol 16:168, 1981.

Goldstein HM, Dodd GD: Double-contrast examination of the esophagus. Gastrointest Radiol 1:3, 1976.

Koehler RE, Weyman PJ, Oakley HF: Single- and double-contrast techniques in esophagitis. AJR 135:15, 1980.

Margulis AR, Koehler RE: Radiologic diagnosis of disordered esophageal motility. Radiol Clin North Am 14:429, 1976.

Moss AA, Koehler RE, Margulis AR: Initial accuracy of esophagrams in detection of small esophageal carcinoma. Am J Roentgenol 127:909, 1976.

Ott DJ, Gelfand DW, Wu WC: Reflux esophagitis: Radiographic and endoscopic correlation. Radiology 130:583, 1979.

Ott DJ, Wu WC, Gelfand DW: Reflux esophagitis revisited: Prospective analysis of radiologic accuracy. Gastrointest Radiol 6:1, 1981.

6

Techniques for Examining the Stomach

Four basic techniques are available for the examination of the stomach: *compression, mucosal relief, double-contrast,* and *filling with barium.* Each requires proper implementation, as well as an appreciation for the particular areas of the stomach well shown and the types of pathology likely to be demonstrated. The regions of the stomach shown well by each of the four modalities are illustrated diagrammatically in Figure 6-1.

Except in the most demanding situation, such as in the search for a strongly suspected early gastric cancer, it is unusual for all four of these techniques to be applied during the same examination. However, a thorough upper gastrointestinal examination will routinely employ two or three of these modalities. For example, a diligently performed conventional upper gastrointestinal series makes considerable use of compression and barium-filled views, supplemented by double-contrast views of much of the stomach. The traditional European examination also includes mucosal relief films. On the other hand, a thorough double-contrast or multiphasic examination makes extensive use of double-contrast filming as well as compression and/or mucosal relief films and barium filling.

COMPRESSION FILMING

The satisfactory compression examination of the stomach requires attention to several matters: the timing of the compression films, the amount and density of the barium suspension, the position of the table, the amount of pressure applied, the use of the spine for counterpressure, and the kilovoltage.

Amount of Barium Suspension

The amount of barium suspension employed greatly influences the success of the compression phase of an examination. The usual mistake made in this regard is use of too small an amount of barium in an attempt to avoid a large collection of barium in the stomach that might be difficult to spread out with compression or to penetrate radiographically. Adequate barium, however, must be present in the stomach to permit the folds to be flattened out somewhat during the examination (Fig. 6-2). With too little barium in the stomach during compression filming, the resulting promi-

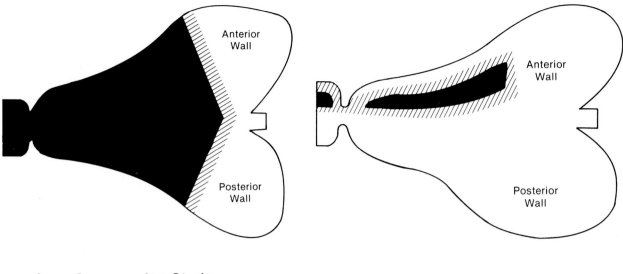

A   Compression Study
Standing Frontal View

B   Mucosal Relief Study
Prone View

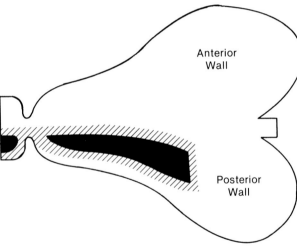

C   Mucosal Relief Study
Supine View

Fig. 6-1 Diagrammatic illustrations of the regions of the stomach shown by each of the four available examination modalities. (A) Compression. The anterior and posterior walls, as well as both curvatures, distal to the rib cage are well demonstrated. Because anterior wall lesions are readily detected on compression films and are easily missed on double-contrast views, the two modalities are often combined. (B) The prone mucosal relief view shows structures on the distal anterior wall well. For this reason, it is often combined with double-contrast views. (C) The supine mucosal relief view shows essentially the same area as the supine double-contrast view but less broadly and possibly with less detail.

nent fold pattern may obscure small lesions. It is thus wise to administer at least 2 to 3 ounces (60 to 90 ml) of barium suspension in preparation for compression filming.

Timing of the Compression Films

Compression views of the distal stomach are best obtained before the barium suspension is able to make its way into the proximal small bowel loops that lie behind the stomach, since barium in those loops may obscure much of the distal stomach. If the examination is a standard, full-column examination, gastroparesis is usually not employed, since compression views can usually be obtained easily and rapidly at the onset of the study. However, if compression films are taken as the initial phase of a multiphasic examination, gastroparesis with gluca-

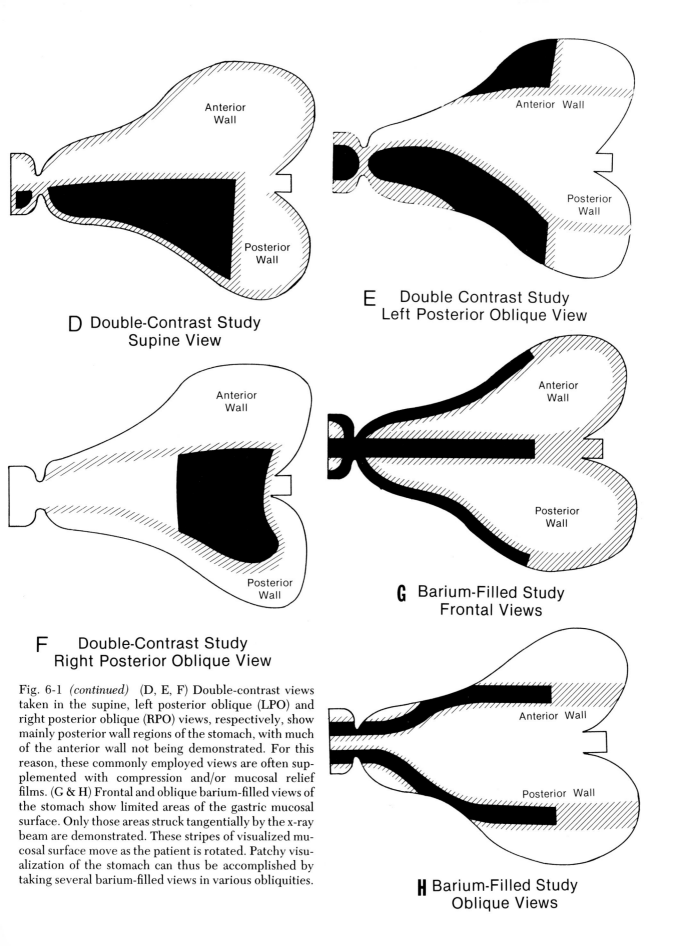

D Double-Contrast Study
Supine View

E Double Contrast Study
Left Posterior Oblique View

F Double-Contrast Study
Right Posterior Oblique View

G Barium-Filled Study
Frontal Views

H Barium-Filled Study
Oblique Views

Fig. 6-1 (continued) (D, E, F) Double-contrast views taken in the supine, left posterior oblique (LPO) and right posterior oblique (RPO) views, respectively, show mainly posterior wall regions of the stomach, with much of the anterior wall not being demonstrated. For this reason, these commonly employed views are often supplemented with compression and/or mucosal relief films. (G & H) Frontal and oblique barium-filled views of the stomach show limited areas of the gastric mucosal surface. Only those areas struck tangentially by the x-ray beam are demonstrated. These stripes of visualized mucosal surface move as the patient is rotated. Patchy visualization of the stomach can thus be accomplished by taking several barium-filled views in various obliquities.

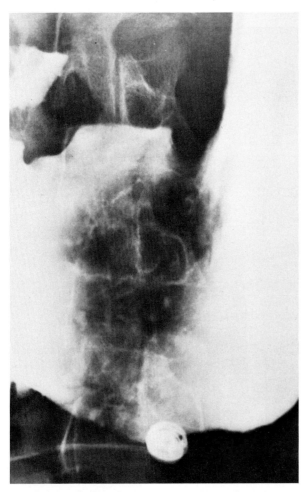

Fig. 6-2 Multiple gastric erosions shown by compression filming during a conventional upper gastrointestinal examination. Note that the vertebral column has been used for counterpressure and sufficient barium has been administered to spread the folds apart, allowing visualization of small lesions that might lie between folds.

gon or Buscopan should be employed to prevent peristalsis from propelling the barium into the small bowel during the compression phase or during the double-contrast filming that follows. Since adequate doses of these gastroparetic agents are effective for 10 minutes or more, it is possible to obtain both compression and double-contrast films of the stomach in most patients before significant small bowel filling takes place.

Density of the Barium Suspension

The density of the barium suspension to a great extent affects the care that must be exercised during compression filming. For the conventional, full-column examination, barium density is usually 60 to 100 percent weight per volume, and moderate pressure is usually successful in thinning out the barium layer sufficiently so that it can be easily penetrated by the x-ray beam (Fig. 6-2). Relatively large amounts of barium can be present in the stomach during the conventional examination and a compression-palpation examination can be successfully performed.

On the other hand, when compression is employed as part of a double-contrast or multiphasic examination, the barium suspension encountered is very dense, up to 250 percent weight per volume. Because of this density, smaller amounts of barium should be employed. Also, because of the difficulty in adequately penetrating a very dense suspension, one must ensure that the layer of barium created during compression filming is sufficiently thin to be easily penetrated radiographically (Fig. 6-3). This requires careful control of the amount of barium present in the stomach, frequent use of the semierect position to spread the barium through the stomach more evenly, and use of the spine for counterpressure.

Position of the Table

The position of the table largely determines the amount of barium present in any particular region of the stomach during compression filming. With the table fully upright, the position usually employed for compression filming during the conventional examination, barium pools in the distal stomach. However, to obtain a more even distribution of barium during compression filming, one may use the semierect position (Fig. 6-4). The inclination of the stomach within the patient's body determines the precise degree of table elevation necessary. The semierect position is particularly helpful in controlling the distribution of the barium when high density barium suspension is being employed during a double-contrast or multiphasic examina-

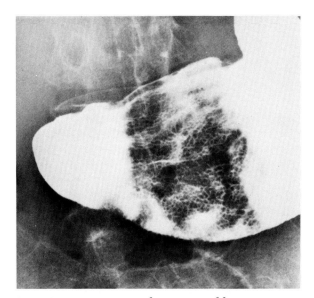

Fig. 6-3 Areae gastricae demonstrated by compression filming employing a high density barium suspension. The vertebral column is used for counterpressure, and the patient has been tilted back to the semierect position to allow excess barium to flow away from the region being compressed.

tion (Fig. 6-3). The semierect position may also be helpful in patients with very long stomachs, in whom it may be otherwise difficult to maintain adequate barium in the midportion of the body of the stomach during compression filming.

Use of the Spine for Counterpressure

The spine should be used for counterpressure, particularly when compression films are made with very high density barium suspensions. The vertebral column prevents the stomach from moving posteriorly in response to the application of compression. The stomach may then be sufficiently compressed to ensure its penetrability by the x-ray beam (Fig. 6-3). For this, it is necessary to position the patient so as to bring the area of the stomach being compressed between the pressure cone and the spine. The overlying vertebral shadows will not interfere with interpretation of the films, since the very dense barium is impossible to confuse with bony structures.

Kilovoltage

Kilovoltage should be kept in the moderate range (100 to 110 kVp) during the compression examination of the stomach, whether part of a standard full-column or multiphasic examination. Contrary to general opinion, increasing the kilovoltage to penetrate a large mass of barium rarely succeeds. Very high kilovoltages simply cause darkening of the barium shadow as a result of scattered radiation. Kilovoltages of 100–110 kVp (using modern three-phase equipment) strike a happy medium between lowering the kilovoltage to minimize scatter and raising the kilovoltage to ensure penetrance of the barium and short exposure times.

Areas Shown by Compression

The area shown well on the compression examination includes mainly the distal half of the stomach (Fig. 6-1). The anterior wall, posterior wall, and greater and lesser curvatures are all well demonstrated in those portions of the stomach that lie below the ribs and are thus amenable to compression filming. In slender patients, most of the stomach will be below the ribs and is easily compressed. In stocky or obese patients, most of the stomach may be up beneath the ribs and will thus be inaccessible. However, the amount of stomach accessible to palpation or compression can sometimes be increased by having the patient take a deep inspiration. The resulting descent of the diaphragm pushes the stomach lower within the abdomen, forcing more of it beyond the lower limit of the ribs.

Pathology shown well on compression films includes virtually all ulcers and masses more than 1 or 2 mm in size in those areas of the stomach that are easily compressible. However, in obese patients or those with extremely strong abdominal musculature, the stomach cannot be easily compressed, and it may be difficult to show lesions of any size. Also, when barium suspensions of moderate density (60 to 100 percent weight per volume) are employed during full-column examination, extremely small lesions such as gastric erosions (Fig.

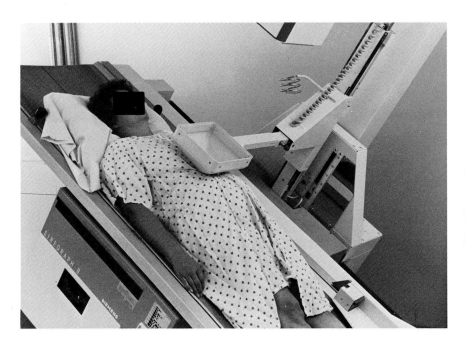

Fig. 6-4 The semierect position may be employed to control distribution of barium within the stomach. In this manner, excess barium may be caused to flow away from the distal stomach, and barium can be maintained in the midbody of the stomach during compression.

6-2) may be difficult to demonstrate with compression filming due to lack of sufficient intrinsic radiographic contrast. On the other hand, the use of high density barium suspensions, as employed during the double-contrast examination, allows demonstration by compression filming of very small structural features, such as the areae gastricae and gastric erosions (Fig. 6-3).

Lesions poorly shown include those that alter the gastric fold pattern in a manner that requires distension of the stomach for the abnormality to be well demonstrated. For example, gastric ulcer scars, whose demonstration usually requires distension of the stomach, are more reliably shown by double-contrast filming. Similarly, certain subtle lesions such as gastric erosions and early gastric cancers, particularly those located on the posterior wall, may not be shown as easily on compression films as on double-contrast films.

Overall, however, compression filming is one of the two most powerful modalities available for the examination of the stomach, approximately equaling double-contrast filming in its overall effectiveness. Furthermore, because most gastric ulcers and erosions occur in the distal stomach where they are accessible to demonstration by palpation and compression, careful use of this modality re-

sults in a very considerable yield of pathology in a Western practice of radiology. It is thus virtually mandatory that compression filming be included in any routine for the radiologic examination of the stomach.

MUCOSAL RELIEF FILMS

Mucosal relief films usually consist of prone (PA) and supine (AP) films of the stomach obtained with an amount of barium just sufficient to demonstrate the gastric folds without appreciably distending the organ (Fig. 6-5). The appearance of mucosal relief films to an extent duplicates that of compression films. Mucosal relief films are usually obtained during the initial phases of the upper gastrointestinal examination, since they require that the stomach not be overfilled with barium suspension.

The usual procedure for obtaining mucosal relief films is to administer 2 to 3 ounces of barium, turn the patient from front to back once or twice to distribute the barium thoroughly throughout the stomach, and then obtain films of the stomach in the prone and supine position. Compression can be applied during the supine (AP) mucosal relief filming of the stomach and may be helpful in demon-

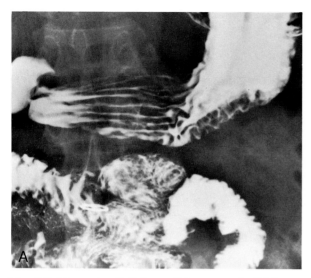 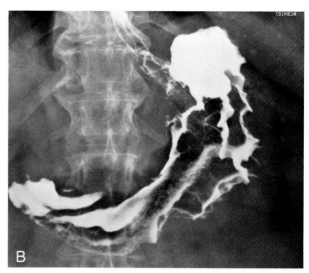

Fig. 6-5 Mucosal relief views of the stomach. (A) Prone mucosal relief view showing the folds in the distal stomach well. This particular view may be employed to demonstrate structures on the distal anterior wall. (B) Supine mucosal relief view in a patient with gastric lymphoma. Because the stomach is not distended, the thickened folds are allowed to project up into the barium, and their abnormal character is well demonstrated.

strating lesions not otherwise visible. If mucosal relief films are obtained as part of a double-contrast examination, it is wise to administer a gastroparetic agent to prevent early filling of the small bowel.

The distal two-thirds of the stomach are well shown on mucosal relief films (Fig. 6-1), with the prone mucosal relief film tending to show well those lesions located on the anterior wall of the distal stomach. As a result, this particular film can be used as a complement to double-contrast films of the stomach to avoid missing anterior wall lesions. Supine mucosal relief films, on the other hand, tend to show lesions located on the posterior wall of the distal stomach.

THE DOUBLE-CONTRAST TECHNIQUE

Double-contrast filming of the entire stomach by the supplemental administration of gas or air into the stomach is a newly evolved and powerful technique. Films of the stomach in the double-contrast mode have now become the heart of what has become commonly known as the double-contrast

upper gastrointestinal series. This examination, although previously known, was perfected in Japan in the early 1960s as a means of detecting early gastric cancer, and it has since been adopted by many radiologists worldwide.

The gas-producing agent is the unique component necessary for a practical routine double-contrast examination. Most gas-producing agents designed for the double-contrast examination are powders, granules, or loosely compacted small tablets containing sodium bicarbonate, a weak acid, and an antifoaming agent. They are designed to dissolve rapidly, releasing 300 to 500 cc of carbon dioxide within the stomach. Many examiners use a small amount of water, typically 10 to 15 ml, to wash down the gas producer. Others administer the gas producer directly with the barium suspension. After administering the barium and gas producer, the patient is rolled 360° two or three times so as to coat the entire stomach with barium, hasten the evolution of gas, and break up any bubbles that may have formed. The patient usually comes to rest on his back, ready for the initial double-contrast film.

The amount of barium administered with the gas-producing agent should be adequate to thor-

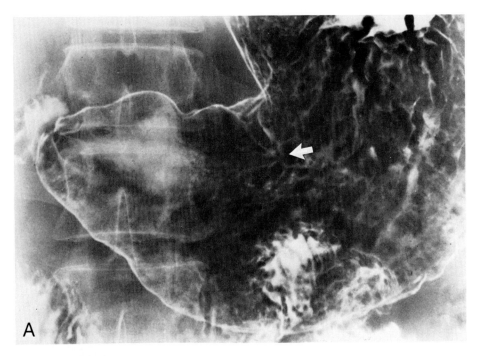

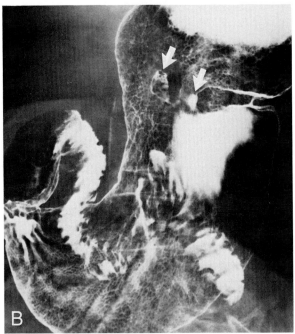

Fig. 6-6 Double-contrast views of the stomach showing exquisite structural detail. Reliable demonstration of pathology is limited, however, to the dependent wall of the stomach, which generally corresponds to the posterior wall. (A) Supine view showing a gastric ulcer scar (arrow) on the posterior wall near the angulus (Gelfand DW, Ott DJ: Gastric ulcer scars. Radiology 140:37, 1981. (B) Right posterior oblique view showing two gastric ulcers (arrows) on the lesser curvature and posterior wall, as well as prominent areae gastricae, a common finding in peptic ulcer disease.

oughly coat the stomach and wash any mucous away from the mucosal surface, allowing the smallest lesions to be seen. Often, there is a tendency to perform the double-contrast examination with an insufficient amount of barium, thinking that a small amount of barium in combination with a large amount of gas will produce a more "elegant" study. However, a generous amount of barium (100 to 150 ml) does not interfere with the double-contrast filming, makes it easier to achieve a thorough coating, and tends to more thoroughly scrub the mucous from the mucosal surface, providing greater surface detail (Fig. 6-6).

High density barium is the second necessary component for a successful double-contrast upper gastrointestinal series. Practitioners of double-contrast radiography have employed barium densities ranging from 100 to 250 percent weight per volume. Densities of 100 to 120 percent weight per volume are generally used in Japan, and higher densities of 200 to 250 percent weight per volume

have been used in the United States and Western Europe. The lower densities make it easier to combine a compression study with the double-contrast films. The higher densities tend to maximize the surface detail shown on double-contrast films. In the generally larger Western patient, the very high densities usually employed are also helpful in maintaining radiographic contrast sufficient to demonstrate fine detail, since large patients tend to generate considerable image-degrading scattered radiation. In the generally much smaller Jap-

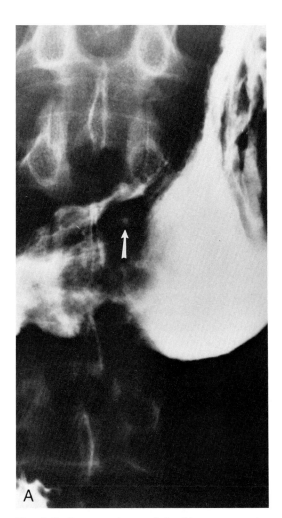
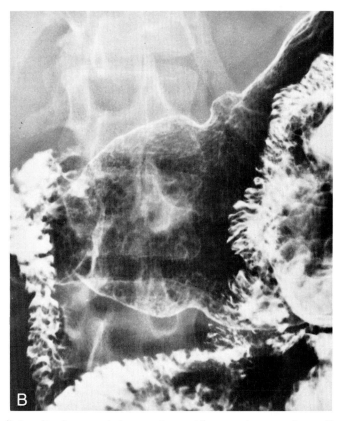

Fig. 6-7 Compression and double-contrast views of the distal stomach in a patient with an active anterior wall gastric ulcer. (A) Compression view showing a small ulcer crater (arrow) surrounded by a mound of edema. (B) Double-contrast view of the same area showing distortion of the lesser curvature, but no direct evidence of the active gastric ulcer. Unless an anterior wall ulcer is deep and/or steep-sided, it is very likely to be undetected on the common double-contrast views.

anese patient, maintenance of good radiographic contrast is an easier matter, even with barium suspensions of lesser density.

Routine films for the typical double-contrast examination of the stomach will include several of the following: supine (AP), left posterior oblique (LPO), right lateral (R Lat), prone (PA), semierect right posterior oblique (RPO), and upright anteroposterior (AP). Several of the foregoing will be taken during any given examination, with some combination of four or five of these views being necessary in most patients.

The area best shown on most double-contrast views is the posterior wall of the distal half of the stomach. This is usually shown in exquisite detail due to the shallow layer or pool of barium that collects on the dependent surface, which in most views corresponds mainly to the posterior wall (Figs. 6-1 and 6-6). The gastric fundus and the greater and lesser curvatures are also coated with barium but are less well shown.

The one area quite difficult to demonstrate on double-contrast films is the anterior wall of the distal half of the stomach (Fig. 6-7). Compression films, prone mucosal relief films, and /or special prone films in double-contrast must be included in the examination to avoid missing lesions in this region. A special double-contrast view of the distal anterior wall, taken in the LAO position with the table in steep Trendelenburg position, can be employed to show the anterior wall in double-contrast (Fig. 6-8), but this view is generally not obtained routinely because of the difficulty it presents to most patients.

Lesions well shown on double-contrast films are those involving minimal elevation or excavation of the gastric mucosal surface and which are located on the dependent wall of that region of the stomach filmed in double-contrast. The shallow pool of barium that forms on the dependent wall tends to outline small elevations and fill small ulcers in an exquisitely detailed manner. Where lesions are not on a dependent wall, however, visibility is confined to those that are steep-sided or cause major changes in the fold pattern of a large portion of the stomach. Thus, deep anterior wall ulcers can be seen as ring shadows but shallow, slope-sided ulcers cannot be seen at all. Polypoid anterior wall lesions are also seen as ring shadows, but plaque-

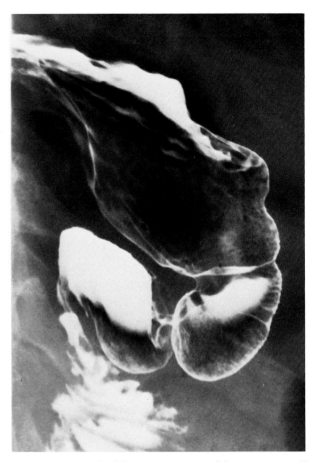

Fig. 6-8 A true double-contrast view of the anterior wall of the distal stomach taken in the left anterior oblique position with the table in Trendelenburg position. Using a remote-control fluroscope, tube angulation has been employed to project the duodenal bulb away from the distal stomach. A gastric ulcer scar is present on the distal lesser curvature and constricts and distorts the antrum.

like lesions with gently sloping sides may be missed completely.

Lesions poorly shown, therefore, include any abnormality on the nondependent walls of the stomach, the sides of which are not steep enough to allow the barium coating to be cut tangentially by the x-ray beam. As a result, lesions ranging from a small gastric erosion to sizeable neoplasms may be undetected unless situated on the dependent wall or detected in profile. Double-contrast films of the stomach, as detailed as they may appear, are thus like a double-edge sword. They are extremely effective at showing very small lesions in certain locations yet may fail to detect sizeable lesions in other regions because of the lesion's configuration and location.

It is also important to note that limited double-contrast filming of the stomach is both possible and desirable during the conventional upper gastrointestinal studies and should be a routine matter. Usually, the gastric antrum and the proximal third of the stomach are well demonstrated in double-contrast on films taken as part of the conventional examination (Fig. 6-9). Since these limited double-contrast views may be helpful in detecting lesions in the regions just mentioned, several steps should be taken to ensure that these areas are seen to best advantage. First, it is necessary to establish a good coating of barium by turning the patient so that the stomach is freshly washed by the barium suspension. Second, a barium of moderately high viscosity and uniform coating properties should be employed to ensure that the coating will be uniformly deposited and sufficiently opaque to be easily visible. Third, it is best to obtain these double-contrast views toward the conclusion of the study when a maximum amount of air has been ingested with the barium suspension. Finally, moderate kilovoltages of 80 to 100 kVp should be employed for the double-contrast views to avoid "burning out" the barium coating and to avoid degradation of the image by excess scattered radiation.

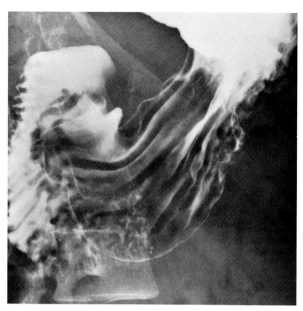

Fig. 6-9 An example of a double-contrast view of the distal stomach obtained during a conventional single-contrast examination. The excellent coating was obtained by using an adequately dense and viscous barium suspension, by freshly washing the distal stomach with barium, and by using a moderate kilovoltage.

BARIUM-FILLED FILMS

All conventional full-column upper gastrointestinal examinations include filming of the stomach filled with barium. Generally, these films are taken at the end of the examination after additional amounts of barium have been administered to the patient in the course of examining the esophagus. The routine views taken as part of a conventional upper gastrointestinal series generally include three or more of the following, all with the table horizontal: supine (AP), LPO, R Lat, right anterior oblique (RAO), and prone (PA).

Abnormalities well shown on barium-filled views of the stomach (Fig. 6-10) include the following: areas of nondistensibility due to extensive scarring or neoplasm, stiffening due to infiltration by tumor, large contour or filling defects caused by the presence of tumors or ulcers of significant size, and small contour changes caused by lesions that are serendipitously projected in profile. Lesions poorly shown include virtually all smaller lesions that are not associated with areas of nondistensibility, small lesions not projected in profile, and many larger lesions hidden by the overlying mass of barium within the stomach. Overall, the yield of lesions on barium-filled films is less than the yield on compression or double-contrast films.

The final integration of the above four modalities into an examination of the stomach is the responsibility of the individual radiologist. Generally, the resulting study follows the rough outlines of either a conventional or "double-contrast" examination, the latter hopefully incorporating compression or mucosal relief phases as well. To date, there is no firm evidence that either of these general forms of examination is superior to the other.

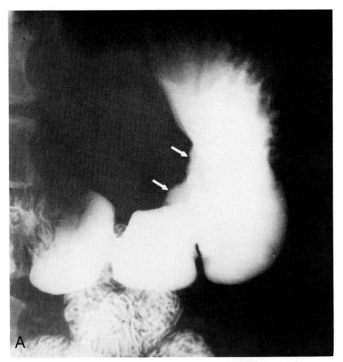

Fig. 6-10 Examples of abnormalities demonstrated on barium-filled views of the stomach. (A) Large carcinoma (arrows) causing stiffening and irregularity of the lesser curvature. (B) Small ulcer (arrow) on the distal lesser curvature that is visible because it is cut tangentially by the x-ray beam and is projected in profile. A good example of Hampton's line is visible at the neck of the ulcer. (C) Moderate-sized benign tumor of the distal stomach shown on a prone barium-filled view. The lesion is large enough to displace most of the barium in its immediate region and can thus be seen en face through the barium column. Visualization of both the lesion and folds in the distal stomach is aided by the compression exerted by the vertebral column.

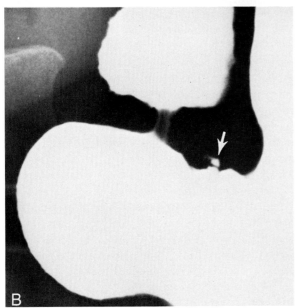

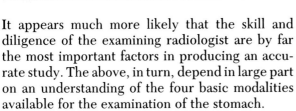

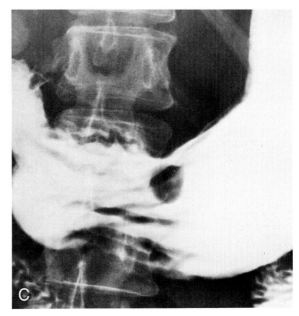

It appears much more likely that the skill and diligence of the examining radiologist are by far the most important factors in producing an accurate study. The above, in turn, depend in large part on an understanding of the four basic modalities available for the examination of the stomach.

The necessity for a dependable and clear demonstration of the mucosal surface of the stomach, and of any pathology present, cannot be overemphasized. Unless the examination is performed dependably and demonstrates the existing abnormalities, the process is essentially a waste and is, in fact, a danger to the patient, since an undetected carcinoma or penetrating ulcer becomes an increasing threat to the patient's well being. Clear and detailed demonstration of a lesion is equally important, since a poorly shown lesion is likely to be overlooked during interpretation of the films, and even if detected its nature may be undeterminable. Dependable, technically excellent examinations are therefore the indispensable basis for the radiologic evaluation of the stomach.

SUGGESTED READINGS

Gelfand DW: The double-contrast examination of the stomach using gas producing granules and tablets. Radiology 93:1381, 1969.

Gelfand DW: High density, low viscosity barium for fine mucosal detail on double-contrast upper gastrointestinal examinations. AJR 130:831, 1978.

Horikoshi H: Characteristics of x-ray examination of the stomach, In Murakami T, ed: Early Gastric Cancer. GANN Monograph on Cancer Research II. Tokyo, University of Tokyo Press, 1971, pp 93–103.

Kawai K, Tanaka H: Differential Diagnosis of Gastric Diseases. Chicago, Year Book 1974, pp 11–53.

Kressel HY, Laufer I: Principles of double-contrast diagnosis. In Laufer I, ed: Double Contrast Gastrointestinal Radiology. Philadelphia, WB Saunders, 1979, pp 21–44.

Op den Orth JO: The standard biphasic-contrast examination of the stomach and duodenum. The Hague, Martinus Nijhoff, 1979, pp 1–21.

7

Techniques for Examining the Duodenum

The four modalities available for the examination of the duodenum include *filling with barium, compression, mucosal relief,* and *double-contrast,* the same employed for the examination of the stomach. Of these techniques, filling with barium, compression, and double-contrast are routinely employed during most upper gastrointestinal studies. Mucosal relief filming is an uncommonly used but useful technique.

BARIUM FILLING

Barium filling is the simplest and most direct method of obtaining films of the duodenum. With the table horizontal, the patient is placed in the right anterior oblique (RAO) or right lateral (R Lat) position after the stomach has been partially or completely distended with barium. Gravity then causes barium to flow into the duodenal bulb each time the pylorus opens. With each wave of relaxation, the duodenal bulb fills with barium, and one or more spot-films of the barium-filled bulb are taken (Fig. 7-1).

Shown well on barium-distended views are any deformities of duodenal outline caused by peptic ulcer disease, large ulcers, smaller ulcers pro-

jected in profile, and filling defects large enough to displace a considerable fraction of the barium in the bulb, such as a large polyp. Shown poorly are all smaller ulcers that are not projected in profile and small tumors insufficient in size to displace a significant amount of the barium in the duodenal bulb.

COMPRESSION TECHNIQUES

In my opinion, examination of the duodenal bulb with compression is the single most productive means of studying the duodenal bulb radiologically. During a standard full-column study, compression filming is usually performed with the patient in the upright position. After compression films of the stomach have been obtained, the patient is asked to drink several more ounces of barium. Peristalsis and the additional volume in the stomach will cause the duodenal bulb to fill in most cases. The bulb is then filmed in compression (Fig. 7-2A).

A further method of obtaining compression films of the duodenal bulb is in conjunction with barium-filled films, with the patient lying in the RAO or prone (PA) position. After the barium-filled

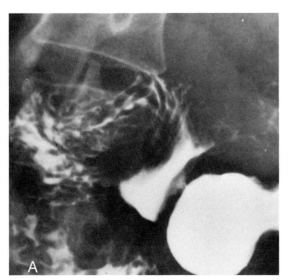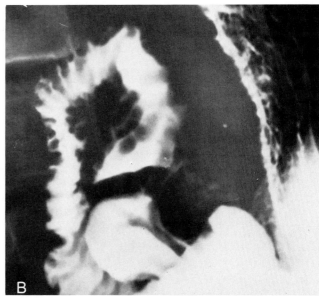

Fig. 7-1 Examples of barium-filled views of the duodenum. (A) Right anterior oblique view showing a barium-filled duodenal bulb of normal contour and normal appearing folds in the postbulbar duodenum. (B) Right anterior oblique view of the barium-filled duodenum demonstrating thick, nodular folds in the proximal duodenum due to duodenitis.

films have been obtained to show the distended contour of the duodenal bulb, an inflatable or padded paddle is inserted under the abdomen directly beneath the bulb. The paddle compresses the barium within the bulb, allowing more certain radiographic penetration of the barium (Fig. 7-2B). This is a very productive examination technique that provides an alternative to upright compression films.

If the duodenal bulb is being compression filmed as part of a double-contrast examination, the compression examination may be performed either at the very beginning or toward the end of the examination. Because of the very dense bariums employed, it is helpful to compress the duodenum between the compression device and the vertebral column, using the spine for counterpressure (Fig. 7-2C). During a double-contrast study employing dense barium, it may be easiest to compress the duodenal bulb in the semiupright position, which more evenly distributes the barium, rather than with the patient fully upright.

Shown well on compression films of the duodenal bulb are virtually all forms of pathology that are commonly encountered. The only restriction to this statement is that subtle erosions and ulcer scars may at times be more easily demonstrated on double-contrast films.

THE MUCOSAL RELIEF TECHNIQUE

The mucosal relief technique entails filling the duodenal bulb with barium in the R Lat position and then turning the patient into a left posterior oblique (LPO) position, causing most of the barium to drain away from the bulb by gravity. The small amount of barium remaining in the duodenal bulb then coats the collapsed duodenal mucosa and forms a mucosal relief image (Fig. 7-3). Generally, films must be taken rapidly, since the air normally present in the gastric antrum will soon enter the duodenal bulb where it forms a double-contrast image. This is virtually the same technique described by Hampton in his description of the recumbent examination of the acutely bleeding patient.

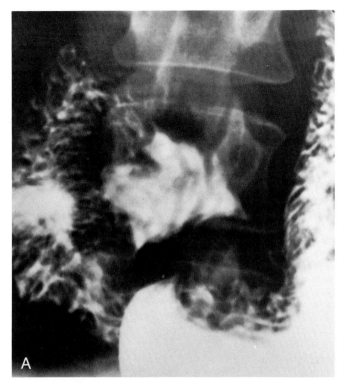

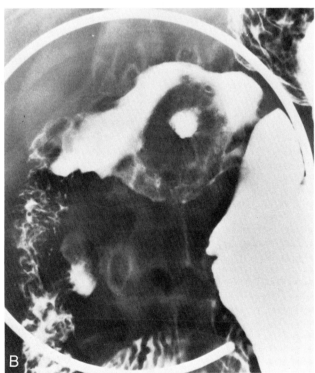

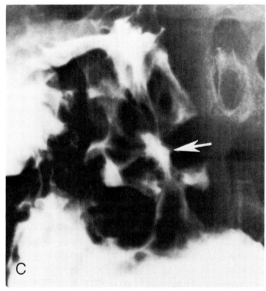

Fig. 7-2 Examples of compression films of the
duodenal bulb using several differing techniques.
(A) Upright compression film demonstrating a
normal duodenal bulb. (B) Large duodenal ulcer
surrounded by a striking mound of edema, demonstrated by compression filming using an inflatable
paddle placed beneath the patient's upper abdomen. (C) An example of a duodenal ulcer (arrow) demonstrated
during a multiphasic examination employing 250 percent weight per volume barium. Note the edema surrounding
the ulcer.

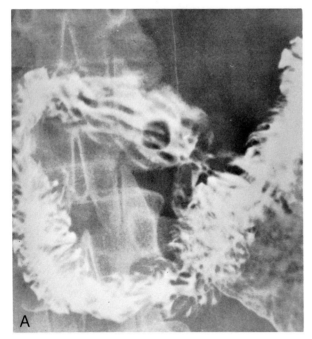
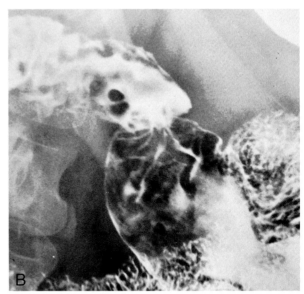

Fig. 7-3 Demonstration of lesions visualized using mucosal relief technique to examine the duodenum. (A) An adenomatous polyp of the duodenal bulb and the mucosal folds of the bulb are clearly seen. Note that air is present in the gastric antrum but has not yet entered the duodenal bulb. (B) Duodenal erosions represented by multiple nodules as demonstrated on mucosal relief film of the duodenal bulb. The air within the gastric antrum has not yet entered the duodenum. At least one gastric erosion is also seen.

Shown well are most forms of duodenal pathology other than anterior wall ulcers. These ulcers may trap air rather than barium during the maneuvers necessary to produce the mucosal relief image and may thus be undetected. However, compression can be applied, expressing any air trapped in the anterior portions of the duodenal bulb and allowing demonstration of anterior wall lesions. Compression-enhanced supine mucosal relief films of the duodenal bulb are an acceptable substitute for the more usual forms of upright or prone compression filming when the latter cannot be obtained.

DOUBLE-CONTRAST TECHNIQUES

When possible, films of the duodenal bulb in double-contrast should be incorporated into every upper gastrointestinal series. The general technique for obtaining good double-contrast films of the duodenum is the same for all types of upper gastrointestinal examinations.

To reliably produce double-contrast films of the duodenum, particularly the duodenal bulb, one first fills the bulb with sufficient barium to ensure that all of its surfaces will be adequately coated. Filling is accomplished by placing the patient in the R Lat position and allowing the bulb to distend with barium. When the proximal duodenum is well-filled with barium, the patient is rapidly turned to the LPO position. The next opening of the pyloric canal will usually allow air from the gastric antrum to enter the duodenal bulb, creating the double-contrast image (Fig. 7-4). Thus, two circumstances are necessary for the successful production of a double-contrast image of the duodenal bulb: first, the bulb must initially be filled and its mucosa thoroughly wetted with barium, and second, there must be sufficient air within the stomach to distend the duodenal bulb. In addition to the above, it is important that the kilovoltage be kept

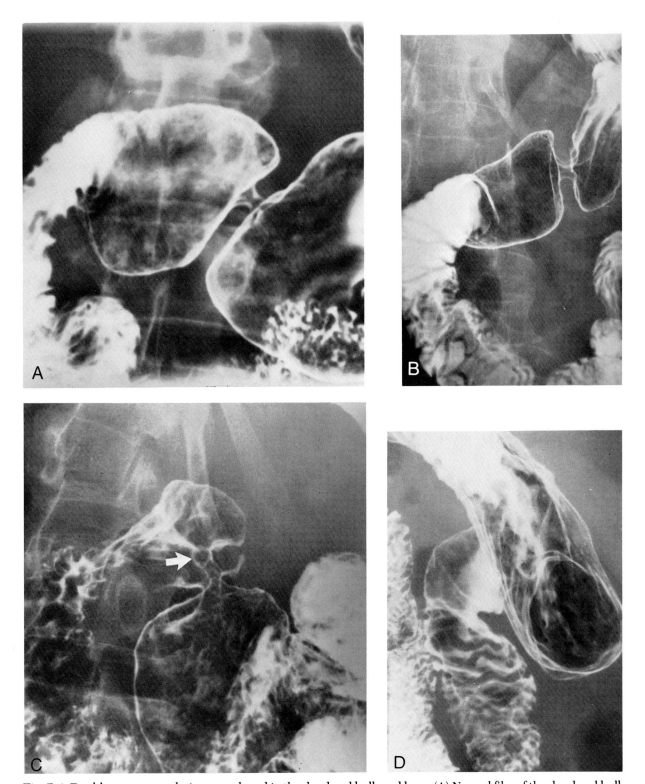

Fig. 7-4 Double-contrast technique employed in the duodenal bulb and loop. (A) Normal film of the duodenal bulb obtained during a double-contrast examination using dense barium. (B) Double-contrast film of the duodenal bulb and distal gastric antrum obtained in the course of a conventional or single-contrast examination. (C) Active duodenal ulcer in a deformed bulb. The ulcer is seen as a ring shadow (arrow) due to location on the anterior wall of the duodenal bulb. In the LPO position employed for this film, the anteriorly located ulcer does not collect barium. (D) True double-contrast view of the anterior wall of the duodenal bulb and postbulbar region obtained in the prone position.

in a moderate range (80 to 110 kVp) to maintain the radiographic contrast necessary for the barium coating to be clearly visible.

Shown well on double-contrast films of the duodenal bulb are those lesions encountered on its posterior wall. The shallow pool of barium accumulating on the posterior wall during double-contrast filming is capable of demonstrating exquisitely small structural detail, normal or abnormal. Since the bulb is distended by air or gas during double-contrast filming, any deformity present will also be demonstrable. Furthermore, because the distension tends to separate the mucosal folds, any nodularity or thickening of these folds is apparent.

Shown poorly are most lesions occurring on the anterior wall. Anterior wall lesions will be completely invisible during double-contrast filming unless their contours are sufficiently steep-sided to cause the barium coating the lesion to be cut tangentially by the x-ray beam. When this is so, a ring shadow or partial outline of the lesion may be visible (Fig. 7-4C). Because one can not readily detect anterior wall lesions on double-contrast films, a technique for demonstrating anterior wall lesions must be used, with the most efficient one being compression. However, a special double-contrast view of the anterior wall of the duodenum may be obtained by keeping the patient on the left side and then quickly rolling him onto his abdomen (Fig. 7-4D). In many patients, this produces a true double-contrast view of the duodenal bulb and loop with the barium layered in a shallow pool on the anterior wall instead of the posterior wall. This technique is excellent for outlining lesions on the anterior wall of the duodenal loop, but often the duodenal bulb, the most frequent site of pathology, will partially fill with barium or will be hidden by overlying shadows of the gastric antrum.

HYPOTONIC DUODENOGRAPHY

Hypotonic duodenography utilizes a paretic agent to halt peristalsis and dilate the duodenum. It was originated as a method of detecting carcinoma of the head of the pancreas, but for that purpose it has been displaced by ultrasound and computerized tomographic scanning. However, it

has proven to be an excellent means of demonstrating almost all intrinsic duodenal lesions and for practical purposes can become a part of any upper gastrointestinal series utilizing a gastroparetic agent.

Hypotonic duodenography, as a specific examination, is best performed by administering 30 mg Pro-Banthine intramuscularly 15 minutes before the procedure. In my experience, Pro-Banthine produces a denser and more reliable duodenal paresis than glucagon. Initial filling of the duodenal loop with barium is accomplished in the R Lat position, the barium flowing from the stomach into the duodenum by gravity. The patient is then

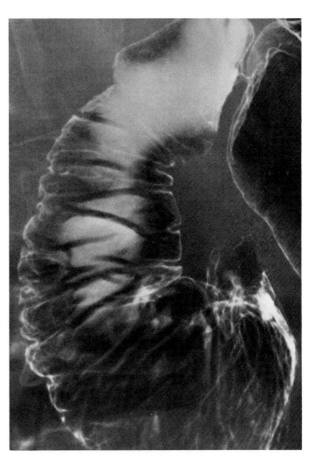

Fig. 7-5 Hypotonic duodenography employing Pro-Banthine as the paretic agent. After barium has filled the duodenum in the R Lat position, the patient has been rotated into an LPO position and gas from the stomach has distended the duodenal loop.

turned to the LPO position and carbon dioxide from the stomach, which has been administered via an effervescent gas-producing agent, rises into the duodenum, distending it fully. At maximum distension, double-contrast films of the duodenal loop are obtained (Fig. 7-5).

Hypotonic duodenography was originally described using duodenal intubation to directly inject barium and air into the duodenum. Since that original description, however, it has become apparent that tubeless hyptonic duodenography, utilizing gas produced within the stomach by effervescent products, is almost equally efficient while being faster and more easily tolerated by the patient.

SUGGESTED READINGS

Akerlund A: Rontgenologische Studien uber den Bulbus duodeni mit besonderer Berucksichtigung der Diagnostik des Ulcus duodeni. Acta Radiol Suppl I:1, 1921.

Bilbao MK, Frische CH, Dotter CT, Rosch J: Hypotonic duodenography. Radiology 89:438, 1967.

George AW, Gerber J: The direct method of diagnosis of duodenal ulcer by means of the roentgen-ray. Am J Roentgenol 1:350, 1913.

Goldstein HM, Zboralske FF: Tubeless hypotonic duodenography. JAMA 210:2086, 1969.

Jacquemet P, Liotta D, Mallet-Guy P: The Early Radiological Diagnosis of Diseases of the Pancreas and Ampulla of Vater: Elective Exploration of the Ampulla of Vater and the Head of the Pancreas by Hypotonic Duodenography. Springfield, IL, Charles C Thomas, 1965.

Martel W: Hypotonic duodenography without intubation. Radiology 91:387, 1968.

Miller RE, Chernish SM, Rosenak BD: Hypotonic duodenography with glucagon. Radiology 108:35, 1973.

Pribram BO, Kleiber N: Ein neuer Weg zur rontgenologischen Darstellung des Duodenums (pneumo-duodenum). Fortschr Rontgenstr 36:379, 1927.

Stein GN, Martin RD, Roy RH, Finkelstern AK: Evaluation of conventional roentgenographic techniques for demonstration of duodenal ulcer craters. Am J Roentgenol 91:801, 1964.

8

Techniques for Examining the Small Bowel

PERORAL METHODS

The peroral small bowel examination is the time-honored and most frequently employed method for studying the small intestine, and consists of simply feeding barium suspension to the patient and radiographing it as it progresses through the small intestine. However, many details of the examination can be varied, and these details determine the effectiveness of the study.

The Small Volume Technique

The small volume technique is an older peroral small bowel examination method that allows the patient to ingest only a small volume of barium suspension, typically 8 ounces or less, at the onset of the examination and none at later stages. Advocates of this method point out that limiting the volume of barium suspension largely avoids the problem of overlapping loops of small bowel obscuring each other during the examination. However, the small volume technique requires that many films be taken as this small volume of barium makes its way through the small bowel. Small volume examinations also tend to progress slowly,

since peristalsis is not stimulated to any extent. Theoretically, there is also a chance that certain areas of the small bowel may not be seen during this examination, the small volume of barium having passed through these segments between films. It is fair to say that this technique has lost popularity in recent years to the large volume technique.

The Large Volume Technique

By a simple response to volume, large volumes of barium suspension have the effect of stimulating small bowel peristalsis. Furthermore, the continuing ejection of barium into the small bowel from the barium-filled stomach tends to force the barium column distally. Thus, the large volume study has the advantages of being more rapid, and it results in opacification of the entire small bowel by the time the column reaches the cecum (Fig. 8-1). It is then possible to spot-film the entire small bowel, taking care to separate and compress each loop of small intestine (Fig. 8-2).

A standard procedure for this examination has evolved: the patient ingests 16 ounces (500 ml) or more of a stable 50 to 75 percent weight per volume barium suspension, usually in conjunction

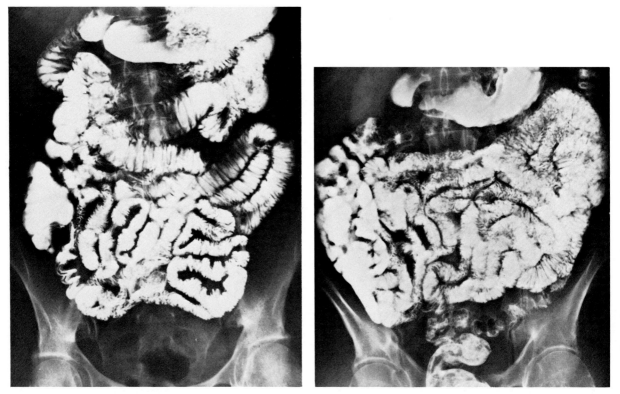

Fig. 8-1 Two examples of opacification of the entire small bowel by barium suspension using the large volume technique. Sufficient barium suspension has been given so that some barium remains in the stomach at the completion of the examination. Note that in both cases the small bowel is partially lifted out of the pelvis by a full bladder, the patient having been told to not void.

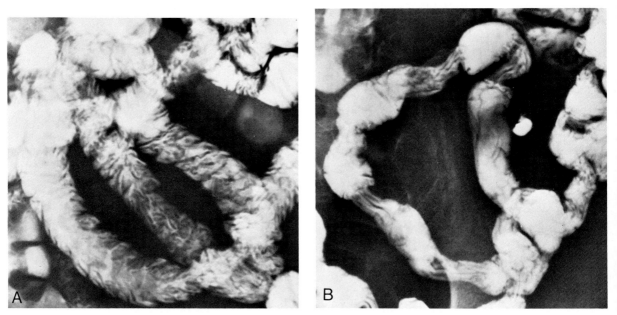

Fig. 8-2 Examples of separation and radiography of individual small bowel loops using compression technique. (A & B) Normal small intestinal loops.

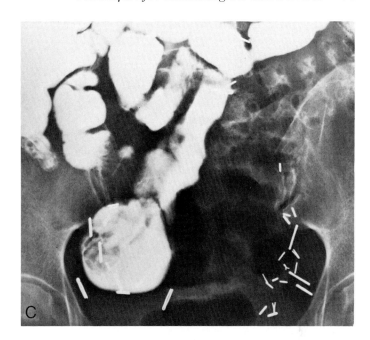

Fig. 8-2 *(continued)* (C) Meckel's diverticulum containing food. (D) Terminal ileum showing moderately advanced Crohn's disease. A small Meckel's diverticulum is also visible. (E) Terminal ileum showing early Crohn's disease.

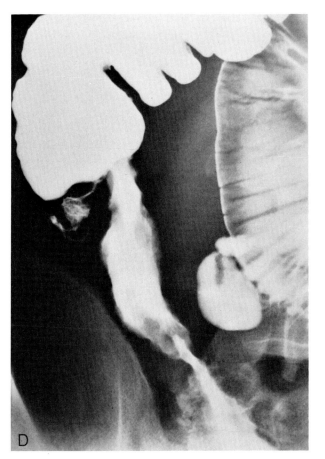

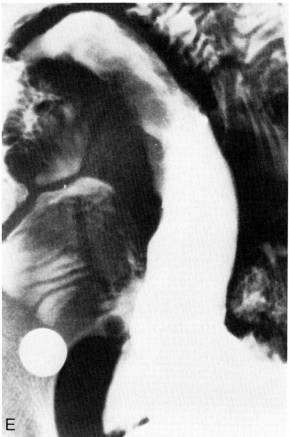

with a prior upper gastrointestinal series. Prone (PA) films of the abdomen are then obtained at the following intervals: 15 minutes, 30 minutes, 1 hour, 2 hours, 3 hours, and 4 hours or until the barium reaches the colon. With modern barium suspensions, the cecum will usually be reached within 1 to 2 hours, although often the examination will be more rapid or of longer duration. During this time, the stomach should be kept full of barium so that barium is constantly being ejected into the small bowel. When the barium suspension has reached the cecum, the patient is placed in the supine (AP) position, and compression films of the entire small bowel are obtained, concluding the examination. Many radiologists, however, restrict compression spot filming to the terminal ileum, since this is the most common site of pathology, namely Crohn's disease. However, failure to show the entire small bowel on spot films means that many localized lesions, such as tumors and Meckel's diverticula, will not be detected. This is probably the greatest contributory factor toward inaccuracy in small bowel radiology. When the entire small bowel has been thoroughly compression spot filmed, the examination can be terminated.

Compression Filming Techniques

Successful compression filming of the entire small bowel is the key to accuracy in all forms of small bowel examination and requires cognizance of two facts. First, the small bowel is extremely mobile within the abdominal cavity, and second, it does not lie in a flat plane across the abdomen.

The mobility of the small intestine allows a compression device to slide one loop of small bowel off another, thus permitting visualization of each loop without encumbering overlying shadows. This technique can be used to isolate groups of small intestinal loops for spot filming (Fig. 8-2). Thorough spot filming of the small bowel usually requires approximately 6 to 8 small films.

The disposition of the small bowel within the abdomen is not planar, but rather a curve that follows the contour of the anterior abdominal wall. As a result, the patient must be turned slightly from side to side during compression filming to obtain en face views of all of the loops of small intestine. If the lateral portions of the small bowel are to be clearly visualized, oblique films must be a part of the examination.

Demonstrating the Terminal Ileum and Pelvic Small Bowel

The distal ileum is of special interest to radiologists because of the prevalence of Crohn's disease and of tuberculosis in developing areas of the world. In a patient with diarrhea or other potential symptoms of Crohn's disease, the small bowel examination can not be considered complete unless detailed films of the terminal ileum have been obtained. Filming the terminal ileum can most easily be accomplished by turning the supine patient to a slightly left posterior oblique (LPO) position while applying compression in the region of the ileocecal valve. In combination, these two maneuvers tend to rotate and/or push out of the way any small bowel loops overlying the terminal ileum, bringing it into clear view (Fig. 8-2E).

Overlapping pelvic small bowel loops can be difficult to radiograph adequately, since they are located where compression is difficult to apply as a means of spreading the loops apart for filming. However, the following methods may be applied to elevate the small bowel loops out of the pelvis, assuming they are not fixed in that location by adhesions. First, the patient may be asked to drink quantities of water and told not to void, the resulting full bladder elevating the small bowel loops out of the pelvis (Fig. 8-1). Alternatively, this may be combined with a water or air enema, filling the rectum and sigmoid and further elevating the small bowel loops from the pelvis. A third method involves applying localized pressure on the anterior abdominal wall in the pelvic region, while simultaneously asking the patient to exhale forcibly several times. With each exhalation, one or more loops of the pelvic small bowel will slide up out of the pelvis until all or almost all of them have left the pelvis (Fig. 8-3). The Trendelenburg position may be used with any of the above maneuvers to further encourage the distal small bowel to move up and out of the pelvis.

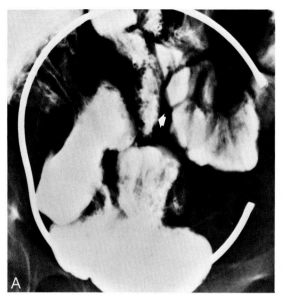

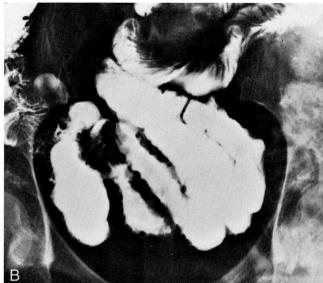

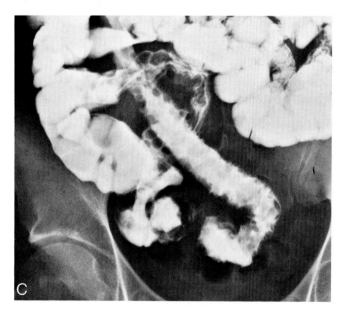

Fig. 8-3 Demonstration of the use of compression to elevate and separate pelvic bowel loops. (A) Prone compression film using an inflatable paddle. Most small bowel loops have been displaced out of the pelvis. The terminal ileum (arrow) can be seen entering the patient's pelvic cecum. (B) Compression being used to displace pelvic small bowel loops away from an abnormal ileum in a patient with Crohn's disease. (C) Use of compression to displace out of the pelvis all small bowel loops except for the patient's terminal ileum, which demonstrates Crohn's disease.

SMALL BOWEL ENEMAS

A variety of methods exist for examining the small bowel via administration of an enema of barium sulfate suspension. These small bowel enemas may be divided into two classes: antegrade examinations administered through a tube advanced into the duodenum or jejunum and reflux small bowel enemas accomplished by retrograde administration of barium suspension through an ileostomy, colostomy, or rectal tube. Enteroclysis is the term now used for antegrade studies, while retrograde methods are often labeled as reflux small bowel enemas.

Enteroclysis

The most common method for enteroclysis is the single-contrast method popularized by Sellink, with earlier contributions by Gershon-Cohen, Scott-Harden, and others. The examination can be divided into three phases: preparation of the patient, intubation of the small bowel, and the radiographic examination itself.

Preparation of the Patient. Enteroclysis requires cleansing of the colon prior to the study. The cleansing flushes any solid material out of the distal ileum and colon, and the empty colon then offers no retrograde pressure that might impede the distal flow of the barium suspension. The procedure for cleansing the colon is that used for preparation of a patient for barium enema.

Intubation. Most radiologists performing enteroclysis examinations employ either the Nolan or Bilbao-Dotter tube, slightly stiff tubes with a guidewire, which are capable of reaching the proximal small bowel. The most straightforward procedure is to use the mouth as the route of intubation, allowing the patient to swallow the tube himself if possible. When the tube has reached the distal esophagus, the guidewire is inserted to almost its full length, allowing the distal few centimeters of the tube to remain flexible. With further intubation, the floppy end of the tube follows the greater curvature of the stomach (Fig. 8-4A), traverses the pylorus, and enters the duodenum. Since the stiff guidewire cannot easily negotiate the duodenal loop, the guidewire is progressively withdrawn while the tube is advanced further into the duodenum (Fig. 8-4B). To avoid reflux of barium into the stomach with subsequent vomiting, it is best to advance the tube into the jejunum when possible (Fig. 8-5). However, successful studies can be performed with the tube in the third or fourth portion of the duodenal loop, although gastric reflux and resultant vomiting are more likely to occur.

Infusion. The examination of the small bowel proceeds with administration of a relatively dilute barium suspension, usually in the range of 20 to 30 percent weight per volume. To stimulate peristalsis, 30 ml of Gastrografin may be added to 800 ml of barium suspension, which is then placed

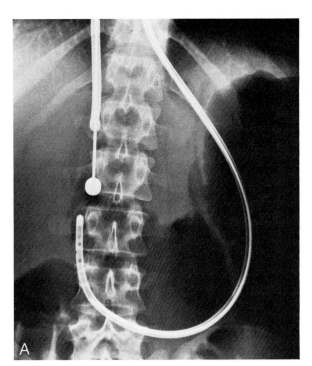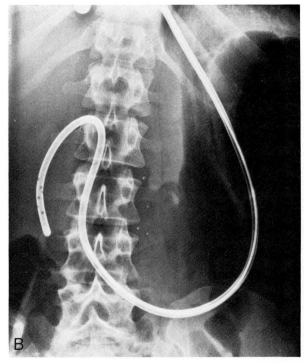

Fig. 8-4 Intubation procedure for enteroclysis. (A) The guidewire has been withdrawn slightly to allow the distal end of the tube to remain flexible. The tube has followed the greater curvature and is about to enter the duodenum. (B) The guidewire has been withdrawn further and the flexible end of the tube has entered the duodenum.

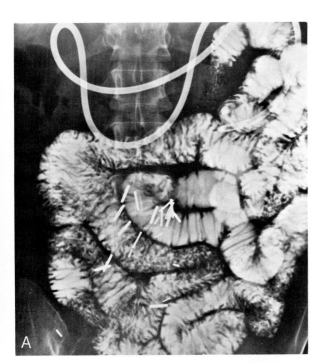

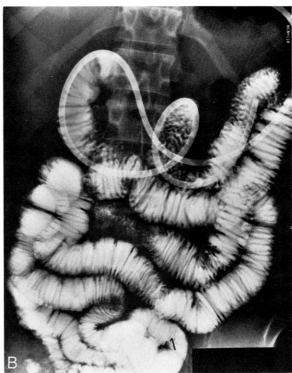

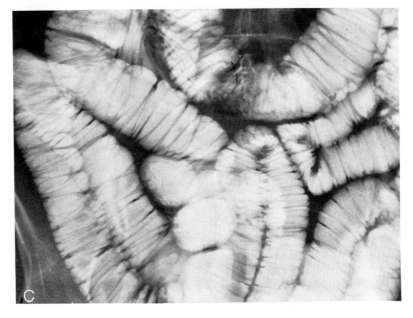

Fig. 8-5 Radiographs of enteroclysis examinations during filling and spot filming. (A & B) Large radiographs taken during filling of the small bowel. The degree of distention being obtained at this stage is correct. (C) Spot film taken at the conclusion of an enteroclysis procedure when additional barium has been used to fully distend the small bowel. Compression is employed to separate the loops for radiographic clarity.

in an enema bag connected to the Bilbao-Dotter tube. Administration of barium then proceeds at a rate of approximately 100 ml per minute, usually accomplished with the bag 18 inches above the table. The proper rate of flow provides considerable distension of the small bowel while peristalsis continues normally and sweeps the barium distally (Fig. 8-5). If barium suspension is administered too slowly, barium is propelled distally by peristalsis before adequate distension can be achieved. If barium suspension is administered at too great a rate, the jejunum becomes overdistended and will be reflexly paralyzed. This usually results in reflux of barium suspension into the stomach, vomiting, and failure of the barium suspension to progress into the distal small bowel. Thus, the examiner must observe the degree of distension and the amount of peristalsis, tailoring the flow rate to give adequate distension without paralyzing the small bowel or causing substantial gastric reflux.

Radiography. During enteroclysis, two types of films are generally obtained. Large prone films, taken in the PA and both anterior oblique positions (RAO and LAO), are used to show large areas of the small bowel (Fig. 8-5); compression spot films, taken in the supine (AP) position, are used to separate and radiograph every loop of small bowel without overlapping barium shadows (Fig. 8-5C). A combination of compression, Trendelenburg position, air enema, and forcible exhalation aid in lifting small bowel loops out of the pelvis to be separated and compressed for better visualization. The examination is complete when all loops of bowel, including the terminal ileum, have been clearly radiographed.

Several *double-contrast variants* of the enteroclysis examination should be briefly mentioned. Air-barium double-contrast enteroclysis may be accomplished by first performing a small bowel enema with 40 to 60 percent weight per volume barium suspension, followed by intravenous administration of glucagon and the inflation of the small bowel with air via the enteroclysis tube. Prone and supine films are then taken, designed to show each portion of the small bowel in double-contrast. Sellink and others performing routine single-contrast enteroclysis often employ a supplemental double-contrast study performed by administration of water after the small bowel has

been filled with barium, the water providing a double-contrast effect due to the laminar flow phenomenon. Double-contrast enteroclysis using barium suspension followed by methylcellulose solution has also been advocated.

Reflux Small Bowel Examinations

Reflux small bowel examinations may be performed via an ileostomy, via a colostomy, or via the rectum following barium enema. All of these examinations may be used to study the entire small bowel, but they are most useful in the examination of the distal regions of the small bowel. It should be noted that reflux examination of the entire small bowel tends to be an uncomfortable procedure, particularly if the examination is being performed via a distal colostomy or via the rectum.

Preparation of Patient. For the reflux examination of the small bowel via an ileostomy, no preparation is necessary, since the ileal contents are usually liquid. However, if the examination is performed via a colostomy or through the rectum, the colon must be clean, since any fecal material in the colon will be refluxed into the small bowel and may simulate the appearance of polypoid neoplasms. In sufficient quantity, fecal material may also mask any small lesions that are present. Thus, the patient requires a vigorous bowel preparation identical to that for a barium enema.

Reflux examination via an ileostomy is performed using a Foley catheter inserted into the ileostomy. It is important that the balloon portion of the catheter is inserted a sufficient distance to have traversed the abdominal wall. The balloon is inflated with several milliliters of air, and traction is exerted on the catheter. The balloon of the catheter then acts as a ball valve where it meets the constricted segment of ileum at the abdominal wall. Approximately 1,000 ml of dilute, 20 to 30 percent weight per volume barium suspension, is placed in an enema bag and its tube is connected to the Foley catheter. The examination per se consists simply of running the barium suspension into the small bowel, which fills slowly in retrograde fashion (Fig. 8-6). Prone and supine films are obtained, with care taken to compress each loop of small bowel. The examination is particularly useful

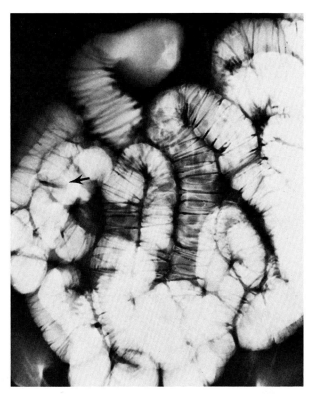

Fig. 8-6 Reflex examination of the entire small bowel via an ileostomy. The balloon of the catheter is visible (arrow). The entire small bowel has been refluxed to the level of the duodenal bulb.

for detection of the adhesions, which may produce partial obstruction or ileostomy dysfunction, and for the detection of Crohn's disease recurrent in the ileum after colonic resection.

Reflux study via a colostomy is performed in much the same manner as the examination via an ileostomy. The examination is straightforward if only a small length of colon lies between the colostomy and the ileocolic junction. However, if a considerable length of colon is present proximal to the colostomy, the examination can be uncomfortable. Also, it may be necessary to switch from infusion of barium suspension to infusion of water at the midpoint of the examination so that the colon is purged of barium that could obscure the underlying small bowel.

Reflux examination of the small bowel via the rectum is the most difficult of the reflux small bowel examinations and the most uncomfortable

for the patient, since an enema of immense volume must be retained. After intravenous injection of 0.5 mg glucagon, the examination commences with a single-contrast barium enema using a barium suspension of approximately 15 to 30 percent weight per volume. The colon is filled with barium and radiographed to the extent dictated by clinical circumstances. When the colon has filled with barium, the barium suspension is stopped and water is then infused, the most convenient arrangement employing two enema bags and a "Y" tube. The water infusion accomplishes two purposes. First, it propels the barium suspension from the colon into the small bowel. Second, it displaces the barium from the distal colon and renders it largely radiolucent, allowing overlying small bowel loops to be more easily radiographed, a matter of particular importance in the pelvic region. It is sometimes helpful to apply intermittent compression to the region of the ileocecal valve, the application and release of pressure promoting initial reflux of bar-

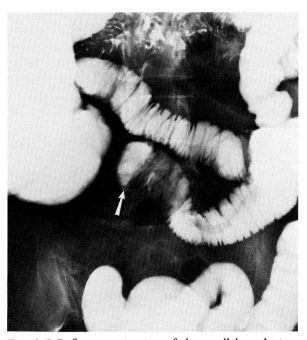

Fig. 8-7 Reflux examination of the small bowel via a barium enema. The barium in the distal small bowel demonstrates an obstruction (arrow) caused by adhesions (Ott DJ, Gelfand DW: Gastrointestinal contrast agents. JAMA 249:2380, 1983. Copyright 1983, American Medical Association.)

ium through the valve. Radiography of the small bowel is accomplished via the various methods described above. This examination appears to be most applicable to the detection of obstructing lesions of the distal small bowel such as adhesions or neoplasms (Fig. 8-7).

SUGGESTED READINGS

Caldwell WL, Floch MH: Evaluation of the small bowel barium motor meal with emphasis on the effect of volume of barium suspensions ingested. Radiology 80:383, 1963.

Ekberg O: Double contrast examination of the small bowel. Gastrointest Radiol 1:349, 1977.

Gelfand DW, Ott DJ: Barium sulfate suspensions: An evaluation of available products. AJR 138:935, 1982.

Gershon-Cohen J, Shay H: Barium enteroclysis. A method for the direct immediate examination of the small intestine by single and double contrast techniques. Am J Roentgenol 42:456, 1939.

Golden R: Technical factors in the roentgen examination of the small intestine. Am J Roentgenol 82:965, 1959.

Herlinger H: A modified technique for the double contrast small bowel enema. Gastrointest Radiol 3:201, 1978.

Marshak RH, Lindner AE: Radiology of the Small Intestines. Philadelphia, WB Saunders, 1976, pp 1–7.

Miller RE: Complete reflux small bowel examination. Radiology 84:457, 1965.

Scott-Harden WG, Hamilton HAR, McCall Smith S: Radiological investigation of the small intestine. Gut 2:316, 1961.

Sellink JL: Radiological Atlas of Common Diseases of the Small Bowel. Leiden, HE Stenfert Kroese, 1976, pp 73–108.

Vallance R: An evaluation of the small bowel enema based on an analysis of 350 consecutive examinations. Clin Radiol 31:227, 1980.

9

Techniques for Examining the Colon

PATIENT PREPARATION

Many radiologists believe that proper preparation of the patient for a barium enema is more important than the exact technique used for the examination itself. The necessity for a thoroughly clean colon, free of solid or slush-like fecal material, is caused by the resemblance of fecal material to polypoid lesions and its ability to hide substantial neoplasms of the colon. In addition, the presence of fecal material coating the mucosa makes it impossible to evaluate the mucosal surface for the presence of inflammatory diseases. Despite occasional statements to the contrary, there is no known barium enema technique with the ability to reliably demonstrate colonic lesions in the presence of retained fecal material.

Virtually all effective colonic cleansing regimens include the following elements: liquid diet for a minimum of 24 hours to reduce the bulk of the stool, sequential administration of two strong laxatives the evening prior to the examination, hydration of the patient, and cleansing enemas the morning of the examination until the return is clear. With the above, a virtually clean colon can be expected in 90 percent or more of patients receiving a barium enema. Each of the elements mentioned above is necessary for proper colon cleansing, and bears further discussion.

Clear Liquid Diet

A clear liquid diet is usually employed for 24 to 48 hours for the purpose of halting the intake of nondigestible fibers, thus causing a decrease in the bulk of the stool. If fruit juices, broths, and gelatins are allowed, a modest protein-sparing caloric intake is provided.

Hydration

Hydration is required for two purposes. First, the diarrhea caused by administration of strong laxatives draws fluid from the body that must be replaced if the patient is to remain comfortable and retain strength. Furthermore, good hydration must be maintained to promote adequate flow of fluid into the bowel, which is necessary to flush the fecal material from the colon.

Laxatives

Laxatives are basic to any barium enema preparation regimen, and their use by knowledgeable gastrointestinal radiologists tends to share certain characteristics. First, sequential administration of two strong laxatives several hours apart has been found necessary for thorough cleansing. The initial laxative administered is usually one that is active primarily in the small bowel, typically causing an inrush of fluid into the small intestine and then into the colon. Thus, a saline laxative such as magnesium citrate, or castor oil on the basis of its irritative effect, may cause fluid to be drawn into the lumen of the small intestine. The second laxative given should promote colonic contraction, causing expulsion of the fluid generated in the small bowel along with the solid colonic contents. The most prevalent combination is magnesium citrate followed by bisacodyl or purified extract of senna, the latter two being strong colonic irritants. My preferred regimen is magnesium citrate followed by castor oil, the latter being a mild colonic irritant as well as a strong small intestinal irritant. Yet another established regimen is castor oil followed by senna extract, the castor oil causing flow of fluid into the small bowel by its irritant action and the senna extract causing colonic contraction. To date, no definite advantage has been established for any one of the combinations just mentioned, and all are effective when followed by cleansing enemas.

Cleansing Enemas

Cleansing enemas are the final and indispensable element of a thorough barium enema preparation and serve at least two purposes. First, the cleansing enema in a well-prepared patient usually succeeds in washing out of the colon the last particles of solid material. Second, the effluent of the cleansing enema indicates whether the patient's initial preparation with diet, hydration, and laxatives has indeed been effective in eliminating most solid material from the colon. If initial preparation has been ineffective, a second day of preparation may be necessary.

Cleansing enemas should consist of nothing more than approximately 1500 ml of warm tap water. The addition of materials such as tannic acid, bisacodyl, or other colonic irritants to the enema is of dubious benefit. The enemas should be administered with the patient lying first prone and then on the right side to ensure that fluid reaches all parts of the colon. If, on expulsion, fecal material is still present in the effluent, a second or third enema can be administered. When the colon is finally clean, a waiting period of 30 to 60 minutes should be allowed for the patient to expel and/or resorb any remaining fluid in the colon, minimizing the amount of retained water in the colon when the barium enema is finally administered. A 1-hour wait is desirable preceding a double-contrast enema, while 30 minutes is sufficient preceding a full column barium enema.

THE CONVENTIONAL, FULL COLUMN BARIUM ENEMA

Although simple in concept, obtaining maximum yield from the conventional, full column barium enema requires attention to detail and a thorough understanding of what renders a small object, such as a polyp, visible or invisible within a column of barium.

The first principle in obtaining a satisfactory full column barium enema examination is to radiograph every portion of the colon in a manner ensuring that it is not superimposed by other barium-filled loops of bowel. Since the colon can be quite tortuous, particularly in the sigmoid region, this may require filming of various segments of the colon from a number of angles to provide an unencumbered image of each segment of the colon. Furthermore, it is desirable that each portion of the colon be seen at least on two films, so that any suspected pathologic entity can be confirmed. This is accomplished by an appropriately planned combination of small spot films, particularly of the more tortuous portions of the colon, plus several large films of the entire colon taken at angles designed to once again show each of its segments.

The second principle in obtaining an effective full column barium enema is the use of compression during spot filming, a technique unfortunately not utilized frequently enough. The necessity of compression-filming the colon arises from the fact

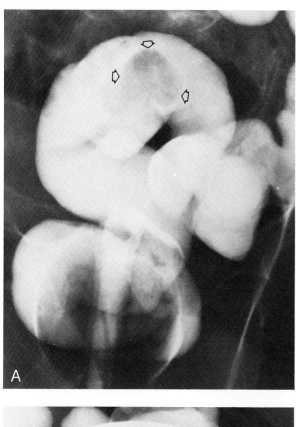

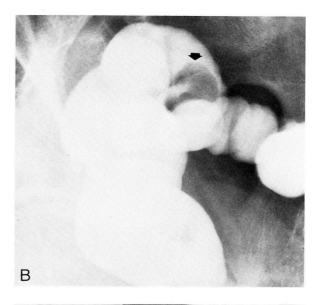

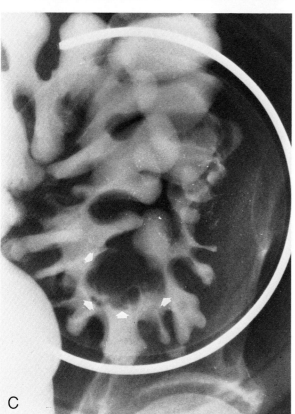

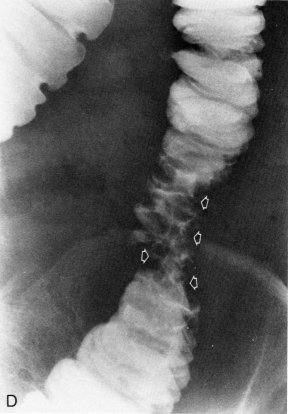

Fig. 9-1 Typical spot films taken during a conventional full column barium enema. Except in the pelvic area, most films have been taken with application of compression. (A) Supine (AP) view of the rectum and sigmoid colon showing a large polyp (arrows) in the sigmoid region. (B) Left posterior oblique view of the rectum and sigmoid colon showing a large sigmoid polyp (arrow). (C) Compression spot film of the descending-sigmoid colon junction showing an intramural inflammatory mass (arrows) due to diverticulitis. (D) Compression spot film of the descending colon circumferential narrowing (arrows) caused by a surrounding inflammatory mass due to diverticulitis. *(Figure continues on next page.)*

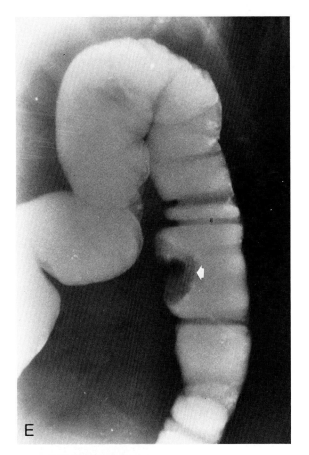

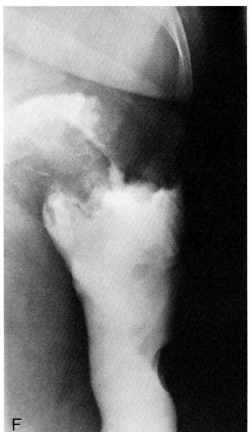

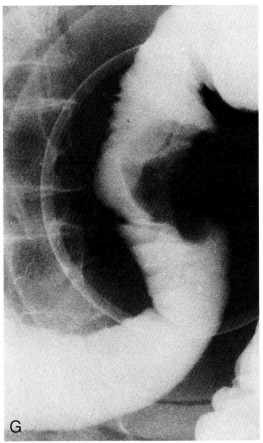

Fig. 9-1 *(continued)* (E) Compression film of the splenic flexure taken in the RPO position showing a villous adenoma (arrow) of the descending colon. (F) Compression film of the splenic flexure of the colon demonstrating a partially obstructing circumferential carcinoma. (G) Compression film of the transverse limb of the splenic flexure demonstrating a sessile polypoid carcinoma.

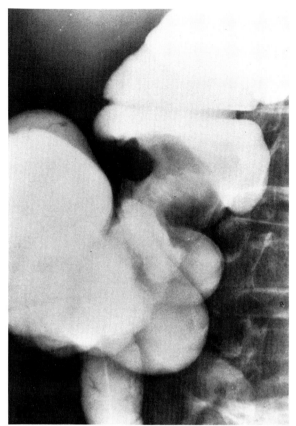

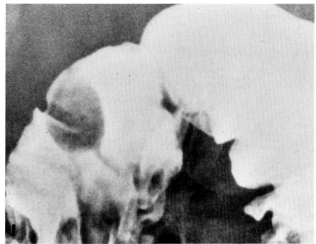

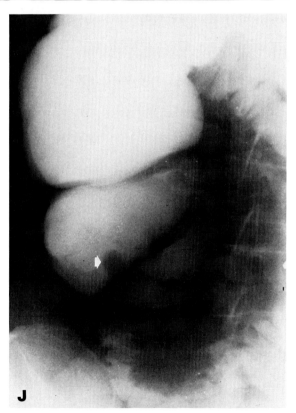

Fig. 9-1 *(continued)* (H) Film of the transverse colon revealing a circumferential carcinoma. (I) Film of the hepatic flexure taken in the LPO position in a patient with carcinoma of the lung metastatic to the colon, presenting as an intramural mass. (J) Compression spot film of the cecum and terminal ileum showing a polypoid mass (arrow) due to an inverted appendiceal stump.

that the colon is a large organ and the barium in a filled colon is capable of masking small filling defects within the lumen. This will be so even when the barium appears to be adequately penetrated by the x-ray beam. The sensitivity of the single-contrast enema for detection of small lesions, such as polyps, is improved several fold by the application of compression, which thins out the barium column so that any mass lesion present occupies a greater fraction of the barium column. This is best accomplished by routinely compression-filming the entire colon in the course of the spot-filming

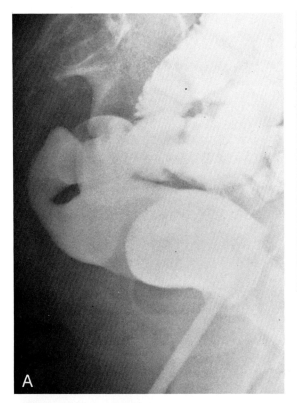

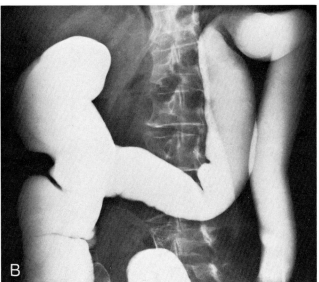

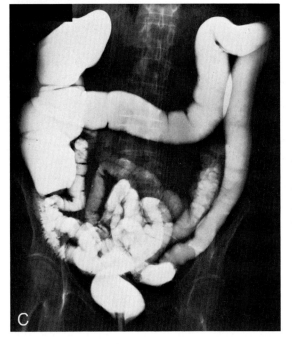

Fig. 9-2 Routine Bucky films of the colon as taken at the conclusion of a single-contrast barium enema. All films are from the same patient, who has uncomplicated diverticulosis of the sigmoid and descending colon. (A) Left lateral film of the rectum. (B) Left anterior oblique film encompassing most of the colon and showing the transverse colon, splenic flexure, and descending colon to good advantage. (C) Prone (PA) film of the entire colon. Note that the barium is thin enough for bone shadows to be visible through the barium column.

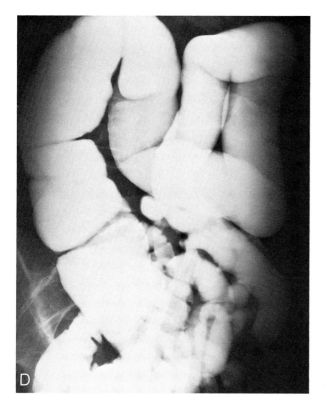

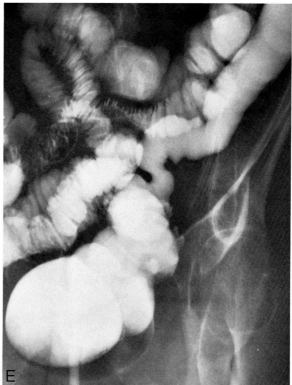

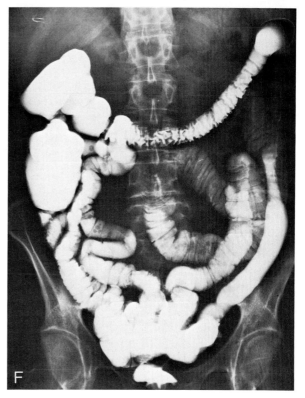

Fig. 9-2 *(continued)* (D) Right anterior oblique film of most of the colon showing the region of the hepatic flexure well. (E) Prone (PA) angled view of the rectum and sigmoid colon. Angulation of the beam toward the feet in the prone position tends to unfold overlapping loops of sigmoid colon. The patient's diverticulosis of the sigmoid colon is visible on this view. (F) Prone (PA) postdrainage view of the colon. The feathery pattern of the transverse colon represents a mucosal relief view of the folds of the collapsed colon.

process. The only portions of the colon that usually cannot be adequately compression-filmed are the rectum and distal sigmoid, due to the overlying bony pelvis. Fortunately, this region is accessible to sigmoidoscopy.

The Film Sequence

The film sequence during a reasonably thorough full column barium enema would be as follows, and is similar for both conventional and remote control apparatuses (Fig. 9-1). The colon is filled with barium with the patient in the supine or left posterior oblique (LPO) position. With the patient in the LPO position, spot films of the sigmoid colon and hepatic flexure are obtained. The cecum is spot filmed with the patient supine (AP). The splenic flexure is then filmed with the patient in the right posterior oblique (RPO) position. If the examination is to be as thorough as possible, the spot films are obtained with compression applied, and the intervening areas of the colon, such as the ascending, descending, and transverse colon, are compression spot-filmed as well. Approximately 6 to 10 films are required to thoroughly spot film the colon in most patients.

When spot filming is completed, the patient is turned to the left lateral (L Lat) position, and at this point the conventional and remote control examinations diverge. With the conventional fluoroscope, the technician uses the overhead tube and table Bucky device to obtain films of the rectum in the L Lat position and of the entire colon in the left anterior oblique (LAO), prone (PA), and right anterior oblique (RAO) positions (Fig. 9-2). An angled view of the sigmoid colon in the RAO or LPO position is also obtained. With a remote control fluoroscope, these films can be taken by the radiologist under direct fluoroscopic control.

The full column barium enema, when performed in a thorough manner, is capable of demonstrating 80 to 90 percent or more of all neoplasms 1 cm in size or greater, and is able to demonstrate the status and extent of inflammatory bowel disease, such as ulcerative colitis or Crohn's disease, in all but its earliest forms. However, even the most carefully performed full column examination, is unlikely to reliably demonstrate small polyps or

other types of lesions much smaller than 1 cm in size. Also, the examination may fail to demonstrate the very earliest changes of ulcerative colitis or Crohn's disease. For demonstration of these latter entities, in my opinion, a double-contrast barium enema should be employed.

Postevacuation Films

Most radiologists supplement the full column films described above with a postevacuation or postdrainage film (Fig. 9-2) obtained after the patient has evacuated or after most of the barium has been drained from the colon by dropping the enema bag to the floor. This produces what is in actuality a mucosal relief film of the colon and allows a view of the colonic mucosa unencumbered by the mass of barium present in the filled colon. The postevacuation film increases the sensitivity of the full column examination for the detection of polyps and for the detection of the relatively early changes of inflammatory bowel disease. Indeed, early inflammatory bowel disease is likely to be visible during a full column examination only on the postevacuation film.

Limited Double-Contrast Examination

The full column examination also may be supplemented by a double-contrast phase to increase its accuracy. In its simplest form, this may consist of draining barium from the colon by dropping the enema bag to the floor for several minutes, followed by insufflation of air by the technician. Prone and supine films of the colon are then obtained. This limited double-contrast examination is useful in that it allows double-contrast visualization of the distal sigmoid and rectum, areas that cannot be thoroughly examined with a full column examination.

Biphasic Barium Enema

The biphasic barium enema is a more elaborate variant of the examination described immediately above. In the biphasic barium enema, a complete single-contrast examination is performed. Following evacuation or drainage of most of the barium, the colon is distended with air. A complete double-contrast second examination of the entire colon is then performed. In capable hands, this examination probably has an unexcelled yield of colonic pathology of all varieties. However, it has the disadvantages of being expensive and time consuming, and of providing a double-contrast phase compromised by use of a barium suspension too dilute for optimal results.

THE DOUBLE-CONTRAST BARIUM ENEMA

The double-contrast enema performed as a primary examination was an outgrowth of the biphasic examination when it was determined that the double-contrast phase of the biphasic examination was capable of showing virtually all of the pathology demonstrated on the biphasic study. It was reasoned that with the use of a dense barium optimal for double-contrast radiography, and by careful filling and positioning of the patient, a double-contrast examination might be developed that might equal the biphasic examination in accuracy with less expenditure of time and film.

Materials

Adoption of the double-contrast examination by large numbers of radiologists has rapidly followed the development of appropriate equipment and barium suspensions for this examination. An accurate double-contrast examination requires coating of the mucosal surface with an opaque, easily discerned layer of barium. In the United States, the most popular barium suspensions for the double-contrast enema are moderately dense and viscous, usually sold as factory-prepared liquids. These have been well designed for their purpose, and possess a uniformity of quality difficult to duplicate by preparation of barium suspensions in the radiology department itself.

Glucagon is administered by many radiologists to relax the colon during performance of a double-

contrast enema. Colonic relaxation helps the patient retain the air and barium, which may otherwise be difficult, and it makes the patient more comfortable during the examination. It also helps a feeble patient retain a single-contrast enema. The typical dose of glucagon for a barium enema is 0.5 mg intravenously.

Performance of the examination is greatly aided by employing the proper tubing and tip. To allow reasonably rapid filling of the colon when employing viscous barium suspensions, most radiologists now use tubing of one-half inch inside diameter. For administration of air, either a "Y" tube or a special air administration tip can be employed. The special tip has the advantage of producing fewer bubbles and allowing more complete drainage of barium from the rectum in the course of the examination.

The Double-Contrast Enema in Two Stages

The earliest form of double-contrast enema was performed in two stages. In this form of the examination, the patient is placed on the table and barium administered to the level of the hepatic flexure. The patient is then allowed to evacuate most of the barium, and the colon is filled with air under fluoroscopic control. After rotating the patient to distribute the barium and coat the mucosa, filming of the colon in double-contrast is performed. This two-stage method has the advantage of simplicity of technique. However, it possesses the disadvantages of requiring inordinate amounts of time; inability to control the amount of barium evacuated by the patient, resulting in overfilled or poorly coated areas of the colon; and often refluxing the terminal ileum during evacuation, obscuring the sigmoid colon.

The Double-Contrast Enema in One Stage

Filling of the colon with barium and air in one stage is now the most common approach. A relatively simple routine is as follows: the patient is placed on the table in the prone position, with the

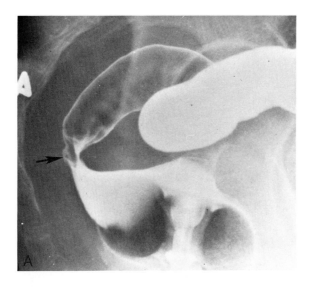

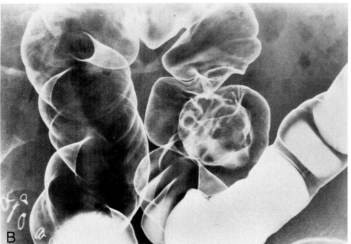

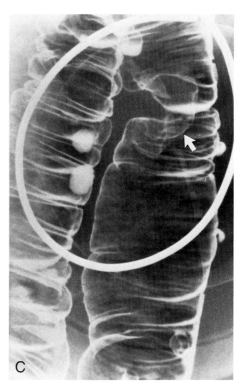

Fig. 9-3 Spot films taken during a typical double-contrast barium enema as performed on a conventional fluoroscope. (A) Left lateral view of the rectum in a patient with ulceration (arrow) and stricture of the rectum of unestablished etiology. (B) Left posterior oblique film of the sigmoid colon showing a polypoid carcinoma. (C) Upright RPO film of the splenic flexure, with compression used to spread the loops apart, revealing a polypoid carcinoma of the descending colon (arrow).

head of the table depressed 15 to 20°. The colon is then filled with barium until the head of the barium column reaches the distal transverse colon. With the patient still in the prone head-down position, air is insufflated, pushing the barium through the transverse colon and around the hepatic flexure into the ascending colon. The table is then elevated 45°, the bag is dropped to the floor, and the excess barium is siphoned from the distal colon

and rectum. With the table brought to the horizontal and the patient still in the prone position, more air is instilled until it is seen fluoroscopically that the colon is entirely distended. At this point, if the patient is fully cooperative, the tip may be removed from the rectum. The patient is then instructed to roll up onto the right side and then into the supine position. Barium will flow from the transverse colon into the right colon, and virtually

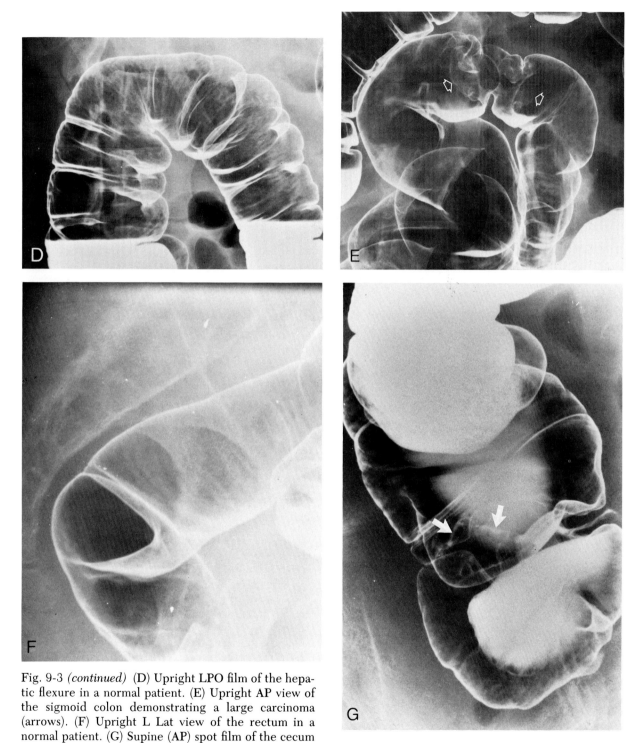

Fig. 9-3 *(continued)* (D) Upright **LPO** film of the hepatic flexure in a normal patient. (E) Upright **AP** view of the sigmoid colon demonstrating a large carcinoma (arrows). (F) Upright L Lat view of the rectum in a normal patient. (G) Supine (AP) spot film of the cecum and ascending colon showing a carcinoma in the region of the ileocecal valve. This anterior wall lesion is seen only faintly (arrows) as a series of faint white lines where the x-ray beam has intercepted the barium-coated edge of the lesion tangentially.

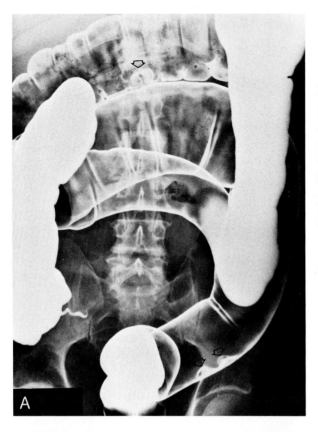

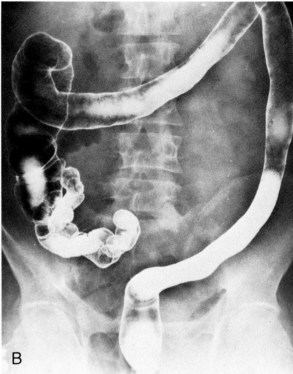

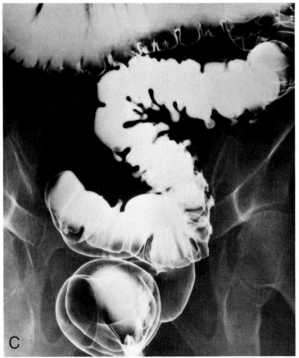

Fig. 9-4 Representative example of Bucky films of the colon taken at the conclusion of a double-contrast enema when performed on a conventional fluoroscope. (A) Supine (AP) view of the colon showing at least three sessile polyps (arrows). A lower abdominal and pelvic mass is elevating the sigmoid colon out of the pelvis. (B) Prone (PA) view of the colon in a patient with quiescent chronic ulcerative colitis. Note the shortening of the colon and total lack of haustral markings. Apart from a gaping ileocecal valve, the distal ileum is normal. (C) Prone (PA) angled view of the sigmoid colon showing extensive diverticulosis.

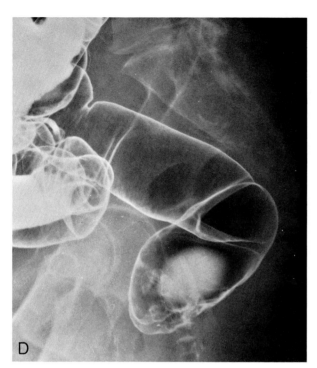

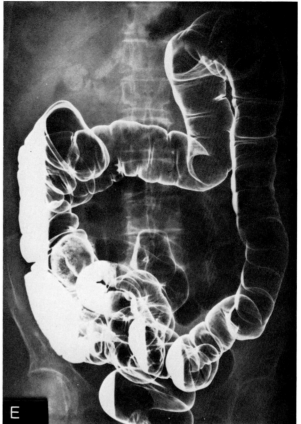

Fig. 9-4 *(continued)* (D) Right lateral film of the rectum in a normal individual. (E) Right lateral decubitus film of the entire colon in a normal patient. (F) Left lateral decubitus film of the entire colon in a normal patient.

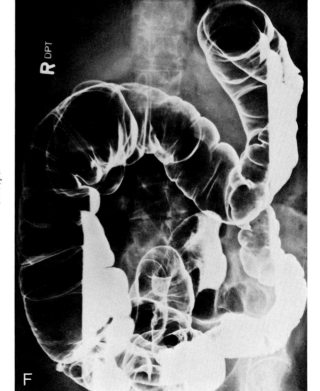

all segments of the colon will contain appropriate amounts of barium and air.

The above routine has several advantages. First, the patient is never moved from the prone position during the entire filling, draining, and reinflating procedure. This speeds the procedure and minimizes the degree of patient cooperation required. Second, the removal of the tip before any patient movement is required further speeds the procedure, makes the examination less cumbersome, and helps the patient retain the enema. Third, the simplicity of the routine makes it suitable for use with remote control fluoroscopes. Finally, it reliably produces a high quality examination.

The films taken for a double-contrast barium enema depend considerably upon whether the examination is being performed on a conventional or remote control fluoroscope. Each sequence is therefore described separately.

Filming Sequence for Conventional Apparatus (Figs. 9-3 and 9-4). With the patient supine and the barium and air properly distributed through the colon, two or three of the following views are taken as necessary to provide complete visualization of the sigmoid colon and rectum: LPO, AP, and L Lat.

The patient is then rolled 360°, in the direction away from the examiner, for purposes of thoroughly coating the entire colonic mucosa. With the patient again supine, the table is brought fully upright and the following spot films are obtained: RPO of the splenic flexure, LPO of the hepatic flexure, AP of the sigmoid colon, and L Lat of the rectum.

The head of the table is then lowered to 15 to 20° Trendelenburg, and a supine (AP) spot film of the cecum is obtained.

The above concludes the spot-filming sequence, and the following large films of the colon are taken by the technician with the table horizontal using the overhead tube and table Bucky apparatus: AP of entire colon, PA of entire colon, PA angled view of sigmoid, and R Lat of rectum.

The patient is then transferred to a stretcher and the following horizontal beam films are obtained employing the Bucky apparatus of the upright table (alternatively the patient may remain on the table and a vertically held grid cassette may be employed): R Lat decubitus of entire colon and L Lat decubitus of entire colon.

Filming Sequence for Remote Control Apparatus. The patient is filled with barium and air and rotated in the manner described above, eventually coming to rest in the supine position. The following films are then taken under fluoroscopic control in the sequence indicated:

1. Supine (AP) or LPO view of sigmoid colon and rectum with tube angulation (Fig. 9-5A).
2. Left lateral view of sigmoid colon and rectum (Fig. 9-5B).
3. Prone (PA) or RAO view of sigmoid colon with tube angulation (Fig. 9-5C).
4. Right lateral view of sigmoid colon and rectum (Fig. 9-5D).

The table is then fully elevated and the following films obtained:

5. Posteroanterior view of entire colon (Fig. 9-5E).
6. Right anterior oblique view of hepatic flexure (Fig. 9-5F).
7. Left anterior oblique view of splenic flexure (Fig. 9-5G).

The table is returned to the horizontal position and the following films obtained:

8. Prone (PA) view of entire colon (Fig. 9-5H).
9. Supine (AP) view of entire colon (Fig. 9-5I).
10. Right posterior oblique view of entire colon (Fig. 9-5J).
11. Left posterior oblique view of entire colon (Fig. 9-5K).
12. Supine (AP) view of cecum with the head of the table depressed 15 to 20° (Fig. 9-5L).

The double-contrast barium enema when properly performed is capable of demonstrating 90 to 95 percent of all neoplasms in the colon, including virtually all large malignancies. It is also capable of demonstrating the earliest colonic changes of ulcerative colitis and Crohn's disease and is useful for demonstrating the earliest changes of Crohn's disease in the terminal ileum if that structure has been refluxed during the study.

The disadvantages of the double-contrast barium enema versus the single-contrast enema are that it is much more uncomfortable for the patient,

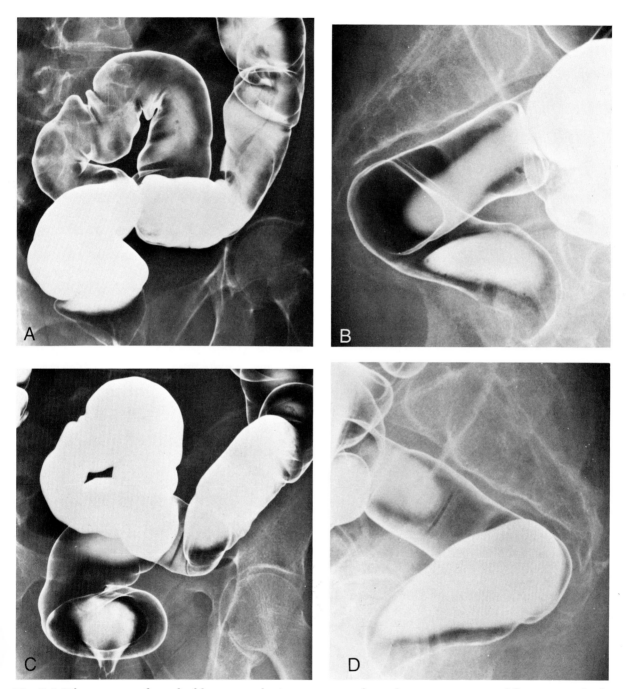

Fig. 9-5 Film sequence for a double-contrast barium enema performed on a remote control fluoroscope. In this example, all of the films are of the same normal patient. (A) Supine (AP) angled view of the sigmoid colon and rectum. (B) Left lateral film of the rectum. (C) Prone (PA) angled film of the sigmoid colon and rectum. Note that in comparison to the supine view, the position of the air and barium has shifted considerably. (D) Right lateral view of the rectum. *(Figure continues on next page.)*

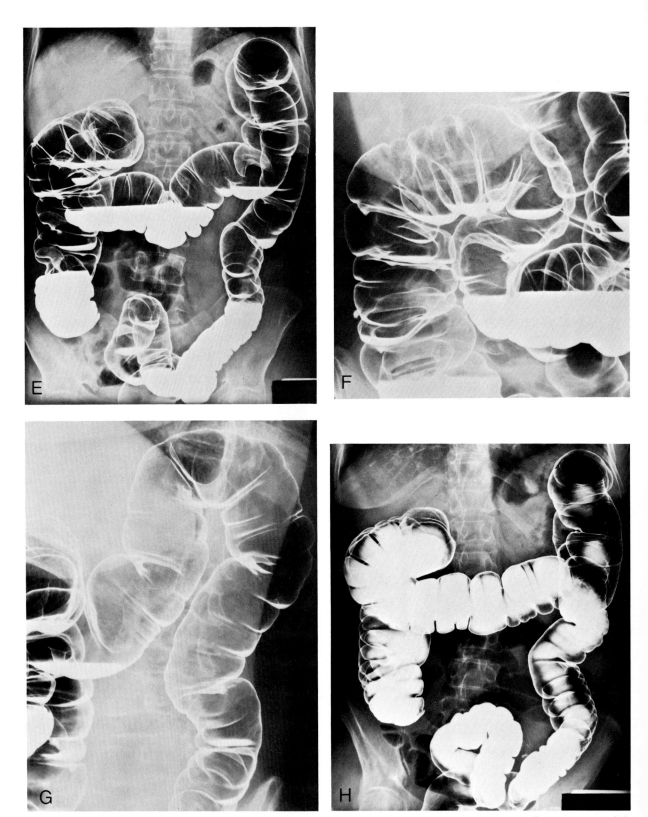

Fig. 9-5 *(continued)* (E) Upright PA film of the entire colon. (F) Upright RAO film of the hepatic flexure region. (G) Upright LAO film of the splenic flexure region. (H) Prone (PA) film of the entire colon.

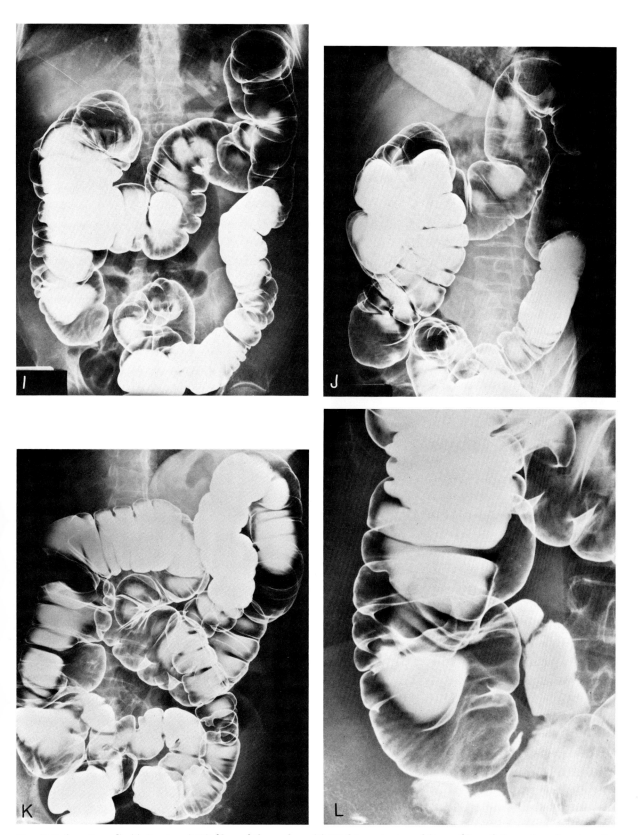

Fig. 9-5 *(continued)* (I) Supine (AP) film of the colon. (J) Right posterior oblique film of the colon showing the splenic flexure region. (K) Left posterior oblique film of the colon showing to advantage the hepatic flexure, ascending colon, and cecum. (L) Supine (AP) film of the cecum taken with the head of the table depressed 20°.

it requires considerably more physician time and room time, it is considerably more expensive, and many patients can not cooperate sufficiently. Many radiologists therefore employ certain criteria to select patients for the double-contrast examination in an effort to minimize the number of these studies performed.

Since the advantages of the double-contrast examination lie mainly in the detection of small polyps and the evaluation of early inflammatory bowel disease, and because the incidence of polyps and carcinoma of the colon is minimal until age 40, the following criteria may be employed in selecting patients for the double-contrast study: over age 40 and able to tolerate the examination, occurrence of rectal bleeding, history of previous colonic neoplasm, and clinical indication of mild or early inflammatory bowel disease.

With the above criteria for selecting patients, approximately 50 percent of patients will be examined using double-contrast technique in a typical radiologic practice. The selection process will ensure that the double-contrast examination is applied to those patients likely to have the types of pathology most readily detected by the double-contrast study.

SUGGESTED READINGS

Christie AC, Coe FO, Hampton AO, Wyatt GM: The value of tannic acid enema postevacuation roentgenograms in the examination of the colon. Am J Roentgenol 63:657, 1950.

Figiel SJ, Figiel LS, Rush DK: Study of the colon by use of high-kilovoltage spot-compression technique. JAMA 166:1269, 1958.

Gershon-Cohen J, Shay H: The colon as studied by double contrast enema. Am J Roentgenol 27:836, 1932.

Gianturco C: High-voltage technique in the diagnosis of polypoid growths of the colon. Radiology 55:27, 1950.

Gianturco C, Miller G: Routine search for colonic polyps by high voltage radiography. Radiology 60:496, 1953.

Hartzell HV: To err with air. JAMA 187:455, 1964.

Laufer I: The double-contrast enema: Myths and misconceptions. Gastrointest Radiol 1:19, 1976.

Margulis AR: Is double contrast examination of the colon the only acceptable radiographic examination? Radiology 119:741, 1976.

Marshak RH: The barium enema in the high risk carcinoma patient (letter to the editor). Radiology 125:549, 1977.

Miller RE: A new enema tip. Radiology 92:1492, 1969.

Miller RE: Examination of the colon. Curr Probl Radiol 5:1, 1975.

Miller RE: The cleansing enema. Editorial. Radiology 117:483, 1975.

Miller RE: Faster flow enema equipment. Radiology 123:229, 1977.

Miller RE, Chernish SM, Skucas J, et al: Hypotonic colon examination with glucagon. Radiology 113:555, 1974.

Welin S, Welin G: The double-contrast examination of the colon: Experiences with the Welin modification. Stuttgart, Georg Thieme, 1976, pp 5–16.

10

Normal Anatomy and Related Considerations

Knowledge of normal anatomy of the gastrointestinal tract is vital to the determination of whether a pathologic condition is present. Moreover, beyond a knowledge of normal radiographic appearances, the examining radiologist must understand the many ways in which the location, orientation, and contours of each organ affect the manner in which it is examined.

Most physicians appreciate the standard nomenclature of the anatomy of the gastrointestinal tract as taught in medical school classes. The following material on the normal anatomy of the gastrointestinal tract reviews that descriptive nomenclature and considers the implications of gastrointestinal anatomy on the radiologic examination and its interpretation.

THE PHARYNX

The pharynx is the segment of the gastrointestinal tract least understood by radiologists, simply because detailed radiologic examinations of the pharynx are seldom conducted. The portion of the pharynx of particular interest to the fluoroscopist is the hypopharynx, which extends from the epiglottis to the esophageal inlet. Its anatomy is most easily discernible on frontal and lateral views when coated with barium in the double-contrast mode (Fig. 10-1).

In the frontal view (Fig. 10-1A), the appearance of the hypopharynx as outlined by barium resembles a laryngogram. Superiorly, the epiglottis is visible as a barium-coated structure with its superior margin forming an arch. The valleculae, formed at the junction of the epiglottis and the tongue, are usually filled with a small amount of barium, forming two inferiorly convex collections. In general, the valleculae present a smooth appearance, although occasional small filling defects appear in the valleculae due to the normal nodularity of the posterior surface of the tongue.

Laterally, the margins of the hypopharynx are smooth and slightly convex outward, being formed by the lateral margins of the piriform sinuses and their upward extensions. Connecting the piriform sinuses are one or more arcuate lines of barium representing the mucosa on the posterior wall of the pharynx and the posterior surface of the larynx. The inferior margin of the hypopharynx seldom retains barium between swallows. It lies below the level of the piriform sinuses and merges into the esophageal inlet at the level of the C6 vertebral body.

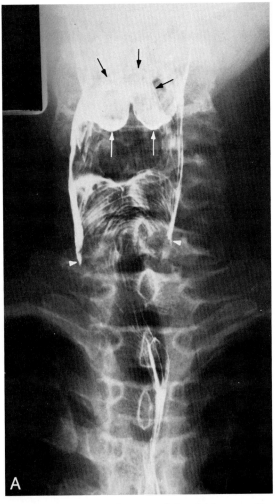

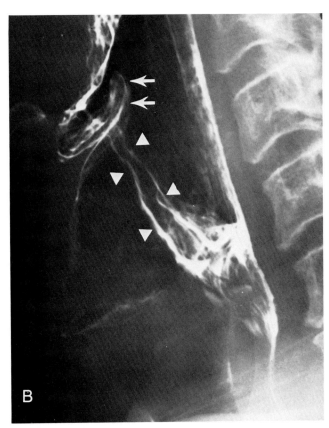

Fig. 10-1 Frontal and lateral views of normal structures in the pharynx and cervical esophagus. (A) Frontal view demonstrating the epiglottis (black arrows), paired valleculae (white arrows), and piriform sinuses (arrowheads). The arcuate lines connecting the piriform sinuses are fine transverse folds in the hypopharynx. The cervical esophagus is seen in mucosal relief as several thin folds coated by barium. (B) Lateral view of the hypopharynx in double-contrast. Major landmarks include the epiglottis (arrows), the superimposed valleculae anterior to the epiglottis, the aryepiglottic folds (arrowheads), and the posterior wall of the pharynx.

On the lateral view of the pharynx (Fig. 10-1B), the posterior wall of the pharynx presents a smooth contour, tracing a line several millimeters anterior to the cervical vertebrae. The hypopharynx is demarcated superiorly by the epiglottis, which projects superiorly and slightly posteriorly from the base of the tongue. The valleculae are visible as superimposed pockets containing barium just anterior to the base of the epiglottis. Starting at the base of the epiglottis, the superior margin of the larynx is outlined by the posteriorly and inferiorly sloping aryepiglottic folds, which are usually almost superimposed on each other.

Abnormalities of structures adjacent to the hypopharynx constitute a considerable portion of the pathology manifested on films of the hypopharynx. The intimate apposition of the posterior pharyngeal wall to the cervical vertebrae determines that any enlargement of the vertebrae (by osteoarthritic spurring, neoplasm, etc.) will cause anterior displacement of the posterior pharyngeal wall. The adjacency of cervical lymph nodes to the pharynx causes the pharynx to be impressed laterally by any metastatic or granulomatous mass that enlarge those lymph nodes. Also, the adjacency of the thyroid and parathyroid glands to the inferior portions of the pharynx allows enlargement of either of these structures to deviate the contours of the pharynx. Finally, because the pharynx incompletely circles the larynx, it is often the site of metastases from laryngeal malignancies.

THE ESOPHAGUS

The esophagus is divisible into cervical and thoracic regions that require different technical approaches for their examination and, with the exception of primary malignancy, present with different constellations of diseases. As a result, the cervical and thoracic esophagus are best considered separately.

The Cervical Esophagus

The cervical esophagus begins at the level of the cricoid cartilage and the C6 cervical vertebra. It terminates at the thoracic inlet at the level of the T1 cervical vertebra, where it merges imperceptively into the thoracic esophagus. When distended by passage of a barium bolus, the cervical

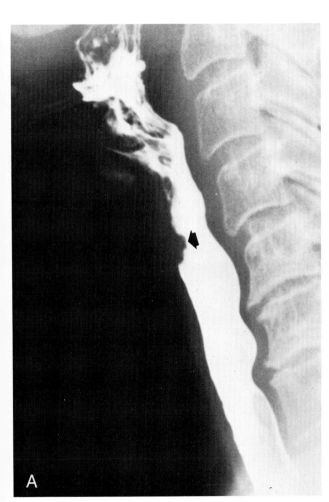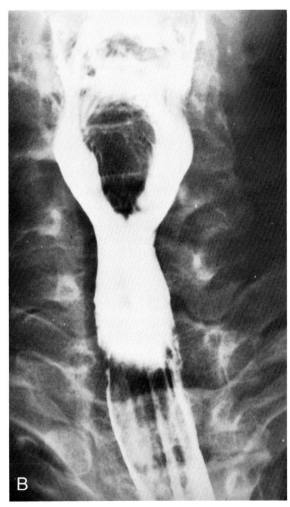

Fig. 10-2 Frontal and lateral views of the hypopharynx and cervical esophagus filled with barium during deglutition. (A) Lateral view demonstrating indentation of the posterior wall of the cervical esophagus by hypertrophic vertebral spurs. The mass-like protrusion on the anterior wall at the pharyngoesophageal junction represents a small submucosal venous plexus, which should not be mistaken for a neoplasm or web. (B) Frontal view showing the oval filling defect commonly produced by impingement of the posterior aspect of the larynx upon the barium stream.

esophagus usually presents the appearance of an almost featureless tube (Fig. 10-2A), with a smooth mucosa. In a minority of patients, however, a small rounded, web-like or plaque-like protrusion may be seen on the anterior wall at the pharyngoesophageal junction, representing a submucosal venous plexus that should not be mistaken for a web or small neoplasm. When collapsed but coated with barium, three or four slender longitudinal folds can be seen coursing the length of the cervical esophagus (Fig. 10-1A).

The inner circular and outer longitudinal muscle coats of the cervical esophagus are of striated muscle, causing peristalsis through the region to be extremely rapid. Because striated muscle is host to a different and less common group of neuromuscular disorders, functional disorders of peristalsis are far less frequent in the cervical esophageal region than in the thoracic esophagus, most of which contains smooth muscle. Furthermore, the rapidity of peristalsis in the cervical esophagus causes it to be difficult to radiograph in the distended state. Motion recording devices are thus particularly helpful in its examination (Fig. 10-2).

The adjacencies of the cervical esophagus are relatively simple. Like the pharynx, it is bordered posteriorly by the cervical spine. Laterally, major structures whose potential disease processes are likely to affect the cervical esophagus include the lobes of the thyroid gland, the inferior pair of parathyroid glands, and the cervical lymph nodes. Deviation of the cervical esophagus is the most common esophageal manifestation of disease in these adjacent organs and results from their neoplastic or granulomatous enlargement.

Thoracic Esophagus

The thoracic esophagus extends from the level of the T1 vertebral body to the esophagogastric junction, which normally lies within the esophageal hiatus of the diaphragm. Its middle and distal thirds are the regions most often involved by disease processes, both intrinsic and extrinsic. Because it courses through the mediastinum, its adjacencies are quite complex.

Apart from the region of the esophagogastric junction, which is described below, the normal appearance of the thoracic esophagus takes the form of a smooth, tube-like structure (Fig. 10-3A). It lies anterior to the thoracic vertebrae and throughout most of its course is slightly to the left of the midline. Three indentations on the thoracic esophagus may normally be seen (Fig. 10-3B). The aortic arch indents its left side and may deviate it slightly to the right. In the occasional patient with a right aortic arch, the imprint of the aorta is on the right side (Fig. 10-3C). Immediately inferior to the aortic arch, the esophagus also may be slightly indented by the crossing of the left lower lobe bronchus. In its distal half, a broad indentation on the anterior and left lateral aspect of the esophagus is caused by the heart, primarily the left atrium and ventricle. When the esophagus is empty but coated with barium, three or more smooth, slender longitudinal folds will be seen running its full length, particularly in the frontal view (Figs. 10-3D and E). Rarely, transverse folds may be seen as a transient contractile phenonenon (Fig. 10-3F). In the absence of disease states, however, the mucosa of the esophagus is smooth.

Peristalsis of the esophagus in young, normal patients takes the form of a primary wave that sweeps a bolus of barium distally in a single, smooth motion (Fig. 10-3E). In elderly individuals this wave may normally be incomplete or accompanied by mild uncoordinated contractile activity known as tertiary contractions. In the proximal fourth of the thoracic esophagus, peristalsis is rapid because of the presence of striated muscle. In the distal three-fourths, however, primary peristalsis is somewhat slower due to the presence of smooth muscle, which cannot contract as swiftly as can striated muscle. Disorders of motility in the distal three-fourths of the thoracic esophagus are relatively common and may cause dysphagia, particularly in the elderly.

The Esophagogastric Junction

The transition zone between esophagus and stomach, often labeled the esophagogastric junction, requires separate discussion because of its moderately complex anatomy and function, and because of its importance in the diagnosis of hiatus hernia and reflux esophagitis. The prevalence of

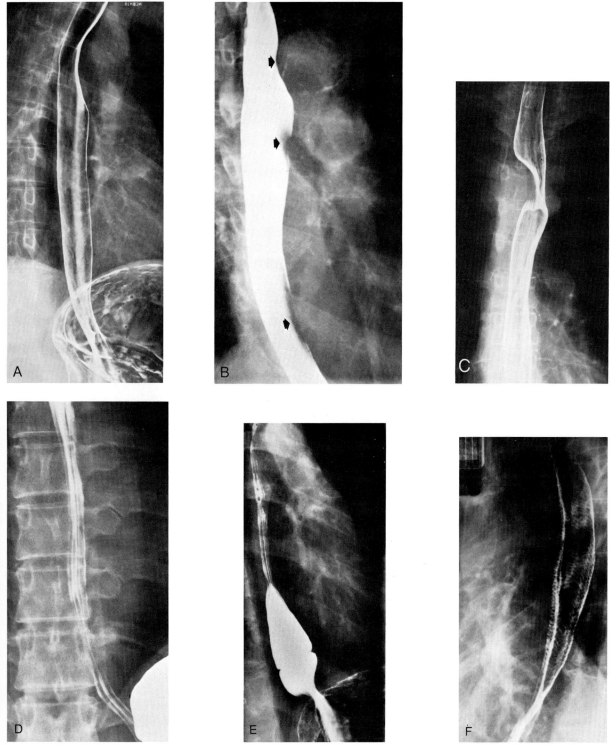

Fig. 10-3 Illustrations of the major anatomic features of the thoracic esophagus. (A) Double-contrast film showing the normally smooth mucosa seen when the esophagus is distended. (B) Three normal indentations on the esophagus (arrows) caused by the aortic arch, left bronchus, and heart. (C) Indentation of the right side of the thoracic esophagus by a right aortic arch. (D) Mucosal relief film showing the normally thin, smooth folds present in the collapsed esophagus. (E) Primary peristaltic wave stripping the barium suspension downward in the thoracic esophagus following deglutition of a single swallow of barium. The patient has a hiatal hernia, and the transverse mucosal fold ("B" ring) is visible above the esophageal hiatus. (Fig. E reprinted by permission of the publisher from Ott DJ: Radiologic evaluation of the esophagus. In Castell DO, Johnson LF, eds: Esophageal Function in Health and Disease. New York, copyright 1983 by Elsevier Science Publishing Co., Inc., pp 211–235.) (F) Transient transverse folds in the thoracic esophagus, which have been reported as a normal finding, as well as in association with esophagitis.

hiatus hernia and reflux esophagitis, the latter being as common a cause of upper gastrointestinal symptoms as peptic ulcer, suggests that a thorough appreciation of the anatomy of this region is indispensible.

The most specific mucosal landmark of the esophagogastric junction is the squamocolumnar junction, also termed the "Z" line. It marks the transition from smooth, squamous esophageal mucosa to columnar gastric mucosa, the latter having a finely nodular surface caused by the areae gastricae (Fig. 10-4A). The "Z" line is normally seen in the region of the esophageal hiatus, and can at times be directly identified on double-contrast and mucosal relief films of the region (Fig. 10-4B). Its upward displacement is a sensitive indicator of hiatus hernia.

The esophagogastric region may be notched laterally by a smooth muscle bundle known as the gastric sling fibers. These originate on the lesser curvature of the stomach and form a relatively discrete bundle that sweeps around the lateral aspect of the esophagogastric junction and then reinserts on the lesser curvature. In patients with

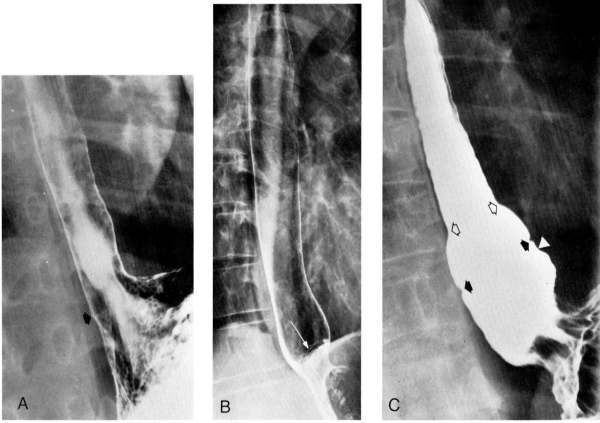

Fig. 10-4 Illustrations of the anatomic features identifying the esophagogastric junction. (A) Esophagogastric junction (arrow) as indicated by transition from smooth esophageal mucosa to nodular gastric mucosa, the nodules being the areae gastricae. (B) Smooth esophageal mucosa meeting irregular gastric mucosa (arrow) at the esophagogastric junction. (C) Barium-filled view showing the classic anatomic landmarks at the esophagogastric junction. The broad upper indentation (open arrows) is caused by the "A" ring. The small notches (closed arrows) represent the transverse mucosal fold, also known as the mucosal ring, or "B" ring. The slightly dilated segment of esophagus between the muscular ring and the mucosal ring is termed the esophageal vestibule. A slight indentation (arrowhead) on the lateral side of the eosphagogastric junction is caused by the gastric sling fibers.

hiatus hernia, when the esophagogastric junction is displaced upward and distended during examination, this discrete muscle bundle may form a notch on the lateral aspect of the esophagogastric junction (Fig. 10-4C).

The muscular coat of the several centimeters of esophagus proximal to the esophagogastric junction is somewhat thicker and more active than the remainder of the esophageal musculature. It is known manometrically as the high pressure zone, and its normal contracted state is one of the major antireflux mechanisms. Patulousness of the distal esophagus where it enters the stomach indicates a disturbance of the high pressure zone and is an important clue that gastroesophageal reflux may be occurring.

Two ring-like landmarks, of muscular and mucosal origin, are important in radiographically determining the location of the esophagogastric junction (Fig. 10-4C). The more proximal, broader "A" ring is of muscular origin and is normally visible several centimeters proximal to the esophageal hiatus. Distal to the "A" ring is a slightly dilated region of the distal esophagus known as the esophageal vestibule.

A second, ring-like landmark at the esophagogastric junction lies distal to the vestibule and is variously known as the transverse mucosal fold, the "B" ring, or the mucosal ring. It generally lies a few millimeters distal to the "Z" line and is present in only one-third to one-half of patients. It can only be seen in the presence of hiatal hernia and when the region is fully distended. In the absence of hiatal hernia, the transverse mucosal fold lies tucked within the esophageal hiatus, and the full distension necessary for its demonstration is prevented. There is reason to believe that the distal esophageal ring described by Schatzki, which may be a cause of dysphagia, is an exaggerated, web-like transverse mucosal fold.

THE STOMACH

The radiographic nomenclature commonly used to describe the several regions of the stomach varies slightly from that found in anatomy texts. Proximal to the incisura angularis, radiographic and anatomic terminology agree on the following descriptions. The fundus is that rounded proximal portion of the stomach lying above a line drawn transversely across the stomach at the level of the esophageal inlet. The area of the stomach surrounding the esophagogastric junction is known as the cardia, because of its proximity through the diaphragm to the heart. The largest segment of the stomach is the body, which lies between the fundus and a line transecting the stomach at the incisura angularis.

Distal to the incisura angularis, anatomic and common radiologic terminology diverge slightly. In anatomy texts, the stomach distal to the incisura angularis is known as the pyloric portion, divided by the sulcus intermedius into the pyloric vestibule and the pyloric antrum. In common radiologic terminology, the entire gastric segment distal to the incisura angularis is termed the gastric antrum, without further subdivision.

The stomach's usual shape is roughly that of the letter *J*. In obese or muscular individuals, the stomach tends to be transversely oriented. In those of slender body habitus, the stomach is more frequently long and vertically oriented.

The position of the stomach within the abdomen is such that the proximal portion of the stomach lies quite posteriorly, adjacent to the retroperitoneal tissues, while the distal portion of the stomach lies anteriorly, adjacent to the anterior abdominal wall. Thus, in saggital section the stomach is tilted. The combination of its hooked, or "J" shape, and its tilt within the abdomen greatly affect the manner in which the stomach is examined radiologically and best visualized by each of the available examination methods.

The mucosal surface of the stomach is dominated by two structures: the easily visualized gastric rugae and the less easily demonstrated areae gastricae, which are of much smaller dimension than the rugae. Although there is considerable variation, the gastric rugae tend to roughly parallel the long axis of the stomach (Figs. 10-5A and B). Normally, they will be approximately 3 to 5 ml in thickness as seen radiographically and are clearly visible when the stomach is partially filled. However, they may be completely effaced by gastric distension, particularly when a gastroparetic agent such as glucagon or Buscopan has been administered.

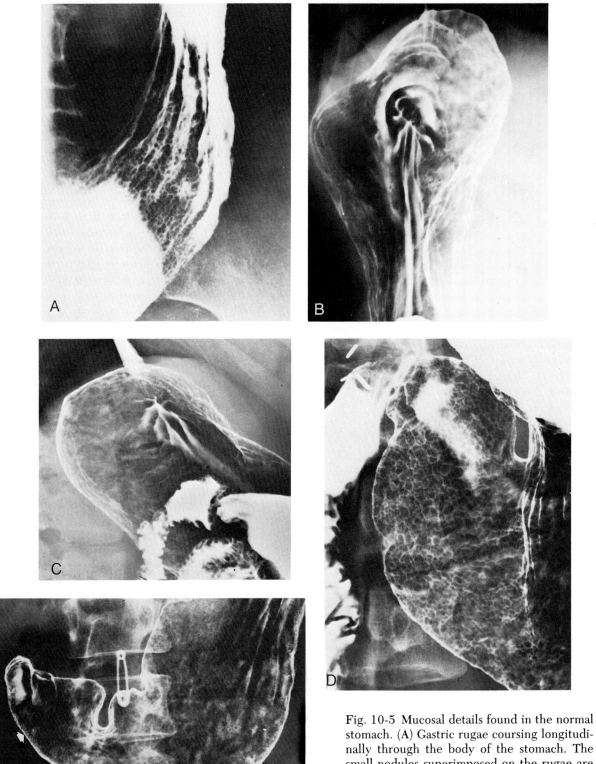

Fig. 10-5 Mucosal details found in the normal stomach. (A) Gastric rugae coursing longitudinally through the body of the stomach. The small nodules superimposed on the rugae are the areae gastricae. (B) Fold pattern at the esophagogastric junction producing a hooded appearance. (C) Stellate fold pattern at the esophagogastric junction imitating a gastric ulcer scar. (D) Areae gastricae visible in the distal stomach. In this example, they are slightly prominent. (E) Transverse mucosal rippling in the gastric antrum, an infrequent finding of uncertain etiology. (Fig. E from Gelfand DW: Japanese style double-contrast examination of the stomach. Gastrointest Radiol 1:7, 1976.)

When the stomach is distended during a double-contrast examination, a stellate or hood-shaped pattern of folds may be created at the esophagogastric junction. These are best seen on right lateral films (Figs. 10-5B and C) and should not be confused with the converging folds produced by gastric ulcers, ulcer scars, and carcinomas.

The areae gastricae are small, nodular tufts on the mucosal surface that are most readily visible on double-contrast examinations (Fig. 10-5A and D). Normally, their diameter does not exceed 2 to 3 mm. Changes in the appearance of the rugae and the areae gastricae are of diagnostic importance, since their absence or unusual prominence may signal the presence of any of several abnormal conditions.

Another mucosal detail occasionally seen in the gastric antrum is fine transverse rippling of the antral surface (Fig. 10-5E). It is seen in a small minority of patients and has been postulated, without any verification, as being due to contractions of the muscularis mucosae.

The muscular coat of the stomach is quite complex, consisting of longitudinal, circular, and oblique muscle fibers, the longitudinal fibers being for the most part external to the two other layers. Peristaltic activity in the stomach is generally absent proximal to the region of the esophagogastric junction. However, peristalsis is usually visible in the body of the stomach and the individual waves slowly progress distally until reaching the pyloric canal. Unlike the esophagus, functional disorders of gastric motility are an uncommon cause of symptoms. However, the presence or absence of normal peristalsis is of considerable radiologic importance in that local or generalized absence of peristalsis is often an important fluoroscopic clue to the presence of an infiltrating malignancy.

A prominent circular muscle is present at the pylorus, constituting the pyloric valve. This muscle indeed acts as an outflow valve, regulating the speed of outflow of gastric contents into the duodenum. Abnormality of this valving action, either in the direction of complete patulousness or persistent spasm, may be an indication of the presence of pathology at the pyloric region, most often a peptic ulcer or other inflammatory lesion.

The adjacencies of the stomach are quite complex and are of considerable use radiologically, since the location of the stomach in the midst of the upper abdominal organs dictates that it will be displaced by their significant enlargement. The liver lies anterior to the stomach. Enlargement of its left lobe pushes the body of the stomach posteriorly and to the left, and enlargement of its right lobe displaces the more distal portions of the stomach posteriorly and inferiorly. The pancreas lies behind most of the distal two-thirds of the stomach. Enlargement of the head or body of the pancreas, as occurs with pancreatic tumor or pseudocyst, displaces the most adjacent portion of the stomach anteriorly and/or superiorly. The periaortic lymph nodes also lie posterior to the distal stomach. Their enlargement by metastatic malignancy or lymphoma presents much the same appearance as displacement of the stomach by a pancreatic mass. The spleen lies posterior to the most proximal portions of the stomach, and its enlargement generally causes anterior and medial displacement of the fundus and body of the stomach. Rarely, a tumor or other mass in the left kidney will displace the body of the stomach anteriorly as well.

Unlike the esophagus, malignancies originating in structures adjacent to the stomach generally do not often invade the stomach wall all the way through to the mucosal surface until very late in their course. Thus, fistulae to adjacent organs as a result of metastatic involvement are rare.

THE DUODENUM

Although the duodenal loop is classically divided into four parts, from the standpoint of its radiologic evaluation it consists of three significant divisions: the duodenal bulb, the segment extending between the apex of the duodenal bulb and the most inferior portion of the duodenal loop, and the remainder of the duodenum to the ligament of Treitz. The duodenal bulb is of importance because of the prevalence of peptic ulcer, and it is always thoroughly examined during an upper gastrointestinal study. The segment of the duodenum between the apex of the duodenal bulb and the duodenum's most inferior extent contains the major and minor papillae and encircles most of the head of the pancreas. It is therefore the portion of greatest interest in patients with potential pan-

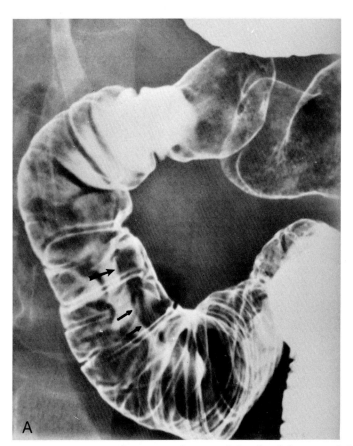
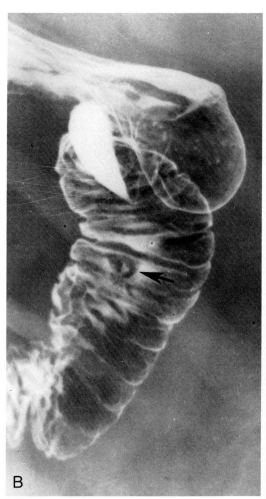

Fig. 10-6 Anatomic features and mucosal details of the normal duodenum. (A) Hypotonic dudenography showing the normal circular folds of the duodenum. The major papilla is visible (upper arrow). The longitudinal fold (lower arrows) extends distally from the major papilla. Note that when fully distended, the duodenal bulb is usually devoid of folds. (B) Minor papilla (arrow) visible on a prone film obtained during hypotonic duodenography.

creatic or biliary tract disease. The remaining segment of the duodenum, which ascends towards the ligament of Treitz, is less frequently the site of pathology, and may be difficult to thoroughly evaluate without resorting to a motion recording medium or to hypotonic duodenography with duodenal intubation.

The mucosal features of the duodenum are of radiologic interest. When distended, the spade-shaped duodenal bulb is often devoid of normal folds (Fig. 10-6A). Beyond the duodenal bulb, however, folds are always present and normally have the character of those present throughout the small bowel, being approximately 2 ml in thickness and circular in orientation. The ampulla of Vater, an oval structure 1.0 to 1.5 ml in length is present on the posteromedial wall of the duodenal loop, usually accompanied by the only consistent longitudinal fold in the duodenal loop (Fig. 10-6A). The minor papilla, generally no larger than 0.5 to 1.0 cm in diameter, tends to be located on the anterior wall of the duodenum and is reliably visible only on prone double-contrast films of the duodenal loop (Fig. 10-6B). On double-contrast

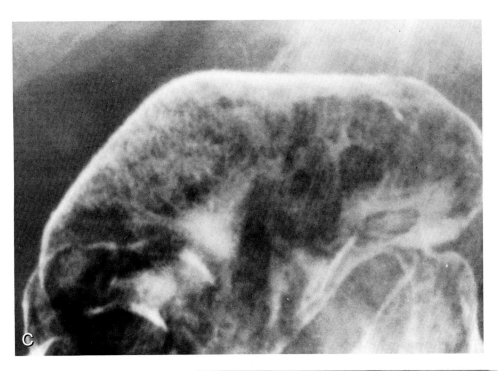

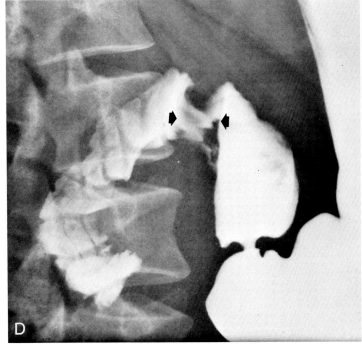

Fig. 10-6 *(continued)* (C) The villi of the duodenal mucosa visible as a velvety pattern. (Fig. C from Gelfand DW, Ott DJ: Radiographic demonstration of small intestinal villi on routine studies. Gastrointest Radiol 6:21, 1981.) (D) Band-like indentation on the proximal duodenum (arrows) caused by the structures of the porta hepatis.

studies, the mucosal villi may occasionally be discerned a fine, velvet-like pattern (Fig. 10-6C).

The muscle coats of the duodenum consist of inner circular and outer longitudinal fibers similar to those found throughout the small intestine. Normal peristalsis usually commences in the duodenal bulb as a continuation of gastric peristalsis and sweeps distally. Also seen normally are limited reverse peristaltic components, which tend to churn the duodenal contents. Abnormalities of peristalsis such as total flacidity, persistent spasm, or extremely rapid peristalsis constitute nonspecific but meaningful clues to the presence of pathologic conditions such as peptic ulcer or duodenitis.

Several adjacencies of the duodenum are noteworthy. The duodenal loop partially encircles the pancreatic head, and tumors or other enlargements of the pancreatic head may cause impressions on its medial contour. The common duct lies just behind the apex of the duodenal bulb, where it may cause a broad, vertical impression up to 1 cm wide (Fig. 10-6D). The quadrate lobe of the liver lies above and in front of the proximal portion of the duodenum, and its enlargement may push the duodenum inferiorly. The gallbladder lies adjacent to the lateral aspect of the duodenal loop and, particularly when enlarged, may indent it. Periaortic lymph nodes lie behind much of the duodenum, and their enlargement by tumor may displace the duodenum anteriorly.

THE MESENTERIC SMALL BOWEL

The jejunum and ileum together constitute the mesenteric small bowel, which may be defined as that segment of intestine extending from the ligament of Treitz to the cecum. The division between jejunum and ileum is arbitrary, with no distinct demarcation between the two. Instead, the appearance of the intestine undergoes a gradual change from the proximal jejunum to the distal ileum.

The radiographic appearance of the small intestinal mucosa is dominated by the presence of the valvulae conniventes. With the bowel distended, these folds are transversely oriented and 1.0- to 2.0-mm thick in normal individuals. In the jejunum the folds are deep and numerous while in the ileum

the folds become sparse. When opacified by orally administered barium, the jejunum is normally almost empty, the folds collapsed upon each other and presenting a feathery pattern (Fig. 10-7A). By comparison, the ileum tends to be partially filled with barium and segments of it may be fully distended. The distal ileal mucosa may also contain small nodular elevations caused by aggregates of lymphoid tissue (Fig. 10-7B)—the Peyer's patches—which are seldom more than 2 mm in diameter and are most often visible in children and young adults.

It has recently been reported that the villi of the small intestinal mucosa may be demonstrated radiographically if sufficient radiographic resolving power is employed. These are seen as small filling defects of fractional millimeter dimension, and are most easily shown on peroral, full column studies (Fig. 10-7C).

The muscular coat of the mesenteric small bowel contains inner circular and outer longitudinal layers. In general, peristalsis consisting of distally propulsive waves is visible throughout the small bowel during fluoroscopy (Fig. 10-7A). Segmental contractions and reverse peristalsis of limited extent may also be seen. As with the duodenum, flacidity, lack of peristalsis, and extremely rapid peristalsis constitute reasonably reliable but nonspecific signs of abnormality. Dilatation to more than 3.0-cm diameter, involving part or all of the small bowel, is a significant sign of a variety of small intestinal abnormalities ranging from nontropical sprue to intestinal obstruction.

The mesenteric small bowel fills much of the abdominal cavity and comes in close approximation to almost all abdominal and pelvic organs. Thus, organ enlargement or abdominal masses will usually displace or compress one or more loops of small intestine.

THE COLON

The colon is the most complex of gastrointestinal organs from the radiologist's standpoint. Because it is the most frequent site of gastrointestinal neoplasm, every centimeter of the colon must be thoroughly examined during a barium enema. However, the colon is 1.5-meters long, is often

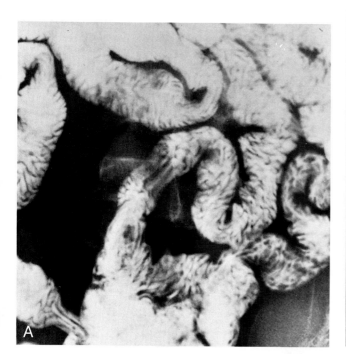

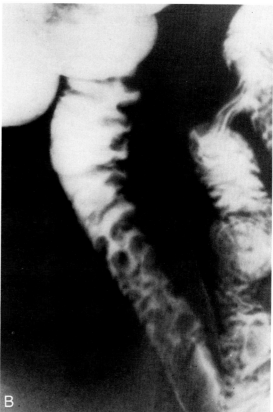

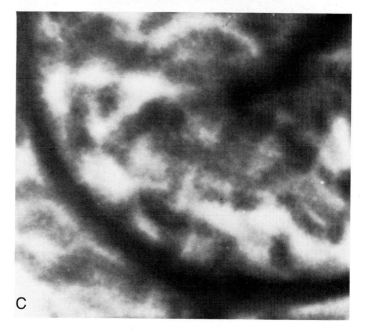

Fig. 10-7 Mucosal details of the mesenteric portion of the small intestine. (A) Feathery pattern of the valvulae conniventes in the mid-small intestine. (B) Film of the terminal ileum with small nodules representing the lymphoid follicles, or Peyer's patches. These are commonly seen in children and young adults, but disappear in older individuals. (C) Small intestinal villi visible as innumerable filling defects and finger-like projections from the mucosal surface. (Fig. C from Gelfand DW, Ott DJ: Radiographic demonstration of small intestinal villi on routine studies. Gastrointest Radiol 6:21. 1981.)

tortuous, and meanders into almost every portion of the abdominal cavity, with certain segments being partially or completely retroperitoneal. Its length and tortuosity thus make its evaluation an everyday challenge to the radiologist. Since the colon is almost always examined in retrograde fashion, the anatomy pertinent to its radiologic examination is described in the same fashion.

The rectum is within the bony pelvis and lies directly anterior to the sacrum. Its distal demarcation is obvious but its proximal limit, the pelvic peritoneal reflection, may be difficult to appreciate radiologically. The pelvic peritoneal reflection is the demarcation between sigmoid colon and rectum, and on a lateral film of the rectum it usually lies close to a line drawn from the junction of the upper and middle thirds of the sacrum toward the pubic symphysis (Fig. 10-8A). The major internal

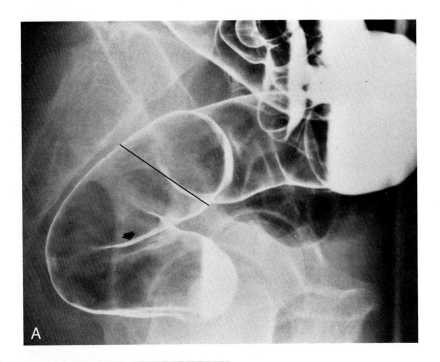

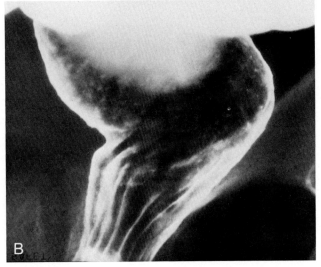

Fig. 10-8 Anatomic and mucosal details of the rectum. (A) Lateral view of the rectum showing a single valve of Houston (arrow). The level of the peritoneal reflection is indicated by the black line. (B) Frontal view of the rectum showing the rectal columns, which contain the hemorrhoidal veins. The small, punctate collections of barium are within dilated mucus glands and are occasionally seen as a normal finding.

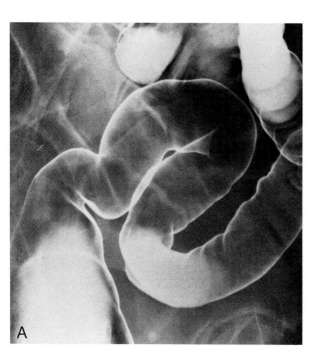

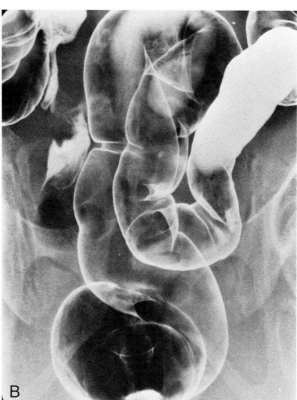

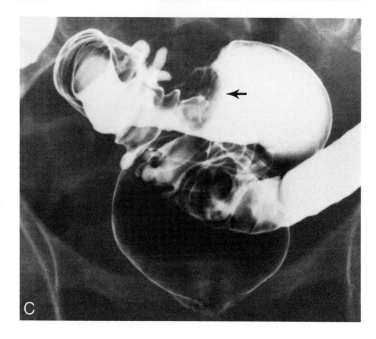

Fig. 10-9 Variable appearances of the sigmoid colon. (A) Classic "S" shape found in patients with a short sigmoid colon. (B) Moderately redundant sigmoid colon with partial overlapping of loops. (C) Considerably tortuous sigmoid colon in a patient with diverticulosis coli as well as a polypoid neoplasm (arrow). This neoplasm was overlooked on the initial reading of the films, probably due to the complexity of overlapping shadows.

features of the rectum are one or more inconstant circular folds known as the valves of Houston (Fig. 10-8A). On double-contrast barium enemas, folds converging toward the anus, the rectal columns, may also be seen; these are more prominent when internal hemorrhoids are present (Fig. 10-8B).

Adjacencies of the rectum are to the sacrum posteriorly and the bladder and reproductive organs anteriorly. The sacrum is an infrequent site of neoplastic enlargement which may displace the rectum anteriorly. On the other hand, the female reproductive organs are common sites of neoplasms and cysts that usually displace the rectum posteriorly. The bladder also lies anterior to the rectum, and its distension may similarly compress the rectum and displace it posteriorly.

The sigmoid colon, because it is on a mesentery of varying length, follows no standard course or contour except that in patients with relatively short sigmoid colons it is usually "S" shaped as classically described (Fig. 10-9A). However, in many patients the course of the sigmoid colon is more complex (Figs. 10-9B and C).

The remaining, more proximal portions of the colon (descending colon, transverse colon, ascending colon and cecum) are disposed in roughly an "M" shape, the upward points of the "M" being the hepatic and splenic flexures. By definition, the cecum is the pouch-like segment situated below the ileocecal valve, its blind end normally directed downward. The appendix opens into the cecum on its inferomedial aspect.

From the radiologist's standpoint, the important aspect of the colonic flexures is that the hepatic flexure is situated obliquely within the abdomen, while the splenic flexure is situated in an almost anteroposterior manner. While most radiologists realize that the hepatic flexure is best radiographed in an oblique position, it is often not appreciated that the most extensive view of the splenic flexure in the majority of patients occurs in what is almost a lateral view.

The interior of the colon is dominated by the sac-like haustrae, which are separated from each other by the semilunar folds (Fig. 10-10). On a smaller scale, however, the normally smooth colonic mucosa may show two additional fine patterns. The first is that of the innominate lines, a network of very fine, transversely oriented

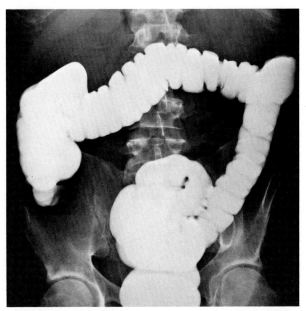

Fig. 10-10 Film of the colon demonstrating a normal haustral pattern. The sac-like haustrae are separated by the semilunar folds. Apart from these folds, the colonic mucosa is usually smooth.

grooves separating small elevations of the colonic mucosa analagous to the areae gastricae (Fig. 10-11A). The second is that of the submucosal lymphoid follicles, which are seen on a minority of double-contrast studies as fine nodular elevations approximately 2.0 mm in diameter (Fig. 10-11B).

Another colon mucosal pattern of considerable importance is that of the collapsed normal mucosa, the so-called postevacuation pattern. This is in essence a mucosal relief view of the colon showing the character of the folds present when the colon is empty. In normal patients this is seen as a feathery pattern (Fig. 10-12), which may be displaced by neoplasms or altered by inflammatory processes.

An anatomic feature of radiographic importance in the right colon is the ileocecal valve, of interest because its variable appearance is capable of simulating a neoplasm. In most patients, the ileocecal valve is seen as a widening of the semilunar fold dividing the cecum from the ascending colon. The lumen of the ileum enters the colon within that fold (Fig. 10-13A). However, in many patients the ileum will prolapse slightly into the colonic lumen, causing a round or oval protuberance which may

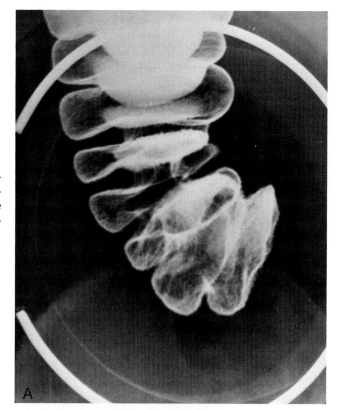

Fig. 10-11 Occasionally seen patterns on the mucosal surface of the colon, best demonstrated on double-contrast films. (A) Network pattern caused by the innominate lines. (B) Small, 1 to 2 mm nodules representing slightly enlarged lymphoid follicles.

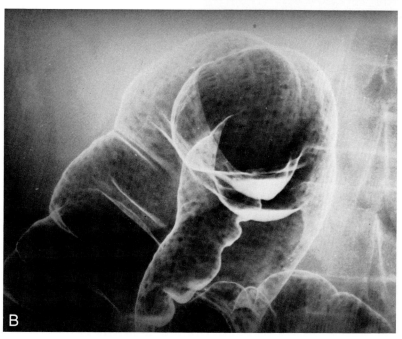

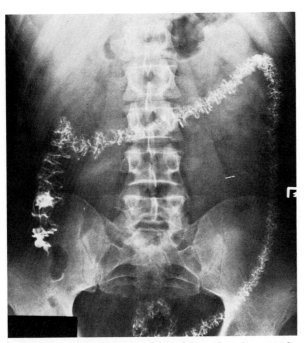

Fig. 10-12 postevacuation film of the colon showing the normal feathery pattern of folds seen in the evacuated colon.

reach 3 or 4 cm in size (Fig. 10-13B). This protuberance is usually smooth in contour and may mimic the appearance of a lipoma or large polyp, both of which occur with reasonable frequency in that region. Usually, it is possible to discern a small collection of barium within the ileum as it opens into the center of the protrusion, confirming that it represents the ileocecal valve. However, when the opening of the valve cannot be seen, or if it is seen at the side of the mass, the possibility of neoplasm must be excluded colonoscopically.

The entry of the appendix into the inferomedial aspect of the cecum has a twofold importance. First, a surgically inverted appendiceal stump may simulate the presence of a small, sessile cecal polyp. Second, in patients with appendicitis, periappendiceal inflammation may indent the inferomedial aspect of the cecum.

The muscular coat of the colon is composed of the usual inner circular and outer longitudinal layers of smooth muscle. However, the gathering of the outer longitudinal muscle into the three distinct bands known as the taeniae coli contrib-

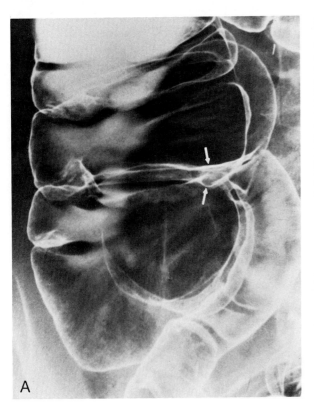

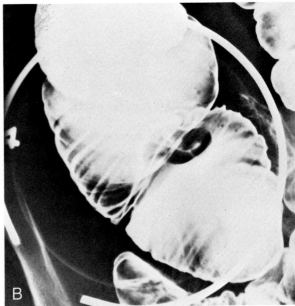

Fig. 10-13 Variable appearance of the ileocecal valve. (A) Slight widening of the semilunar fold at the ileocecal valve, the most common appearance. (B) Prominent normal ileocecal valve. The entrance of the ileum is seen as a barium-filled slit on the surface of the protuberance.

В44

В4ВВ

utes to the formation of the sac-like haustrae. The diagnostic importance of this arrangement is that in the presence of inflammatory disease the haustrae often disappear in the affected portion of the colon, producing a featureless, tube-like contour. This phenomenon may be reversible, the normal contours of the colon being partially or wholly restored after cure or remission.

Peristalsis in the colon usually consists of a contraction that begins near the cecum and progresses distally in a well-coordinated effort to expel the colonic contents. However, nonperistaltic segmental contractions may occur and be visible during barium enema, particularly in the sigmoid colon. In certain disease processes, such as ulcerative colitis and diverticulosis, irritability of the colon may be greatly increased, and spastic contractions may be frequent and persistent, even after attempted paralysis of the colon by glucagon or other paretic agents. In ulcerative colitis, severe spasticity of the colon may be one of the earliest radiologic signs, preceding the appearance of ulcerations.

Adjacencies of the colon are important in detection of abdominal organ enlargement and masses. The relation of the sigmoid colon to the bladder and female reproductive organs anteriorly and inferiorly is such that their enlargement tends to displace the sigmoid colon posteriorly and superiorly, often elevating it out of the pelvis. Enlargement of the spleen tends to push the splenic flexure inferiorly. The right lobe of the liver lies immediately above the hepatic flexure, and hepatic enlargement thus displaces the hepatic flexure of the colon inferiorly.

SUGGESTED READINGS

The Esophagus

Clements JL, Cox GW, Torres WE, Weens HS: Cervical esophageal webs: A roentgen-anatomic correlation. Am J Roentgenol 121:221, 1974.

Dodds WJ: Current concepts of esophageal motor function: Clinical implications for radiology. Am J Roentgenol 128:549, 1977.

Friedland GW: Historical review of changing concepts of lower esophageal anatomy. 430 BC–1977. AJR 131:373, 1978.

Gelfand DW, Ott DJ: Areae gastricae transversing the esophageal hiatus: A sign of hiatal hernia. Gastrointest Radiol 4:127, 1979.

Gohel VK, Edell SL, Laufer I, Rhodes WH: Transverse folds in the human esophagus. Radiology 128:303, 1978.

Wolf BS: The inferior esophageal sphincter — anatomic, roentgenologic and manometric correlation, contradictions, and terminology. Am J Roentgenol 110:260, 1970.

The Stomach

Gelfand DW: High density, low viscosity barium for fine mucosal detail on double-contrast upper gastrointestinal examinations. AJR 130:831, 1978.

Koga M, Nakata H, Kiyonari H, et al: Minute mucosal patterns in gastric carcinoma. Radiology 120:199, 1976.

Kreel L: The surface pattern of the stomach. Proc Roy Soc Med 68:111, 1975.

Mackintosh CF, Kreel L: Anatomy and radiology of the areae gastricae. Gut 18:855, 1977.

Rose CP, Stevenson GW: Correlation between visualization and size of the area gastricae and duodenal ulcer. Radiology 139:371, 1981.

The Duodenum

Eaton SB, Ferrucci JT: Radiology of the Pancreas and Duodenum. Philadelphia, WB Saunders, 1973, pp 109–113.

Ferrucci JT, Benedict KT, Page DL, et al: Radiographic features of the normal hypotonic duodenogram. Radiology 96:401, 1970.

Stevenson GW, Somers S, Virjee J: Routine double-contrast barium meal: Appearance of normal duodenal papillae. Diagn Imaging 49:6, 1980.

The Mesenteric Small Bowel

Gelfand DW, Ott DJ: Radiographic demonstration of small intestinal villi on routine clinical studies. Gastrointest Radiol 6:21, 1981.

Sellink JL: Radiological Atlas of Common Diseases of the Small Bowel. Anatomy. Leiden, HE Stenfert Kroese, 1976, pp 3–25.

The Colon

Cole FM: Innominate grooves of the colon: Morphological characteristics and etiologic mechanisms. Radiology 128:41, 1978.

Farrar CW: Patterns of the sigmoid colon and their implications for barium-enema radiography. Med Radiog Photo (Kodak) 55:2, 1979.

Kelvin FM, Max RJ, Norton GA, et al: Lymphoid follecular pattern of the colon in adults. AJR 133:821, 1979.

Matsuura K, Nakata H, Takeda N, et al: Innominate lines of the colon. Radiology 123:581, 1977.

11

Radiologic Manifestation of Gross Pathologic Changes

Most radiologic evaluation of gastrointestinal disease depends on recognition of one or more of a limited number of radiologic signs of gross pathologic change. Recognizing their presence indicates that the area in question is not normal and initiates the process of arriving at a diagnosis. In many instances, location, specific appearance, and clinical background will be sufficient to allow a definitive diagnosis to be made. In other instances, however, the changes seen radiologically will be rather nonspecific, and there will be several entities to be considered that might be capable of producing the particular abnormal appearance.

Several general classes of gross pathologic change visible radiologically are discussed in this chapter, with a limited number of examples. The full range of gastrointestinal pathology is dealt with in greater detail in the subsequent chapters, which describe the specific disease entities of each of the gastrointestinal organs.

EDEMA

Bland edema of the gastrointestinal tract, unaccompanied by inflammation, is most often seen as a consequence of hypoalbuminemia. When the serum albumin level is sufficiently low (less than 2.5 mg percent) that the osmotic pressure of the blood cannot prevent loss of water and electrolytes from capillaries into the extracellular space, many tissues, including the gut, become waterlogged. Edema of the small intestine and colon may also be seen in severe congestive failure, in which capillary hydrostatic pressure exceeds serum osmotic pressure and serum escapes through the capillary walls. Edema may also be the result of permeation of the bowel by an adjacent inflammatory process. The radiologic manifestations of gastrointestinal edema vary from organ to organ, but its most frequent appearance is that of thickening of mucosal folds.

The diagnosis of intestinal edema is most likely to be made in the mesenteric small intestine for two reasons. First, in most of the diseases likely to cause edema—hepatic cirrhosis, congestive failure, protein-losing enteropathy—the mesenteric small bowel will become edematous. Second, it is relatively easy to detect changes in the rather uniform and delicate-appearing valvulae conniventes, which become thickened in the presence of edema. Thus, valvulae conniventes thicker than

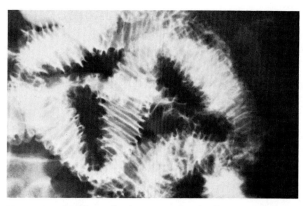

Fig. 11-1 Diffuse thickening of valvulae conniventes due to intestinal edema in a patient with renal failure.

2.0 mm, or whose contour in profile has become rounded or clubbed, are indicative of intestinal edema (Fig. 11-1). In addition, films taken during a small bowel study may provide further clues to the existence of edema, in the form of enlargement of the liver and/or spleen, or the presence of ascites.

In the colon, edema may be more difficult to detect because of the lack of a generalized fold pattern. When the colon is distended during barium enema examination, there may be virtually no manifestations of colonic edema visible. On postevacuation films, however, the folds visible in the collapsed colon may appear thicker and more coarse than normal. However, the wide range of normal for the fold pattern seen on postevacuation films of the colon somewhat discourages the diagnosis of edema by this means. In practice, the diagnosis of intestinal edema is usually made on the basis of radiologic findings in the small bowel rather than in the colon.

INFLAMMATION

Inflammation unaccompanied by ulceration is a common and varied finding throughout the intestinal tract. As with edema, its general manifestation is that of thickening of folds, and it often may be difficult to differentiate the appearance of inflammation from that of bland edema. In many locations in the gut, the appearance of inflammation is nonspecific, and one may be faced with a

long differential diagnosis without being able to arrive at a definite diagnosis.

The Esophagus

In the esophagus, inflammation is most often the consequence of reflux esophagitis. As viewed on mucosal relief films, the usual manifestation of esophageal inflammation are thickening and/or irregularity of the mucosal folds (Fig. 11-2A). On double-contrast films, inflammation may be seen as a granular mucosal pattern (Fig. 11-2B) as compared to the normally smooth appearance of the esophageal mucosa. When inflammatory changes are confined to the distal esophagus, they almost always represent reflux esophagitis, particularly if accompanied by hiatal hernia. On the other hand, inflammation of the esophageal mucosa due to candidiasis or herpetic infection tends to be more diffuse and may be seen anywhere along the course of the esophagus (Fig. 11-2C). Thus, inflammatory changes located well above the esophagogastric junction should suggest a cause other than reflux esophagitis.

The Stomach

In the stomach, the radiologic signs of inflammation are poorly defined, partly because the pathologic classification of the various types of gastritis is based on histologic findings rather than gross morphologic or endoscopic appearances. However, certain forms of gastritis are generally recognized to have identifiable radiologic manifestations.

Most cases of atrophic gastritis exhibit a gastric mucosa that is almost totally devoid of folds (Fig. 11-3A) and, in its final stages, also lacking the normal areae gastricae (although in occasional cases these may become unusually prominent during a particular phase of the disease). Hypertrophic gastritis, a hypersecretory condition not properly classifiable as a gastritis per se, is manifested as thickening of the folds and/or unusual prominence and size of the areae gastricae (Fig. 11-3B). Chemical gastritis due to aspirin or alcohol is often seen as gastric erosions (Fig. 11-3C).

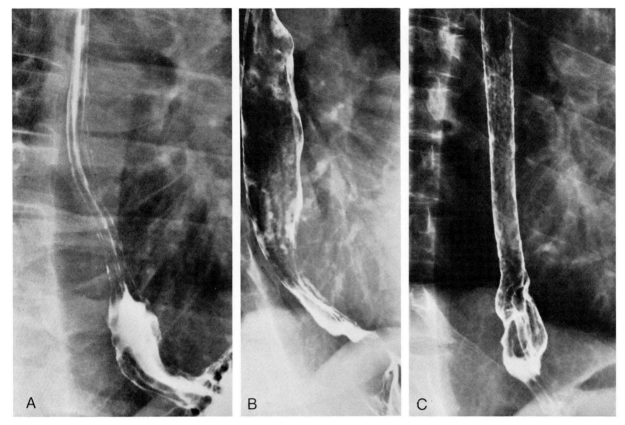

Fig. 11-2 Varied manifestations of inflammation in the esophagus. (A) Thickened, slightly irregular folds in a patient with reflux esophagitis, as seen on a collapsed mucosal view. (Ott DJ, Gelfand DW, Wu WC: Sensitivity of single contrast radiology in esophageal disease. Gastrointest Radiol 8:105, 1983.) (B) Diffuse mucosal irregularity of the distal esophagus in a patient with reflux esophagitis, as seen on a double-contrast film. (C) Double-contrast film showing strikingly granular changes throughout the length of the esophagus in a patient with candidiasis. (Fig. C from Gelfand DW, Ott DJ: Anatomy and techniques in evaluating the esophagus. Semin Roentgenol 16:168, 1981.)

The Duodenum

Nonspecific duodenitis, unaccompanied by ulcer, occurs at least as frequently as peptic ulcer and probably represents a distinct entity. Its usual radiologic manifestations are thickening of folds, often with a distinctly nodular component (Fig. 11-4), and occasional erosions.

The Mesenteric Small Bowel

In the mesenteric small bowel, nonulcerating inflammation is most often the result of parasitic infestation. Irregular thickening of folds may be widespread, but seldom involves the entire small bowel as uniformly as bland edema. Crohn's disease, however, rapidly progresses to the ulcerating phase, and only rarely is a patient examined radiologically early enough in the course of the disease to demonstrate inflammatory thickening of folds unaccompanied by ulceration.

The Colon

In the colon, the appearance of nonulcerating inflammation has been best documented in the case of early ulcerative colitis. Early in this disease, prior to the onset of ulceration, inflammation is

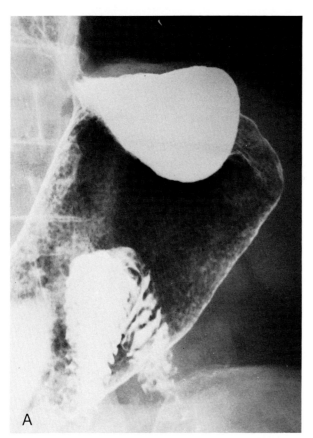

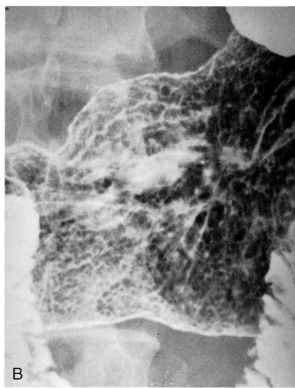

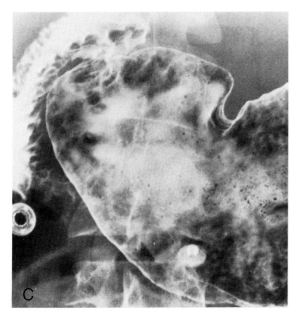

Fig. 11-3 Examples of recognized radiologic manifestations of inflammatory changes in the stomach. (A) Total lack of gastric rugae in a patient with atrophic gastritis. Small, prominent, widely separate areae gastricae are also visible in this particular case. (B) Gastric ulcer scar plus prominent, slightly enlarged areae gastricae in a patient treated for gastric ulcer. (C) Gastric erosions visible as punctate collections of barium surrounded by a radiolucent halo. The location of these erosions in the distal antrum is typical of erosive gastritis caused by aspirin or alcohol.

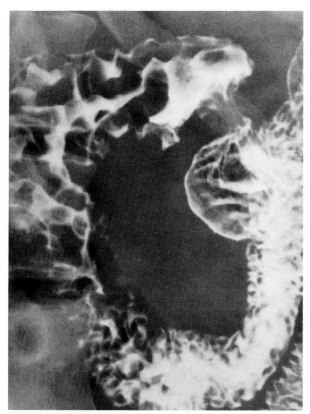

Fig. 11-4 Greatly thickened folds in a patient with nonspecific duodenitis.

seen as a granular appearance on double-contrast and postevacuation films (Fig. 11-5A) or as a slight marginal irregularity visible on full column radiographs. Similar changes also may be seen in other nonulcerating colonic inflammations, such as mild bacillary dysentery.

A nonspecific manifestation of inflammation unique to the colon is the disappearance of its haustral markings in the area involved by the inflammatory process (Fig. 11-5B). This may occur very early in the course of colonic inflammatory diseases, being radiographically visible in ulcerative colitis before ulceration is seen endoscopically. It is similarly seen in patients with Crohn's disease and with dysenteries of several varieties.

ULCERATION

Ulcers may be classified into three broad categories: discrete benign ulceration, diffuse ulceration, and malignant ulceration. Recognition of one of these three forms very quickly directs diagnostic considerations toward specific disease entities.

Discrete Benign Ulceration

The classic example of discrete ulceration is peptic ulcer of the stomach or duodenum, which represents a considerable fraction of the pathology encountered radiologically in the gastrointestinal tract. However, other notable forms of localized ulceration occur and include jejunal ulcer due to potassium tablets, tuberculous ulcers of the ileum, and stercoral and solitary ulcers of the colon.

Discrete ulcers are often surrounded by an area of edema that lies beneath and adjacent to the ulcer. In the case of peptic ulcer of the stomach or duodenum, the edema surrounding the ulcer can be considerable, causing an elevated surround known as the *ulcer mound* (Fig. 11-6). In benign ulceration, the inflammatory mass associated with the ulcer is covered by mucosa and is smooth and gently rounded, differentiating it from the more irregular, nodular surface usually found adjacent to a malignant ulcer.

Very small ulcerations and erosions in the gastrointestinal tract also tend to be surrounded by a small halo of adjacent induration (Fig. 11-3C). Certain of these have been termed *aphthoid* ulcers because of their resemblance to the aphthous herpetic ulcers commonly occurring in the mouth. Aphthoid ulcers are small collections of barium 2 or 3 mm in greatest diameter, surrounded by a narrow halo of radiolucency caused by the slightly raised adjacent area of inflammation. While originally purported to be unique to Crohn's disease, it now appears almost certain that any disease process capable of causing small ulcerations or erosions in the gastrointestinal tract will be found capable of producing aphthoid ulcers.

Diffuse Ulceration

Occurring less frequently than discrete ulceration, diffuse ulceration is more typically associated with entities such as ulcerative colitis, Crohn's disease, ischemia of the bowel, and trauma due to corrosive agents. In most of the inflammatory diseases causing diffuse ulceration, the pro-

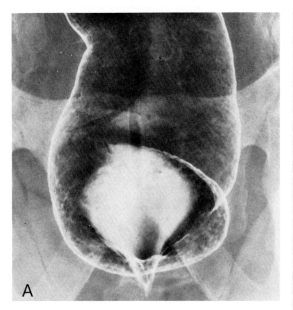

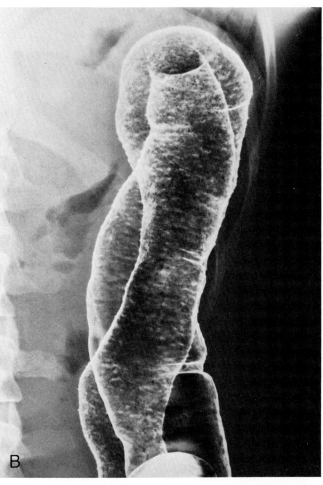

Fig. 11-5 Colonic inflammatory changes as exhibited in two patients with ulcerative colitis. (A) Granularity of the rectum plus loss of the valves of Houston. (B) Granularity, numerous small, shallow ulcers, and loss of haustration.

cess begins as multiple discrete ulcers that enlarge and merge to produce large areas of ulceration. The diffuse ulceration seen in severe ulcerative colitis or Crohn's disease is the consequence of this series of events. On the other hand, the diffuse ulceration associated with ischemia and chemical trauma tends to follow necrosis of broad areas of the mucosal surface in which the mucosa sloughs, leaving an extensive denuded surface.

The radiologic appearance of diffuse ulceration usually depends on which of the above two processes has taken place. In the case of many small and merging localized ulcers, there are often elevated islands of mucosa remaining, surrounded by the merging areas of ulceration (Fig. 11-7). Usually quite inflamed, these islands of mucosa may form polypoid filling defects known as *pseudopolyps* in

ulcerative colitis or *cobblestones* in Crohn's disease. Eventually ulceration may become complete, leaving an amorphous, granular surface.

In the case of diffuse ulceration following ischemia or ingestion of caustic materials, the initial appearance may be that of an extremely edematous, nodular mucosal surface. However, very quickly the mucosa becomes necrotic and begins to slough, allowing barium to flow between the mucosa and the remaining wall of the bowel. The necrotic mucosa is then seen as a radiolucent line separated from the margin of the barium column by 1 or 2 mm (Fig. 11-8A). This may be the initial radiographic appearance of the esophagus in a patient who has swallowed lye, and is also seen in colitis due to antibiotic therapy.

When a mucosal surface has become completely

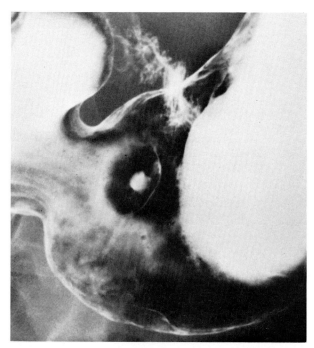

Fig. 11-6 Discrete, benign gastric ulcer sitting on a distinct mound of inflammatory edema. The smooth character of the mucosal surface surrounding the ulcer is indicative of its benign nature.

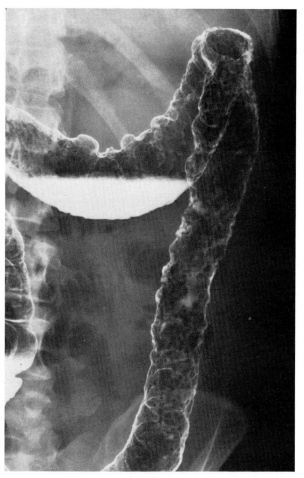

Fig. 11-7 Diffuse ulceration and pseudopolyps in a patient with well-developed acute ulcerative colitis.

ulcerated, the wall of the bowel presents an amorphous, slightly granular or nodular appearance characteristic of the interior surface of bowel devoid of mucosa (Fig. 11-8B). This is most often seen in advanced Crohn's disease of the distal ileum.

Malignant Ulceration

Malignant ulceration describes a malignant neoplasm, usually an adenocarcinoma, presenting as an ulcerating lesion. The ulcer is the result of partial necrosis of the underlying infiltrating or mass-like malignancy. The malignant ulcer is particularly a lesion of the stomach, where the digestive process encourages excavation of a partially necrotic neoplasm. Most malignant gastric ulcers are associated with a mass or an irregular, nodular surround (Fig. 11-9) in contrast to the usually smooth surround of a benign gastric ulcer. Malig-

nant ulcers and their differentiation from benign ulcers are described more thoroughly in Chapter 14, Abnormalities of the Stomach.

BENIGN STRICTURES

The frequent sequel to discrete or diffuse ulceration is stricture. Strictures form as a result of the ulcerated surface producing granulation tissue, which is then converted into collagen-containing connective tissue that contracts as it matures, producing the stricture.

Radiologically, benign strictures tend to have tapering, funnel-shaped margins that are often not clearly demarcated from the adjacent normal seg-

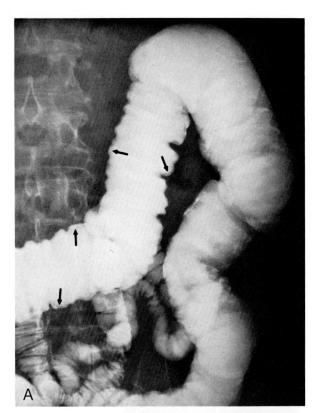

Fig. 11-8 Two differing manifestations of diffuse ulceration. (A) Necrotizing enterocolitis due to antibiotic administration. The mucosa is beginning to slough, as indicated by thin radiolucent lines (arrows) separated from the wall of the colon by a small amount of barium. (B) Distal ileum almost devoid of mucosa, as indicated by the diffusely granular and slightly nodular amorphous appearance in a patient with Crohn's disease.

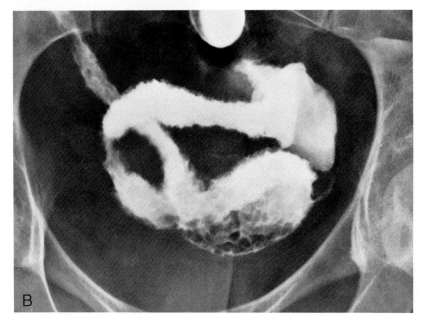

finely nodular margin typical of a diffusely ulcerated surface will be seen. Thus, the appearance of the mucosal surface in the region of the stricture will often indicate whether the ulcerative process that caused the stricture is still active.

CIRCUMFERENTIAL MALIGNANT LESIONS

Circumferential malignant lesions must at times be differentiated from benign stricture. In a circumferential malignancy, the neoplasm has encircled and partially occluded the lumen. Radiologically, the mass itself is usually obvious and there is in addition a well-defined, angular demarcation between the lesion and the adjacent normal areas of the bowel. The lumen through the lesion is ragged due to destruction of the mucosal surface and its replacement by tumor (Fig. 11-11). In the case of the classic circumferential lesion of the esophagus or colon, there is little problem in determining that the abnormality represents a malignancy. However, occasional circumferential carcinomas have a tendency to infiltrate the bowel wall rather than form a discrete mass. These tumors may have tapering margins very similar to those of a benign stricture and are particularly likely to be seen with carcinoma of the esophagogastric junction region, carcinoma of the gastric antrum, and carcinoma of the colon developing in ulcerative colitis. In these cases, it may be difficult to determine by radiologic appearances alone whether the stricture is benign or malignant, and endoscopy with biopsy is warranted.

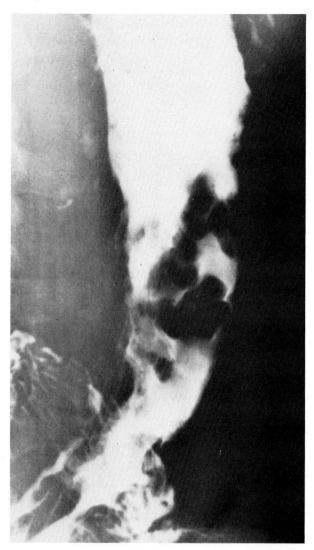

Fig. 11-9 Malignant ulcer of the stomach. Its irregular contour and nodular surround are indicative of malignancy.

ments of bowel (Fig. 11-10). This is in contrast to circumferential malignant lesions, which usually have clearly demarcated, sharply angled margins.

The mucosa in the region of a benign stricture may be intact or ulcerated (Fig. 11-10). If the mucosa is intact, the margin of the barium column will be relatively smooth through the region of the stricture. However, strictures are often accompanied by active ulceration, and either a discrete ulcer or the amorphous, slightly irregular and

INFILTRATION

Any substance introduced diffusely into the wall of a segment of bowel can be said to be infiltrating the wall. Benign materials ranging from blood to amyloid may constitute the infiltrating substance. Also, primary and metastatic malignant neoplasms of the bowel may be capable of infiltrating the bowel wall in a similar manner. In the case of benign infiltration, thickening of folds and "thumbprinting" are the usual radiologic findings

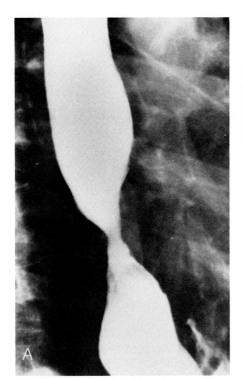

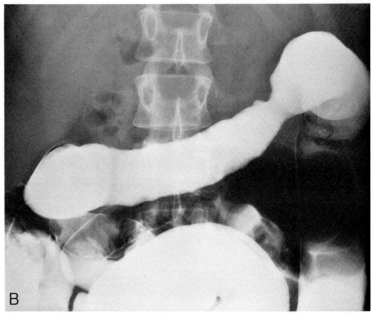

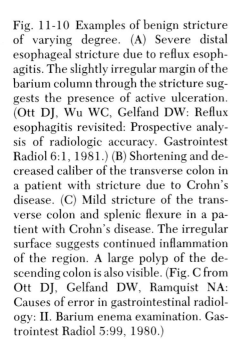

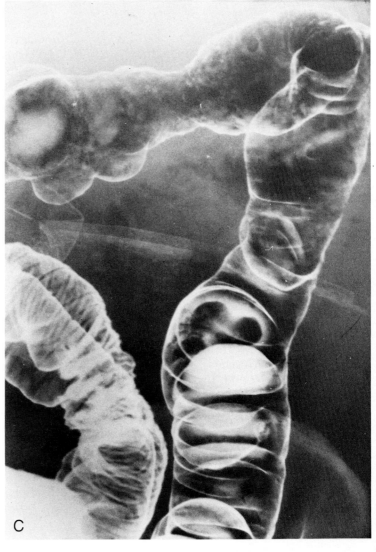

Fig. 11-10 Examples of benign stricture of varying degree. (A) Severe distal esophageal stricture due to reflux esophagitis. The slightly irregular margin of the barium column through the stricture suggests the presence of active ulceration. (Ott DJ, Wu WC, Gelfand DW: Reflux esophagitis revisited: Prospective analysis of radiologic accuracy. Gastrointest Radiol 6:1, 1981.) (B) Shortening and decreased caliber of the transverse colon in a patient with stricture due to Crohn's disease. (C) Mild stricture of the transverse colon and splenic flexure in a patient with Crohn's disease. The irregular surface suggests continued inflammation of the region. A large polyp of the descending colon is also visible. (Fig. C from Ott DJ, Gelfand DW, Ramquist NA: Causes of error in gastrointestinal radiology: II. Barium enema examination. Gastrointest Radiol 5:99, 1980.)

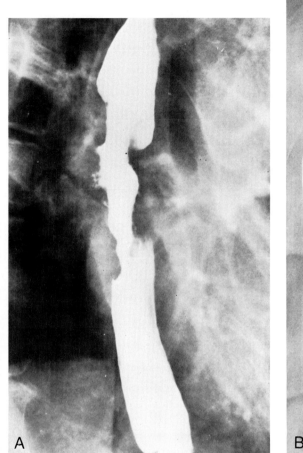 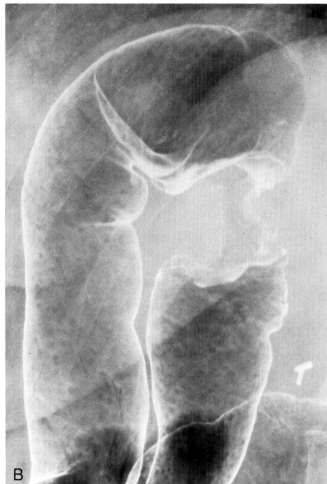

Fig. 11-11 Two examples of circumferential carcinomas in typical locations. (A) Carcinoma of the midesophagus with abrupt margins and a narrowed, irrregular passage through its lumen. (B) Typical "apple core" lesion of the colon at the splenic flexure. Note the overhanging distal margin of the lesion.

(Figs. 11-12A and B). In malignant infiltration, similar findings may be present (Fig. 11-13A), but there may be irregularity, nodularity, and formation of discrete masses as well. Unfortunately, many of the disease entities causing infiltration of the gut bear considerable resemblance to each other, and their radiologic evaluation often involves an extensive differential diagnosis.

Benign diseases capable of infiltrating the bowel wall occur most frequently in the small intestine, where they tend to involve long segments. In most cases, the benign infiltration is relatively uniform throughout the area affected. A typical example of

benign infiltration of the bowel is that of bleeding into the wall of the small intestine occurring in patients receiving anticoagulant medication or in patients with small bowel ischemia. In this circumstance, the valvulae conniventes will be thickened and blunted throughout the involved small bowel segment (Fig. 11-12A).

Malignant infiltration occurs with reasonable frequency in both the stomach and small bowel. Carcinoma of the stomach is particularly apt to infiltrate large areas of the gastric wall in the form of the disease known as linitis plastica, thickening the wall and destroying the normal fold pattern

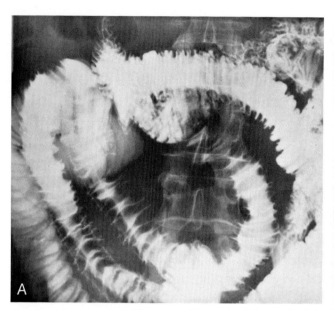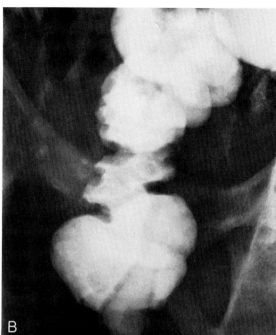

Fig. 11-12 Examples of benign infiltration of the wall of the bowel by blood and edema. **(A)** Small bowel ischemia with marked segmental thickening of the valvulae conniventes. **(B)** Ischemic changes in the distal colon and rectum as manifested by "thumbprinting" visible at the margins of the barium column.

(Fig. 11-13A). In both the stomach and the small bowel, lymphoma may also take the form of an infiltrating lesion. Its typical radiologic appearance is that of thickening of folds (Fig. 11-13B) but often with an irregularity and nodule formation not usually seen in benign diseases. The latter two findings, when they occur, are due to localized growth of the tumor.

MASS LESIONS

The radiographic appearance of a mass lesion is largely determined by its origin: mucosal, intramural, or extrinsic. Within this classification, a lesion must also be subclassified as to whether its appearance suggests a benign entity or a malignancy.

Mucosal Lesions

Mucosal lesions are by definition masses located in or taking origin from the mucosal layer of the bowel wall. Typically, a mucosal mass protrudes into the lumen of the bowel, assuming a spherical, hemispherical, or plaque-like appearance (Figs. 11-14 and 11-15). The edge of such a lesion, when seen in profile, tends to form an acute or right angle with the normal surrounding bowel wall. Lesions most commonly presenting as mucosal lesions include adenomatous polyps, polypoid carcinomas, and occasional benign tumors of mesenchymal origin such as lipomas and leiomyomas.

Because malignancies constitute a substantial fraction of mucosal tumors, one must attempt to determine whether a mucosal lesion is benign or malignant. The criteria for differentiating between benign and malignant lesions of mucosal origin include size, rate of growth, shape, surface characteristics, and the character of the attachment to the bowel wall. Size is important because the rapid growth of malignant lesions tends to ensure that they will be considerably larger than benign lesions when initially discovered. Since benign lesions tend to grow very slowly, appreciable growth on serial examinations is almost always considered a sign of malignancy. Lesions of smooth contour,

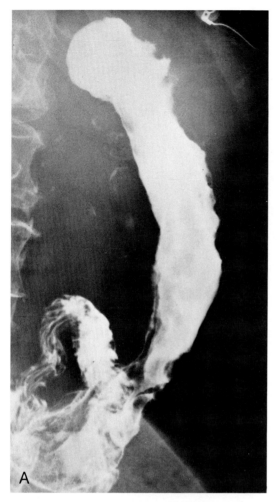

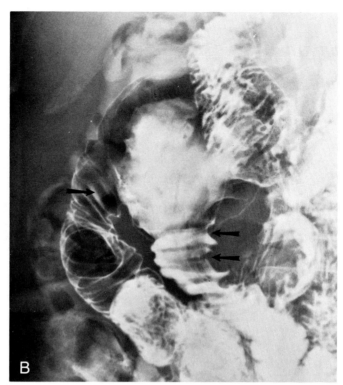

Fig. 11-13 Examples of malignant infiltration of the stomach and small bowel. (A) Linitis plastica involving the proximal half of the stomach. (B) Non-Hodgkin's lymphoma of the small intestine with localized aneurysmal dilatation. The infiltrating lymphoma has greatly thickened the folds in the region (arrows).

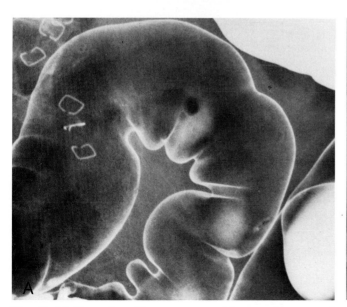

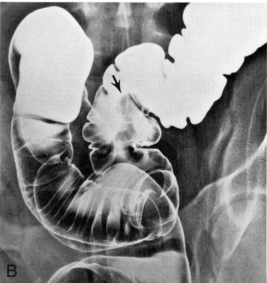

Fig. 11-14 Examples of benign mucosal lesions. They are characterized by smoothness of outline and a rounded shape. (A) Small, round, benign polyp of the colon. (B) Moderate-size polyp (arrow) of the sigmoid colon on a distinct stalk. The exquisitely round head and generous pedicle strongly suggest a benign lesion.

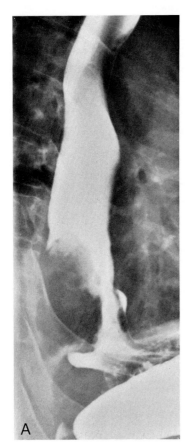

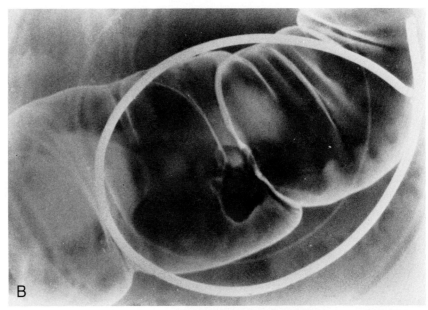

Fig. 11-15 Typical sessile polypoid malignancies exhibiting the expected characteristics. (A) Adenocarcinoma of the distal esophagus forming a broad-based mass of slightly irregular contour. (B) Irregular, plaque-like lesion of the transverse colon that proved to be an adenocarcinoma. (C) Malignant villous adenoma showing the typically lobulated contour of these lesions as seen on double-contrast studies.

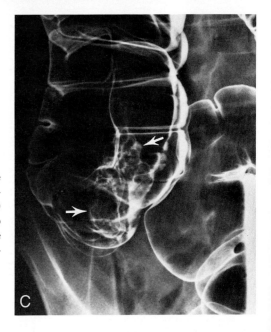

either round or oval (Fig. 11-14), tend to be benign while those of irregular shape (Fig. 11-15) carry a high probability of malignancy. An exquisitely smooth surface indicates that the mucosa over the lesions is intact and is an indicator of a benign lesion (Fig. 11-14), since malignancies usually destroy the overlying mucosa and thus present with an irregular surface (Fig. 11-15). A distinct pedicle or stalk favors benignancy (Fig. 11-14B) while a

sessile lesion is more likely to be malignant (Fig. 11-15).

Intramural Lesions

Intramural lesions tend to be of mesenchymal origin, most commonly leiomyomas. Radiographically, their appearance is characterized by a smooth, rounded, somewhat hemispherical shape (Fig. 11-16). Typically, the angle formed between the surface of the tumor and the surrounding normal mucosa approximates 90° and is well defined.

Most intramural tumors encountered in radiological practice are benign. Occasionally, however, one encounters a malignancy of mesenchymal origin, usually a leiomyosarcoma. Interestingly, although a discrete ulceration may be present, leiomyosarcomas usually do not destroy the overlying mucosal surface and thus tend to present as smooth hemispherical masses similar to the benign lesion. The best means of differentiating this malignancy from its related benign tumor is by size, with a large lesion likely to be a leiomyosarcoma.

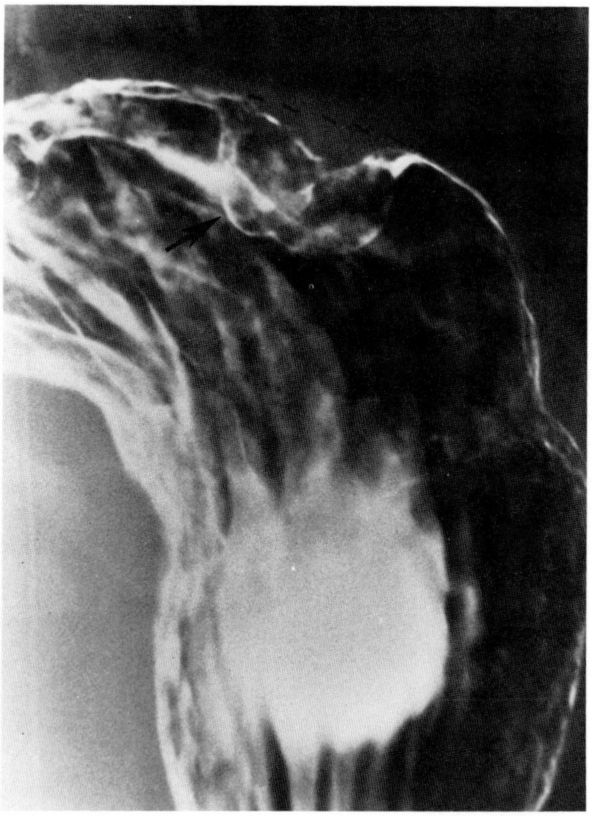

Extrinsic Lesions

Extrinsic lesions are detectable by virtue of the impression they produce on the bowel wall. Usually, extrinsic lesions produce a broad, obviously extrinsic impression with gently curved margins. However, a more complex situation occurs when an extrinsic mass invades or becomes adherent to the wall of the bowel. Under this cir-

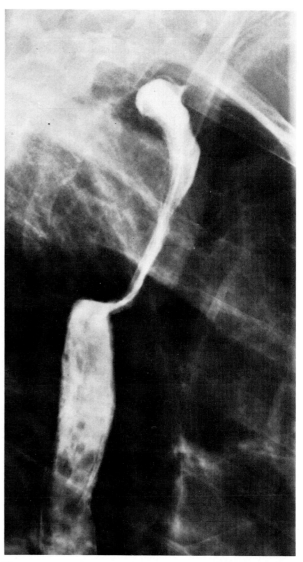

Fig. 11-16 Leiomyoma of the fundus of the stomach presenting as a hemispherical lesion. Note that the margins of the lesion make approximately a 90° angle with the adjacent gastric wall.

Fig. 11-17 Metastatic carcinoma in mediastinal lymph nodes broadly displacing the proximal thoracic esophagus. The sharp angulation at the inferior margin of the lesion suggests that it may be adherent to the esophagus.

cumstance, a more distinct angle develops at the extremity of the lesion, simulating an intramural lesion (Fig. 11-17). Indeed, the lesion in a sense is intramural by virtue of its invasion or adherence. When an extrinsic malignancy very occasionally invades the full thickness of the bowel wall and penetrates the mucosa, it presents as an ulcerated or irregularly polypoid mass resembling a malignancy of mucosal origin.

Metastatic Malignancies

Metastatic malignancies produce the entire gamut of appearances associated with mass lesions or infiltrating neoplasms. If metastatic by direct invasion, they may present as extrinsic, intramural, or mucosal lesions depending on the depth of invasion. Blood-born metastases growing in the bowel wall may present as smooth intramural or irregular mucosal lesions depending on whether the growth of the metastatic nodule has destroyed the overlying mucosa. If the overlying mucosa has remained intact, such metastases appear as smooth, rounded intramural lesions. If the mucosa has been destroyed, the lesions will mimic an irregular polypoid primary carcinoma. The major clue to the metastatic nature of a mass is the patient's clinical history and the possible multiplicity of the lesions. Finally, certain metastatic neoplasms, particularly carcinoma of the breast, may infiltrate the bowel wall in a manner simulating infiltration by a primary neoplasm such as lymphoma or gastric carcinoma.

SUGGESTED READINGS

Edema

Farthing MJG, McLean AM, Bartram CI, et al: Radiologic features of the jejunum in hypoalbuminemia. AJR 136:883, 1981.
Marshak RH, Khilnani M, Eliashoph J, Wolf BS: Intestinal edema. Am J Roentgenol 101:379, 1967.

Inflammation

Andren L, Theander G: Roentgenographic appearances of esophageal moniliasis. Acta Radiol 46:571, 1956.
Goldberg HI, Dodds WJ: Cobblestone esophagus due to monilial infection. Am J Roentgenol 104:608, 1968.
Kressel HT, Glick SN, Laufer I, Banner M: Radiologic features of esophagitis. Gastrointest Radiol 6:103, 1981.
Laws JW, Pitman RG: Radiological features of pernicious anemia. Br J Radiol 3:229, 1960.
Laufer I: Air contrast studies of the colon in inflammatory bowel disease. CRC Crit Rev Diagn Imaging 9:421, 1977.
Op den Orth JO, Dekker W: Gastric erosions: Radiologic and endoscopic aspects. Diagn Imaging 45:88, 1976.
Ott DJ, Wu WC, Gelfand DW: Reflux esophagitis revisited: Prospective analysis of radiologic accuracy. Gastrointest Radiol 6:1, 1981.
Rose C, Stevenson GW: Correlation between visualization and size of the areae gastricae and duodenal ulcer. Radiology 139:371, 1981.
Schulman A, Morton PCG, Dietrich BE: Eosinophilic gastroenteritis. Clin Radiol 31:101, 1980.
Walk E: Erosive gastritis. Digestion 84:87, 1955.

Ulceration

Allan AC, Boley SS, Schultz C, Schwartz S: Potassium induced lesions of the small bowel. II. Pathology and pathogenesis. JAMA 193:1001, 1965.
Carlson HC: Localized non-specific ulceration of the small intestine. Radiol Clin North Am 7:97, 1969.
Carrera GF, Young S, Lewicke AM: Intestinal tuberculosis. Gastrointest Radiol 1:147, 1976.
Freeman AH, Berridge FR, Dick AP, et al: Pseudopolyposis in Crohn's disease. Clin Radiol 51:382, 1978.
Haudek M: Zur rontgenologischen Diagnose der Ulcerationen in der pars media des Magnes. München Med Wschr 57:1587, 1910.
James EM, Carlson HC: Chronic ulcerative colitis and colon cancer. AJR 130:825, 1978.
Marshak RH, Lindner AE: Radiology of the Small Intestine. Philadelphia, WB Saunders, 1976, pp 179–300.
Max RJ, Kelvin FM: Nonspecificity of discrete colonic ulceration on double-contrast barium enema study. AJR 134:1265, 1980.
Nelson SW: The discovery of gastric ulcers and the differential diagnosis between benignancy and malignancy. Radiol Clin North Am 7:5, 1969.
Nolan DJ, Gourtsoyiannis NC: Crohn's disease of the small intestine: A review of the radiological appearances in 100 consecutive patients examined by a barium infusion technique. Clin Radiol 31:597, 1980.
Williams HJ, Stephens DH, Carlson HC: Double-contrast radiography: Colonic inflammatory disease. AJR 137:315, 1981.

Mass Lesions

Bruneton JN, Drouillard J, Roux P, et al: Leiomyoma and leiomyosarcoma of the digestive tract — a report of 45 cases and review of the literature. Eur J Radiol 1:291, 1981.

Davies PM: Smooth muscle tumors of the upper gastrointestinal tract. Clin Radiol 29:407, 1978.

Dodds WJ: Clinical and roentgen features of the intestinal polyposis syndromes. Gastrointest Radiol 1:127, 1976.

Fork FT: Double-contrast enema and colonoscopy in polyp detection. Gut 22:971, 1981.

Gloyna RE, Zoronoza J, Goldstein HM: Primary ulcerative carcinoma of the esophagus. Am J Roentgenol 129:599, 1977.

Lebshitz HI, Lindell MM, Dodd GD: Metastases to the hollow viscera. Radiol Clin North Am 20:487, 1982.

Marshak RH, Wolf BS, Eliasoph J: Roentgen findings in lymphosarcoma of the small intestine. Am J Roentgenol 86:862, 1961.

Op den Orth JO, Dekker W: Gastric adenomas. Radiology 141:289, 1981.

Schatzki R, Hawes LE: The roentgenologic appearance of extramucosal tumors of the esophagus. Am J Roentgenol 48:1, 1942.

Shirakabe H, Frishizawa N, Maruyama M, Kobayashi S: Atlas of X-Ray Diagnosis of Early Gastric Cancer. 2nd Ed. Tokyo, Igaku-Shoin, 1982.

Zornoza J, Dodd GD: Lymphoma of the gastrointestinal tract. Semin Roetgenol 15:272, 1980.

12

Abnormalities of the Hypopharynx

The brevity of this chapter on hypopharyngeal disorders reflects the general paucity of knowledge concerning the radiologic appearances of abnormalities of this region. Since direct visual inspection is possible, few radiologists routinely examine the hypopharynx as part of an esophagogram or upper gastrointestinal series. Increasing attention is being paid, however, to the analysis of swallowing disorders, in which radiologic analysis plays a crucial diagnostic role.

STRUCTURAL ABNORMALITIES

Normal Variants

Two normal anatomic structures are of specific radiologic importance in the hypopharynx. First, in many individuals there is a slight web-like protuberance of the anterior wall of the pharyngoesophageal junction caused by the presence of a submucosal venous plexus (Fig. 12-1). This structure is somewhat flexible, and may be web-like, rounded, or plaque-like. It should not be confused with cervical esophageal web, a pathologic entity capable of causing dysphagia, or with a neoplasm. Second, the posterior hypopharyngeal wall is often indented just above the esophageal inlet, at the C6 vertebral level, by the cricopharyngeus muscle. When of moderate degree, the cricopharyngeus impression is a normal finding. However, hyperactivity of the cricopharyngeus muscle, causing a marked indentation of the barium column (Fig. 12-2), may act as a partial functional obstruction. It may produce symptoms of dysphagia and may be associated with formation of a Zenker's diverticulum.

Hypopharyngeal webs are somewhat infrequent in occurrence, usually being seen in the region of the pharyngoesophageal junction (Fig. 12-3). They generally take origin from the anterior and lateral walls and are usually singular, but multiple webs have been reported. Invariably, their presenting symptom is dysphagia. They should not be confused with the normal, occasionally web-like indentation on the anterior wall of the pharyngoesophageal junction caused by the submucosal venous plexus, since this latter structure is not thought to cause dysphagia.

In the past, hypopharyngeal webs have been considered part of the so-called Plummer-Vinson syndrome, which consists of glossitis, anemia, and pharyngeal or proximal esophageal webs. However, in recent years the existence of webs as part

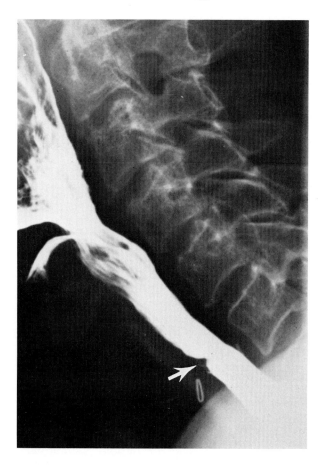

Fig. 12-1 Impression on the anterior aspect of the pharyngoesophageal region due to a normally occurring venous plexus. This should not be confused with a web in the same location.

of this syndrome has been challenged, since it has been demonstrated that the vast majority of pharyngeal or cervical esophageal webs are not associated with anemia or glossitis. It has similarly been conjectured that the Plummer-Vinson syndrome predisposed such patients to an unusual incidence of carcinoma of the pharyngeal region, but this also has been disproven more recently by careful review of data.

Diverticula are abnormal outpouchings from the lumen of the pharynx and are best considered in terms of their location: anterior, lateral, and posterior. For purposes of radiologic diagnosis, it matters little whether the diverticula are congenital or acquired.

The most important anterior diverticulum presenting in the region of the hypopharynx, the laryngocele, is not actually of pharyngeal origin. The opening to a laryngocele is situated within the larynx, and as a result it does not fill with barium.

Instead, it presents as an air-filled, cyst-like structure that may distort the pharynx by compression. By comparison, true pharyngeal diverticula invariably fill with barium at some point during an examination.

Diverticula taking origin from the lateral aspects of the hypopharynx are of two basic types. The first is a broad evanescent or fixed outpouching of the lateral pharyngeal wall noted during deglutition of the barium suspension. In elderly individuals, or in patients who are glass blowers or trumpet players, these outpouchings can become quite large and may become permanent in the case of the latter two examples. The outpouching occurs in the region of the cricothyroid membrane, an area of the lateral wall of the pharynx not invested by the pharyngeal musculature, and therefore an area of potential weakness. Unless the bulging is marked or permanently fixed, this variety of lateral diverticulum is seldom a source of symptoms.

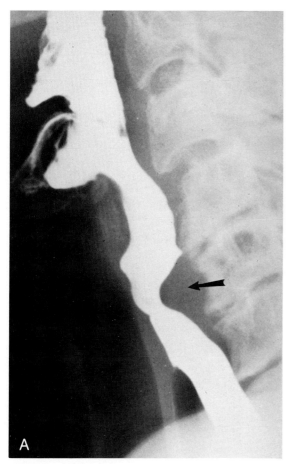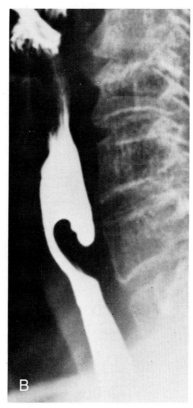

Fig. 12-2 (A) Accentuated indentation on the posterior aspect of the hypopharynx caused by a hyperactive cricopharyngeus muscle (arrow). (B) Hyperactive cricopharyngeus muscle with beginning formation of a Zenker's diverticulum.

A second general class of lateral diverticula is related to the embryonic branchial clefts and may be fixed or may appear only during deglutition. The fixed diverticula take origin from the lateral aspect of the piriform sinuses (Fig. 12-4A), which in themselves are of branchial cleft origin, and represent branchial cleft cysts or sinuses that communicate with the pharyngeal lumen. An evanescent variety of lateral diverticulum also originates in the region of the piriform sinuses and is generally seen only during deglutition. These are the most common of lateral pharyngeal diverticula and take the form of paired or multiple small outpouchings that bulge outward during deglutition in response to increased pressure within the lumen. They appear to be elastic structures pushing into the areas of weakness in the lateral pharyngeal wall corresponding to the original location of the internal orifices of the third and fourth branchial clefts (Figs. 12-3A and 12-4B).

Virtually all posterior hypopharyngeal diverticula are termed *Zenker's diverticula.* They are the most common form of hypopharyngeal diverticulum, and project through the gap in the posterior pharyngeal musculature known as the triangle of Lannier or Killian's dehiscence. The opening of a Zenker's diverticulum is invariably located at the superior aspect of the protuberance of the posterior pharyngeal wall caused by the cricopharyngeus muscle.

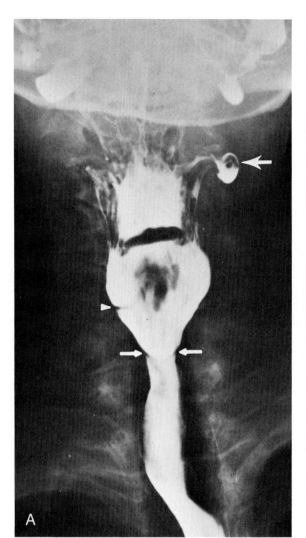 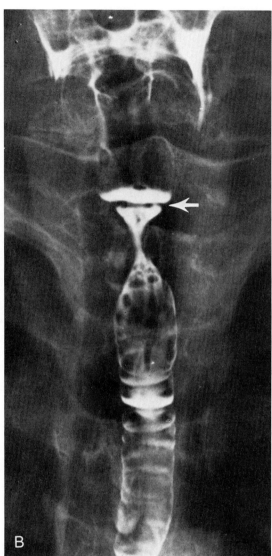

Fig. 12-3 (A) Hypopharyngeal webs. A circumferential web of the pharyngoesophageal junction (arrows) is faintly visible as laterally situated notches. A unilateral partial web is situated more proximally on the right side (arrowhead). A lateral pharyngeal diverticulum is visible on the left (upper arrow). (B) Marked web (arrow) at the pharyngoesophageal junction in a patient who also has multiple webs of the esophagus. (Fig. B reprinted by permission of the publisher from Shiflet DW, et al: Multiple esophageal webs. Gastroenterology 77:556, 1979. Copyright 1979 by The American Gastroenterological Association.)

Zenker's diverticula range in size from a small pinpoint outpouching to a gigantic food-filled sac occupying a considerable portion of the cervical region (Figs. 12-2B and 12-5). In its earliest and smallest stages, Zenker's diverticulum is seen as a small pointed outpouching no more than a millimeter or two in size anterior to the C5-C6 interspace. As it expands beyond the muscular wall it

begins to widen into a sac-like projection. At this stage, however, it is still directed posteriorly. While still small, a Zenker's diverticulum may not be a fixed structure and may appear only during deglutition, disappearing seconds later. As it enlarges, however, a Zenker's diverticulum becomes a fixed structure, and further posterior progress is interrupted by the cervical vertebrae. The diver-

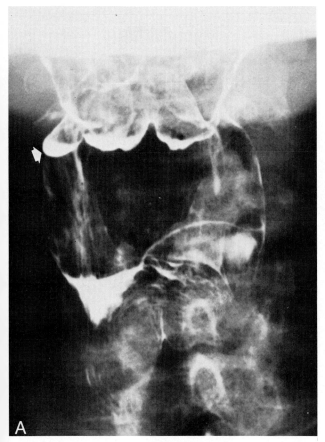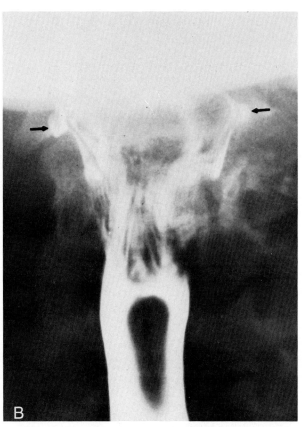

Fig. 12-4 (A) Lateral pharyngeal diverticulum (arrow) in a patient who also has asymmetry of the pharyngeal structures in the region of the piriform sinuses due to asymmetrical pharyngeal dysfunction caused by cerebral ischemia. (B) Evanescent pharyngeal diverticula visible only during deglutition (arrows) in their most typical location.

ticulum may now become laterally or anteriorly directed as it continues to grow in size. Thus, very large Zenker's diverticula are often seen projecting anterolaterally from their origin on the posterior hypopharyngeal wall. Only occasionally does one encounter the classically shown huge pouch lying directly behind the posterior hypopharyngeal wall.

INFLAMMATORY DISEASES

Inflammatory diseases of the mucous surfaces of the hypopharynx are seen by the radiologist only in isolated instances. Most of these diseases are amenable to diagnosis by direct visual inspection,

since much of the wall of the hypopharynx is visible through the oral cavity. The radiologic appearance of esophageal candidiasis is well described. Although not specifically described in the hypopharynx, it can be assumed that the same patchy, irregular, widely distributed plaques and small ulcerations would be visible on double-contrast films of the pharynx. Rarely, other mycoses capable of infesting the gastrointestinal tract will also be found in the hypopharynx.

An extremely rare hereditary disease, the dystrophic form of *epidermolysis bullosa*, may cause extensive lesions in the pharynx, which then cause scarring, webs, and obstruction. *Benign pemphigoid* of the mucous membranes may cause similar constrictions of the hypopharynx and pharyngo-

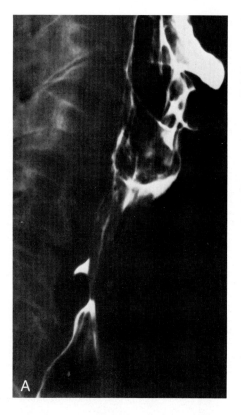

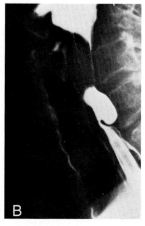

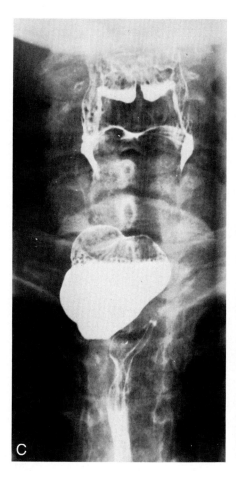

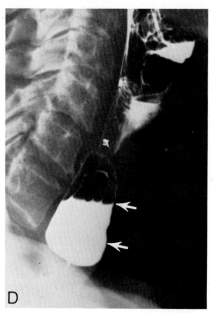

Fig. 12-5 (A) Very early Zenker's diverticulum lying immediately ante-rior to the C5-C6 interspace. These diverticula form due to weakness of the posterior pharyngeal wall, which at this point (Killian's triangle) is not invested by musculature. (B) Zenker's diverticulum somewhat larger than that in Fig. A, now beginning to assume its typical sac-like configuration. (C & D) Large Zenker's diverticulum retaining barium after swallowing. Because of its size, the diverticulum is extending to the right and partially anterior to the cervical esophagus (arrows).

esophageal region. Other rare diseases specifically capable of causing inflammatory lesions of the pharyngeal mucosa include *Behcet's disease* and *lichen planus.*

Acute epiglottitis is a disorder that may rarely cause edema and inflammation of hypopharyngeal strictures in adults (it is common in children). The swelling of the epiglottis and arytenoid cartilages are best appreciated on lateral soft-tissue plain films of the neck.

NEOPLASMS

The majority of neoplasms presenting in the pharynx are primary squamous cell carcinomas taking origin in the pharyngeal mucosa (Fig. 12-6).

Benign tumors and sarcomas are rare. Carcinoma of the larynx spreading directly into the surrounding areas of the pharynx is a second, important source of malignant tumors presenting in the pharynx (Fig. 12-7).

Primary carcinoma of the pharynx may be found in almost any location within the pharynx. The tumor may take any of the common forms in which a malignancy presents, except that circumferential tumors are almost unknown. Thus, a primary pharyngeal carcinoma may be seen as a small polyp or plaque, a larger polypoid lesion, a subtle infiltration of the wall, or some combination of the above.

Fortunately for the early detection of carcinoma, malignancies originating in the pharynx and larynx cause symptoms at an early stage. As a result, however, the radiographic evidence of malig-

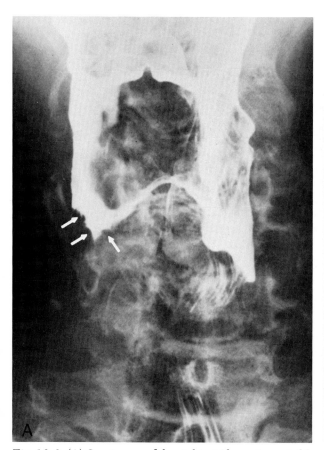 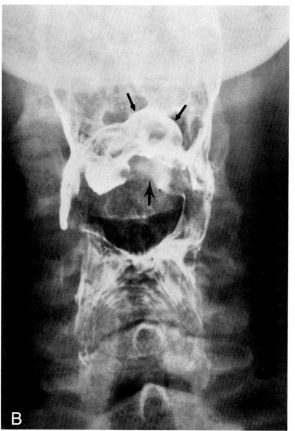

Fig. 12-6 (A) Carcinoma of the right piriform sinus visible as an interruption of the normal configuration of the sinus with resulting asymmetry (arrows). (B) Carcinoma of the epiglottis and base of tongue swelling the shadow of the epiglottis (upper arrows) and filling in the left vallecula (lower arrow). Complete obliteration of a vallecula is almost always a sign of a mass in the tongue or epiglottis.

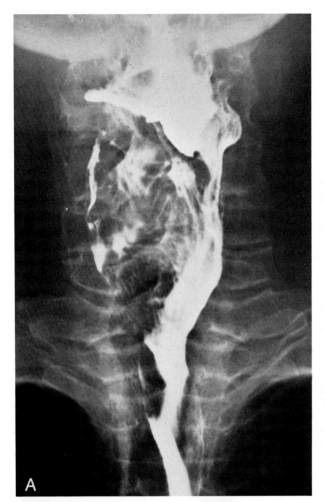

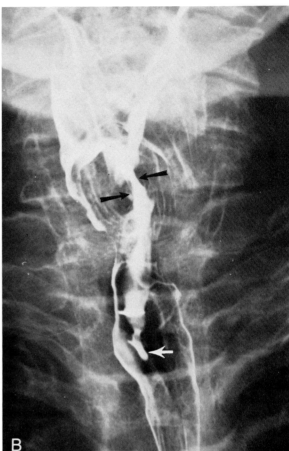

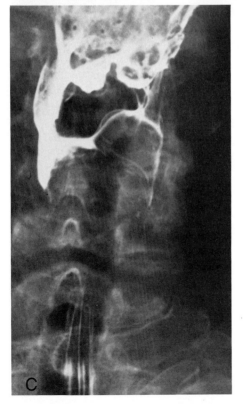

Fig. 12-7 (A) Carcinoma of the larynx metastatic to the cervical soft tissues and obliterating the right-sided pharyngeal structures. (B) Carcinoma of the larynx outlined by barium suspension traversing the laryngeal tumor (upper arrows). Enlargement of laryngeal structures severely distorts the pharynx. Aspirated barium can be seen running into the trachea (lower arrow). (C) Carcinoma of the larynx enlarging the left arytenoid cartilage. The resulting mass fills the left piriform sinus.

nancy may occasionally be quite subtle. The earliest radiographic signs of pharyngeal malignancy may be only an unexpected asymmetry of normally symmetrical bilateral structures, particularly the piriform sinuses and valleculae, or lack of distensibility of a portion of the pharynx when the patient exhales against pursed lips. It should be noted, however, that large anterior cervical osteophytes may indent the posterior pharyngeal wall asymmetrically, to a certain extent simulating the pharyngeal distortions caused by neoplasms.

FUNCTIONAL DISORDERS

Pharyngeal dysfunctions leading to dysphagia or aspiration are common complaints requiring radiologic investigation. Proper pharyngeal function depends on the movement of several structures in a delicately coordinated manner. Disruption of any of these muscular efforts may result in dysphagia, aspiration of swallowed material into the trachea, or regurgitation of material into the nose.

Normal pharyngeal function may be described as a series of sequential and partially simultaneous movements of structures in the region of the pharynx that may be summarized as follows:

1. Initially, the tongue moves upward and posteriorly, squeezing the bolus backward along the palate until it rests in the hypopharynx.
2. The soft palate simultaneously moves posteriorly toward the posterior pharyngeal wall, sealing the opening from the oral cavity into the nose and preventing nasal regurgitation of the swallowed material (Fig. 12-8A).

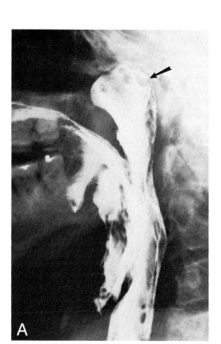 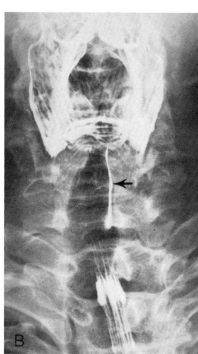 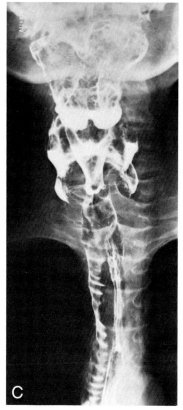

Fig. 12-8 (A) Nasal regurgitation of barium suspension (arrow) in a patient with amyotrophic lateral sclerosis. (B) Slight aspiration of barium (arrow) in a patient with Parkinson's disease. (C) Massive aspiration of barium suspension into the trachea in a patient with bulbar palsy due to cerebral ischemia. (Fig. C from Gelfand DW: Complications of gastrointestinal radiologic procedures. I. Complications of routine fluoroscopic studies. Gastrointest Radiol 5:293, 1980.)

3. As the bolus passes into the hypopharynx, it pushes the epiglottis posteriorly over the entrance of the larynx, preventing food from entering the larynx or trachea (Figs. 12-8B and C). This is aided by the even more vital closure of the supraglottic musculature of the larynx.

4. A combination of posterior movement of the distal third of the tongue and anterior movement of the pharyngeal constrictors pushes the bolus further into the hypopharynx.

5. A reflex relaxation of the cricopharyngeus muscle allows final passage of the bolus into the cervical esophagus, where esophageal peristalsis is initiated and propels the swallowed material distally.

Several disease entities, centered primarily elsewhere in the body, are capable of causing pharyngeal dysfunction on the basis of either neurologic deficit or generalized muscle disease. Table 12-1 lists neurologic and muscle disorders known to cause pharyngeal dysfunction and amenable to radiologic diagnosis or confirmation. The following are specific characteristics of the most common of these entities.

Cerebral Ischemia

Cerebral ischemia is a common cause of pharyngeal dysfunction in the elderly. The most severe deficit is usually noted in the function of the tongue. These patients often have difficulty in forming a bolus between the tongue and the palate

Table 12-1. Neuromuscular Disorders Affecting the Pharynx

Common
  Cerebral ischemia
  Parkinson's disease
  Cricopharyngeal achalasia
Uncommon
  Cranial tumors
  Myasthenia gravis
  Multiple sclerosis
  Poliomyelitis
  Pseudobulbar palsy
  Familial dysautonomia
  Amyotrophic lateral sclerosis
  Neuritis
  Dermatomyositis
  Myotonic dystrophy

and similar difficulty in passing the bolus posteriorly into the hypopharynx. Often, the neurologic deficit results in unilateral hypopharyngeal dysfunction, which results in asymmetry of pharyngeal structures on radiographs (Fig. 12-4A). Clinically, many of these patients will have obvious neurologic deficits characteristic of their cerebral disease.

Parkinson's Disease

Parkinson's disease is an almost equally frequent cause of swallowing difficulty in the elderly. Parkinson's disease is characterized by hesitancy and quivering in the initiation of voluntary movements. When the pharynx is fluoroscoped in the lateral position, this can be seen as quivering and inability to initiate movement of the tongue. These patients inevitably have other, more obvious signs of Parkinson's disease, and the function of the radiologist is to confirm that the swallowing dysfunction is due to the patient's neurologic disorder and not due to an undiagnosed neoplasm or stricture.

Myasthenia Gravis

Myasthenia gravis is most properly described as a disease of the neuromuscular junction. Its overall effect is a generalized weakness of striated muscle. In the radiologic evaluation of the pharynx in these patients, virtually all of the muscular functions involved in correctly passing a bolus into the esophagus are affected. The examination reveals difficulty in forming a bolus and passing it posteriorly, the difficulty increasing with repeated efforts. If the bolus is passed into the pharynx, aspiration into the nose or trachea may be seen due to failure of the muscular structures guarding these portals to function properly.

Dysfunction of the Cricopharyngeus Muscle

Dysfunction of the cricopharyngeus muscle is a not uncommon cause of dysphagia of a peculiar sort, namely the feeling that food is sticking in the throat. This is what occurs in many cases, since the usual dysfunction of the cricopharyngeus muscle is a failure to relax, causing temporary retention of the bolus in the hypopharynx. The characteristic radiologic finding is an exaggerated and persistent impression on the posterior wall of the pharynx caused by a prominent cricopharyngeus muscle (Fig. 12-2) that fails to relax and allow passage of the bolus. This dysfunction has been termed *cricopharyngeal achalasia*. It has been shown that dysfunction of the vagus nerve can cause cricopharyngeal achalasia, and the disorder has in fact been noted in patients who have had a transection of the vagus nerve.

Anterior Cervical Osteophytes

Anterior cervical osteophytes are a structural, nonfunctional cause of cervical dysphagia seen with moderate frequency in the elderly. These patients can sense the abnormal bony mass that displaces the posterior hypopharyngeal wall anteriorly. The large bony spurs usually occur at the C5-C6 level and cause a fixed indentation of the barium column, as opposed to the transient indentation associated with cricopharyngeus muscle activity.

SUGGESTED READINGS

Structural Abnormalities: Hypopharyngeal Webs

Clements JL, Cox GW, Torres WE, Weens HS: Cervical esophageal webs—a roentgen-anatomic correlation. Am J Roentgenol 121:221, 1974.

Friedland GW, Filly R: The postcricoid impression masquerading as an esophageal tumor. Am J Dig Dis 20:287, 1975.

Miller JDR, Lewis RB: Esophageal webs in men. Radiology 81:498, 1963.

Pitman RG, Fraser GM: Postcricoid compression on the esophagus. Clin Radiol 16:34, 1965.

Seamen WB: The significance of webs in the hypopharynx and upper esophagus. Radiology 89:32, 1967.

Waldenstrom J, Kjellberg SR: Roentgenologic diagnosis of sideropenic dysphagia (Plummer-Vinson's syndrome). Acta Radiol 20:618, 1939.

Structural Abnormalities: Diverticula

Ardran GM, Kemp FH, Lund WS: The aetiology of the posterior pharyngeal diverticulum: A cineradiographic study. J Laryng 78:333, 1964.

Bachman AL, Seamen WB, Macken KL: Lateral pharyngeal diverticula. Radiology 91:774, 1968.

Gray ED: Radiological demonstration of potential pharyngeal diverticulum. Br J Radiol 5:640, 1932.

Kattan KR, Muhammad AZ: Laryngocele. Radiological diagnosis. JAMA 244:1617, 1980.

Kaufman SA: Lateral pharyngeal diverticula. Am J Roentgenol 75:238, 1956.

Lindell MM, Jing BS, Fischer EP, et al: Laryngocele. AJR 131:259, 1978.

McMyn JK: Lateral pharyngeal diverticula. J Fac Radiologists 8:421, 1957.

Norris CW: Pharyngoceles of the hypopharynx. Laryngoscope 89:1788, 1979.

Perrott JW: Anatomical aspects of hypopharyngeal diverticula. Aust New Zeal J Surg 31:307, 1962.

Raven RW: Pouches of the pharynx and oesophagus with special reference to the embryological and morphological aspects. Br J Surg 21:235, 1931.

Ward PH, Fredrickson JM, Strandjord NM, Valvassori GE: Laryngeal and pharyngeal pouches: Surgical approach and the use of cinefluorography and other radiologic techniques as diagnostic aids. Laryngoscope 73:564, 1963.

Inflammatory Diseases

Alpert M: Roentgen manifestations of epidermolysis bullosa. Am J Roentgenol 78:66, 1957.

Kabakian HA, Dahmash NS: Pharyngoesophageal manifestations of epidermolysis bullosa. Clin Radiol 29:91, 1978.

Karasick S, Mapp E, Karasick D: Esophageal involvement in benign mucous membrane pemphigoid. J Can Assoc Radiol 32:247, 1981.

Schabel SI, Katzberg RW, Burgener FA: Acute inflammation of epiglottitis and supraglottic structures in adults. Radiology 122:601, 1977.

Smith JMB: Mycosis of the alimentary tract. Gut 10:1035, 1969.

Neoplasms

Fabrikant JI, Dickson RJ: The use of cinefluorography for the radiological examination of the larynx and hypopharynx in cases of suspected carcinoma. Br J Radiol 38:28, 1965.

Howell TR, Gildersleeve GA, King ER: The role of roentgenographic studies in the evaluation and staging of malignancies of the larynx and pharynx. Am J Roentgenol 102:138, 1968.

Schnier BR: Pseudotumors of the hypopharynx and larynx due to anterior cervical osteophytes. Am J Roentgenol 115:544, 1972.

Seamen WB: Contrast radiography in neoplastic disease of the larynx and pharynx. Semin Roentgenol 9:301, 1974.

Functional Disorders

Bosma JF, Brodie DR: Disabilities of the pharynx in amyotrophic lateral sclerosis as demonstrated by cineradiography. Radiology 92:97, 1969.

Donner MW, Selbiger ML: Cinefluorographic analysis of pharyngeal swallowing in neuromuscular disorders. Progress in medical science. Am J Med Sci 251:600, 1966.

Donner MW, Siegel CI: The evaluation of pharyngeal neuromuscular disorders by cinefluorography. Am J Roentgenol 94:299, 1965.

Ekberg O, Nylander G: Cineradiography of the pharyngeal stage of deglutition in 150 individuals without dysphagia. Br J Radiol 55:253, 1982.

Ekberg O, Nylander G: Cineradiography of the pharyngeal stage of deglutition in 250 patients with dysphagia. Br J Radiol 55:258, 1982.

Ekberg O, Nylander G: Pharyngeal constrictor paresis patients with dysphagia: A cineradiographic study. Clin Radiol 33:253, 1982.

Ekberg O, Sigurjonsson SV: Movement of the epiglottis during deglutition. Gastrointest Radiol 7:101, 1982.

Facer JC: Osteophytes of the cervical spine causing dysphagia. AMA Arch Otolaryng 86:341, 1967.

Grunebaum M, Salinger H: Radiologic findings in polymyositis-dermatomyositis involving the pharynx and upper oesophagus. Clin Radiol 22:97, 1971.

Hilding DA, Tachdjian MO: Dysphagia and hypertrophic spurring of the cervical spine. N Engl J Med 263:11, 1960.

Murray JP: Neuromuscular and functional disorders of the pharynx. J Fac Radiologists 9:135, 1958.

Redmond P, Berliner L, Ambas M, Horowitz L: Radiological assessment of pharyngoesophageal dysfunction with emphasis on cricopharyngeal myotomy. Am J Gastroenterol 77:85, 1982.

Seamen WB: Cineroentgenographic observations of the cricopharyngeus. Am J Roentgenol 96:922, 1966.

Seamen WB: Functional disorders of the pharyngoesophageal junction. Achalasia and chalasia. Radiol Clin North Am 7:113, 1969.

Selbiger ML, Pikielney R, Donner MW: Neuromuscular disorders affecting the pharynx. Invest Radiol 2:442, 1967.

Skolnick ML, Glaser ER, McWilliams BJ: The use and limitations of the barium pharyngogram in the detection of velopharyngeal insufficiency. Radiology 135:301, 1980.

Zaino C, Jacobson HG, Lepow H, Ozturk C: Pharyngoesophageal sphincter. Radiology 89:639, 1967.

13

Abnormalities of the Esophagus and Esophagogastric Junction

STRUCTURAL ABNORMALITIES

A variety of diseases present in the esophagus that are neither inflammatory, neoplastic, nor functional in nature, and yet may be the source of disturbing or even life-threatening symptoms and events.

THE HIATUS HERNIA COMPLEX

The radiologic diagnosis of hiatus hernia is of importance in that hiatus hernia appears to play a considerable permissive role in the generation of reflux esophagitis, a common and often distressing clinical problem. The normal anatomy of the esophagogastric junction region is discussed in detail in Chapter 10 and should be reviewed in relation to the radiologic signs of hiatal hernia. Structures important for the radiologic diagnosis of hiatus hernia include the A ring, the esophageal vestibule, the B ring or transverse mucosal fold, the submerged segment, the sling fibers of the stomach, and the areae gastricae. The examination for hiatus hernia should be performed with full

column technique and in the prone or prone oblique position to raise intraabdominal pressure and encourage migration upwards of the herniating portion of the stomach.

Hiatus Hernia

Hiatus hernia may be diagnosed radiologically when one or more of the following alterations of the normal anatomy is seen (Figs. 13-1A–F).

1. The B ring or transverse mucosal fold visible above the esophageal hiatus indicates hiatus hernia, since below these structures lies gastric mucosa (Figs. 13-1A and 13-2).
2. A Schatzki ring (lower esophageal web) seen above the esophageal hiatus is a sign of hiatus hernia, since a Schatzki ring usually lies at or very near the junction of esophageal and gastric mucosa (Figs. 13-1B and 13-3).
3. A notch on the lateral side of the lumen seen above the hiatus, caused by the muscular sling fibers of the stomach, indicates that muscular ele-

(Text continues on page 160.)

155

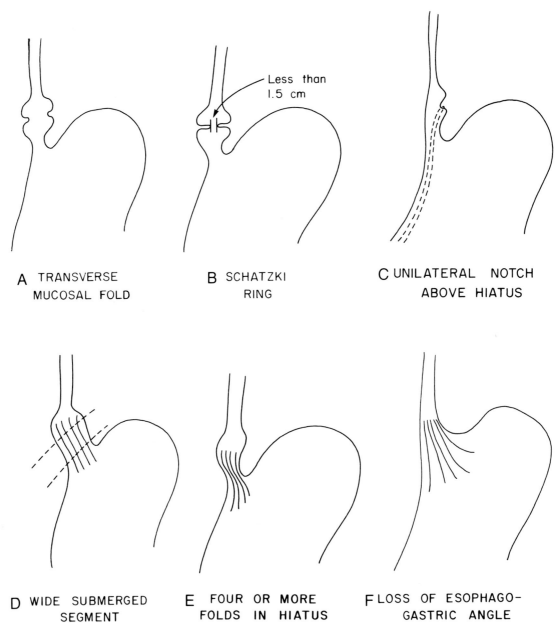

A   TRANSVERSE
MUCOSAL FOLD

B   SCHATZKI
RING

C   UNILATERAL   NOTCH
ABOVE HIATUS

D   WIDE   SUBMERGED
SEGMENT

E   FOUR OR MORE
FOLDS   IN   HIATUS

F   LOSS OF ESOPHAGO-
GASTRIC ANGLE

Fig. 13-1 (A) Transverse mucosal fold causing indentations at the esophagogastric junction above the diaphragm. (B) Schatzki ring, a diaphragm-like structure with a central opening of less than 1.5 cm. A Schatzki ring is in many regards similar to the transverse mucosal fold, but with a more restricted opening. (C) Unilateral notch on the lateral aspect of the esophagogastric junction, caused by the gastric sling fibers, when seen above the hiatus is an indication of hiatal hernia. (D) A widened submerged segment, that portion of the esophagogastric junction traversing the esophageal hiatus, is a sign of hiatus hernia when the width of the submerged segment equals or exceeds its length. (E) Four or more thick folds in the hiatal region is a reasonable presumptive sign of hiatus hernia that should be corroborated. (F) Loss of the esophagogastric angle, the normally acute angle made at the junction of the distal esophagus and fundus of the stomach, is a reasonable sign of hiatus hernia. It is often seen in conjunction with widening of the submerged segment.

Fig. 13-2 (A) Indentations at the esophagogastric junction caused by the proximal wide muscular ring and the narrower transverse mucosal fold distally. Herniated stomach lies between the transverse mucosal fold and the diaphragm. (B) Well-defined transverse mucosal fold demarcating the esophagogastric junction in a patient with hiatus hernia. Note the smooth esophageal mucosa above the transverse mucosal fold and the more granular-appearing gastric mucosa below. (C) Varying appearances of the esophagogastric junction region during differing phases of peristalsis. A transverse mucosal fold is seen on both frames, as notches on the left and as a true fold-like structure on the right. The submerged segment is widened, and there has been loss of the normal esophagogastric angle.

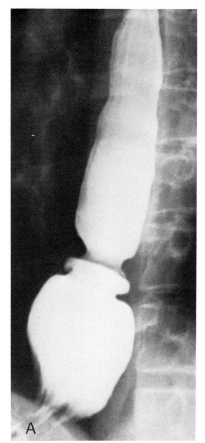
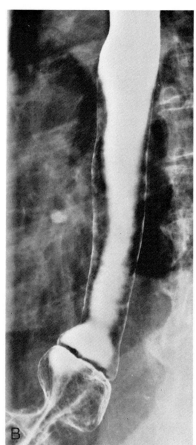
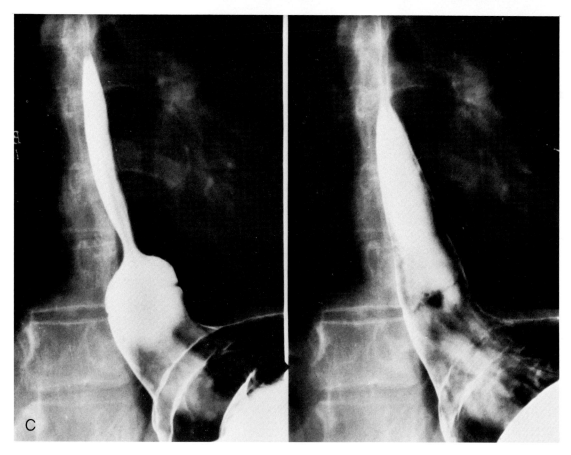

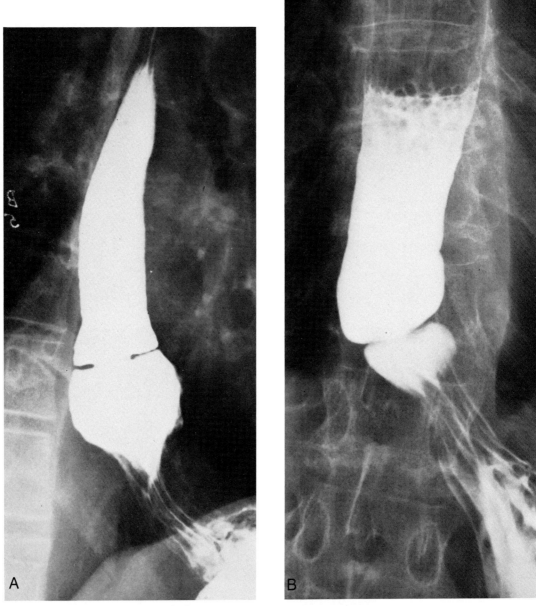

Fig. 13-3 (A & B) Two cases of Schatzki's ring, showing the restricted opening through the web-like structure. In Fig. B, the opening is sufficiently small as to cause restriction of flow of barium, and dilatation of the esophagus above.

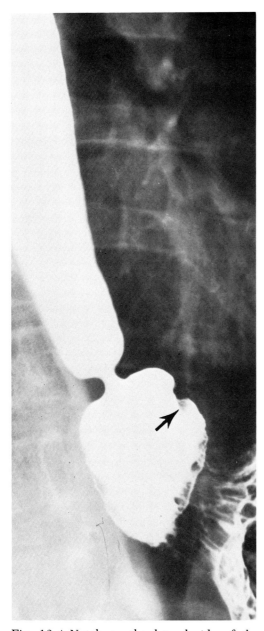

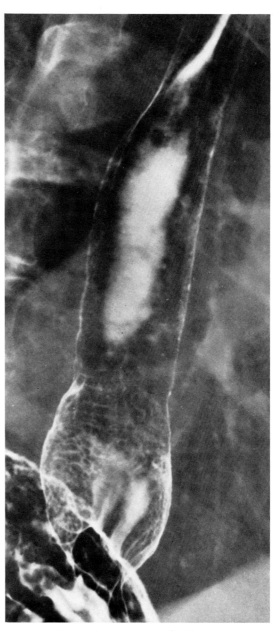

Fig. 13-4 Notch on the lateral side of the esophagogastric junction caused by the gastric sling fibers. The notch marks the esophagogastric junction. The esophageal vestibule lies between the notch and the muscular ring seen above it. (Gelfand DW, Ott DJ: Anatomy and techniques in evaluating the esophagus. Semin Roentgenol 16:168, 1981.)

Fig. 13-5 Hiatus hernia as signified by areae gastricae visible above the diaphragm. The transition from esophageal to gastric mucosa is clearly seen. (Gelfand DW, Ott DJ: Anatomy and techniques in evaluating the esophagus. Semin Roentgenol 16:168, 1981.)

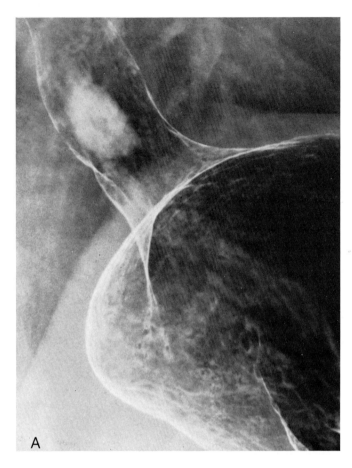

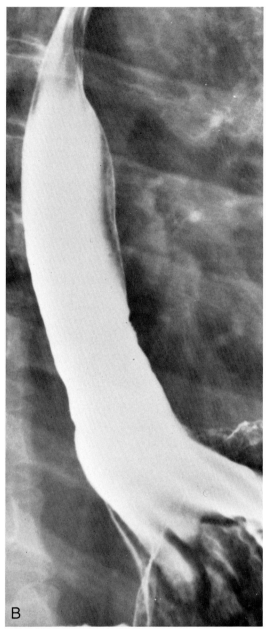

Fig. 13-6 (A & B) Widened submerged segments and loss of the esophagogastric angle as signs of hiatus hernia. Fig. B clearly shows five gastric folds traversing the hiatus (Fig. B from Ott DJ, Gelfand DW, Wu WC: Sensitivity of single contrast radiology in esophageal disease. Gastrointest Radiol 8:105, 1983.)

ments of the stomach lie above the hiatus (Figs. 13-1C and 13-4).

4. Areae gastricae visible above the esophageal hiatus indicate that the mucosal junction lies above the hiatus (Fig. 13-5).

5. A submerged segment wider than it is long suggests that the high pressure zone of the esopha-gus is above its normal location (Figs. 13-1D, 13-2C, and 13-6).

6. Four or more folds traversing the hiatus suggest that gastric mucosa is traversing the hiatus (Figs. 13-1E, 13-3, 13-4, and 13-6B).

7. Loss of the normal acute angle between the esophagus and the fundus of the stomach is a strong

presumptive sign of hiatus hernia and is usually seen in conjunction with widening of the submerged segment (Figs. 13-1F and 13-6).

8. Spontaneous gastroesophageal reflux of significant proportions filling the esophagus to the carina suggests hiatal hernia, which should be confirmed by other more definitive signs.

Signs 1 through 4 are virtually absolute for the diagnosis of hiatal hernia. The remaining signs should be considered presumptive and need corroboration by other radiologic findings or by endoscopy.

Paraesophageal Hiatus Hernia

Paraesophageal hiatus hernia by definition occurs when the esophagogastric junction remains in the abdomen while the fundus of the stomach slides up through the hiatus adjacent to the esophagus. Hiatal hernia in this form is a very uncommon entity. More frequently encountered is the large hiatus hernia with a partial paraesophageal component (Fig. 13-7).

Esophageal Varices

A varix may be defined as a dilated and tortuous vessel, usually a vein. Esophageal varices occur in two distinct varieties — varices of the lower esophagus and downhill varices — each with its set of likely causes.

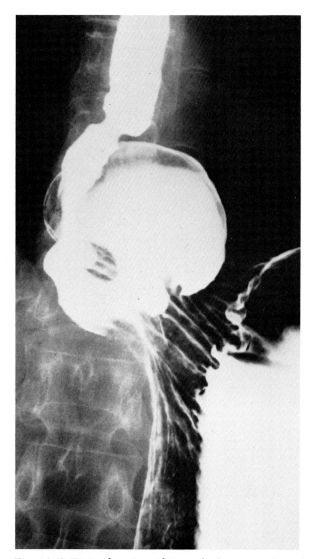

Fig. 13-7 Hiatus hernia with a marked paraesophageal component.

Varices of the Lower Esophagus

Varices of the lower esophagus are the type most commonly encountered and are usually the result of alcoholic cirrhosis of the liver. Other major causes include biliary cirrhosis and thrombosis of the portal or hepatic veins. The varices, or dilated esophageal veins, form one of the potential anastamotic pathways between a partially obstructed portal vein and the systemic venous system.

Radiologically, lower esophageal varices appear as irregular, widened, serpiginous folds coursing through the distal half of the esophagus (Fig. 13-8). The folds vary in caliber from point to point

and may have a somewhat beaded appearance. Irregularity and change in the caliber of the folds are better criteria for making the diagnosis than the width of the folds, since esophageal varices may vary considerably in size. When particularly large, esophageal varices may simulate carcinoma.

Downhill Varices

Downhill varices are a less common form of varices occurring in the midesophagus when the supe-

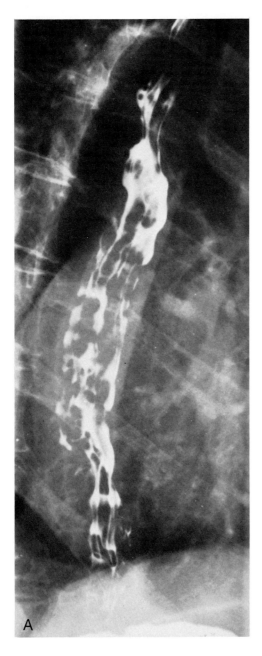

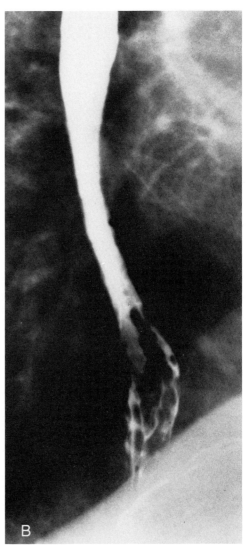

Fig. 13-8 (**A & B**) Esophageal varices visible as enlarged, serpiginous, beaded esophageal folds. (Fig. A from Gelfand DW, Ott DJ: Anatomy and techniques in evaluating the esophagus. Semin Roentgenol 16:168, 1981.)

rior vena cava is occluded. The superior vena caval obstruction is usually due to one of two causes: invasive tumor of the superior mediastinum, usually carcinoma of the lung, or mediastinal fibrosis resulting from chronic mediastinitis, usually tuberculosis or histoplasmosis.

The differential diagnosis of varices includes several entities. Reflux esophagitis may irregularly thicken the folds of the esophagus causing a varicoid appearance. A carcinoma infiltrating submucosally may similarly cause an irregular thickening of esophageal folds. Finally, the presence of gastric mucosa in an undistended hiatus hernia may dupli-

cate the appearance of varices of the distal esophagus.

The reliability of the radiologic diagnosis of varices in the distal esophagus is very dependent upon proper examination technique. Mucosal relief films, best obtained in the left or right posterior oblique (LPO or RPO) views, are most likely to demonstrate lower esophageal varices. To encourage relaxation of the esophagus and filling of the varices, 30 mg of Pro-Banthine (propantheline chloride) should be administered intramuscularly prior to the examination. The taking of many films, combined with Valsalva and Mueller maneuvers, may be required for their demonstration.

WEBS

Upper Esophageal Webs

Upper esophageal webs usually occur just proximal to the thoracic inlet. These are true web-like structures encircling and constricting the esophageal lumen (Fig. 13-9). They are capable of obstructing the esophagus to the passage of solid foods when the diameter through the web is sufficiently small, usually less than approximately 1.0 cm. Note, however, that a web-like indentation is normally seen on the anterior wall of the cervical esophagus in many normal individuals. It is related to a venous plexus present at that location and does not cause dysphagia.

Lower Esophageal Webs

The lower esophageal web, or "Schatzki ring," is by definition associated with hiatus hernia. As described by Schatzki, the ring occurs at the junction of the squamous esophageal and columnar gastric epithelium. Thus, it marks the esophagogastric junction. The Schatzki ring is visible only when the presence of hiatus hernia displaces the esophagogastric junction above the hiatus and only when the distal esophagus is dilated to a diameter greater than the internal diameter of the web (Fig. 13-1B and 13-3). Patients may experience dysphagia when the internal diameter of the ring is less than 1.5 cm as measured radiologically, and vir-

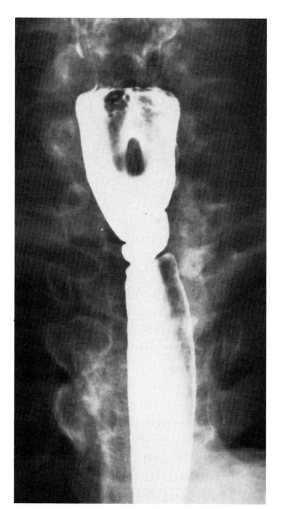

Fig. 13-9 Webs at the pharyngoesophageal junction. The illustrated degree of constriction is sufficient to cause dysphagia.

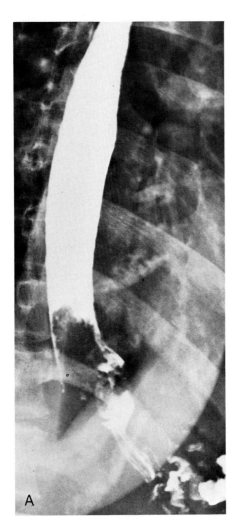

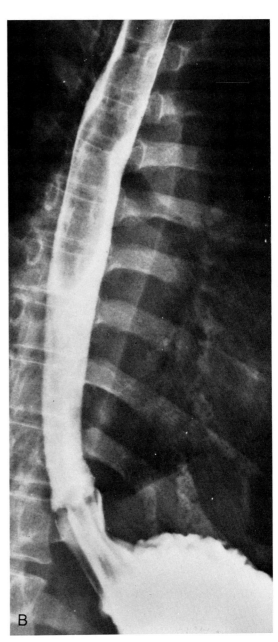

Fig. 13-10 (A) Meat impacted above a Schatzki ring; endoscopic removal was required. (B) Schatzki ring at the esophagogastric junction, the cause of the meat impaction illustrated in Fig. A.

tually all have symptoms when the passage is less than 1.0 cm. A Schatzki ring with a small orifice may be the point of impaction of a food bolus (Fig. 13-10).

Multiple Webs

Multiple webs of the distal esophagus may occur in a manner similar to the single web of the Schatzki ring (Fig. 13-11). Whether these constitute a variant of the Schatzki ring or an unusual form of stricture due to reflux esophagitis is not certain.

PERFORATION

Perforation of the esophagus may occur spontaneously as Boerhaave's syndrome, which results from forcible vomiting, occasionally self-induced, as in the case of Dr. Boerhaave's original patient. The perforation characteristically occurs in the distal half of the esophagus. Usually, free air is visible in the mediastinum or in the pleural cavity. If esophageal perforation is suspected and further radiologic confirmation is desired in the form of demonstration of the actual point of perforation, the esophagus should be examined with water soluble contrast material rather than barium to avoid barium mediastinitis and fibrosis.

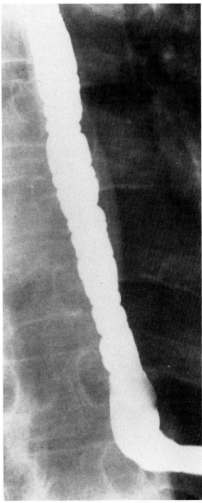

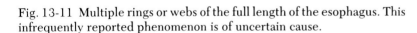

Fig. 13-11 Multiple rings or webs of the full length of the esophagus. This infrequently reported phenomenon is of uncertain cause.

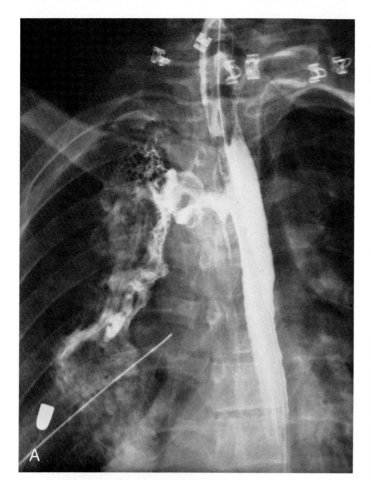

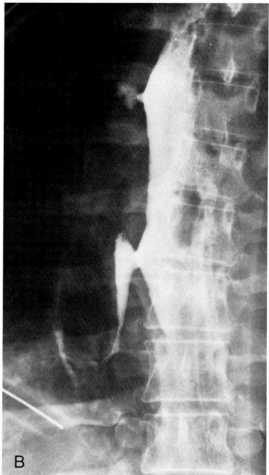

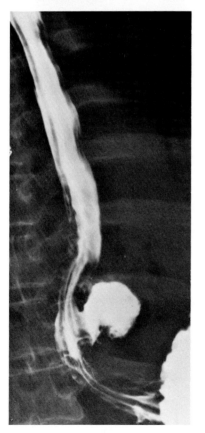

Fig. 13-12 (A) Esophageal perforation caused by a bullet wound. (B) Two esophageal perforations resulting from a swallowed chicken bone. A tract to a right lower lobe bronchus is visible. (Fig. B from Gelfand DW: Complications of gastrointestinal radiologic procedures: I. Complications of routine fluoroscopic studies. Gastrointest Radiol 5:293, 1980.) (C) Perforation of an epiphrenic diverticulum following instrumentation. Mediastinal emphysema is seen surrounding the diverticulum.

The esophagus may also be perforated by a swallowed sharp foreign object (Fig. 13-12), by medical instrumentation, or by a knife or gunshot wound. In the case of endoscopy, the presence of an esophageal diverticulum is a particular hazard, since entry of the instrument into a diverticulum frequently results in perforation.

The *Mallory-Weiss syndrome* consists of a partial thickness tear of the lower esophagus and/or the cardia of the stomach. Its usual cause is forcible or repeated vomiting, and the most common clinical sign leading to its diagnosis is hematemesis. Due to the shallow tear involved, radiologic demonstration of this entity is rare (Fig. 13-13) and the diagnosis is usually established at endoscopy.

IMPACTION

Foreign objects impacted in the esophagus are most often composed of solid food, commonly a poorly chewed piece of meat (Fig. 13-10). The usual site of impaction is the distal esophagus. The most common causes of impaction are stricture due to reflux esophagitis, a Schatzki ring with a limited orifice, or a circumferential carcinoma. Because of the often serious underlying pathology, the esophagus must be thoroughly examined radiologically and/or endoscopically after an impacted food bolus has been retrieved. The examination should be pursued until the cause of the impaction has been established.

DIVERTICULA

Esophageal diverticula are of two common forms: traction-pulsion diverticula and epiphrenic diverticula; a third form — intramural diverticula — is rare.

Traction-Pulsion Diverticula

Traction-pulsion diverticula usually occur near the carina and have traditionally been thought to be the consequence of inflammatory involvement of the wall of the esophagus by tuberculous or fungal infection of adjacent lymph nodes. As the

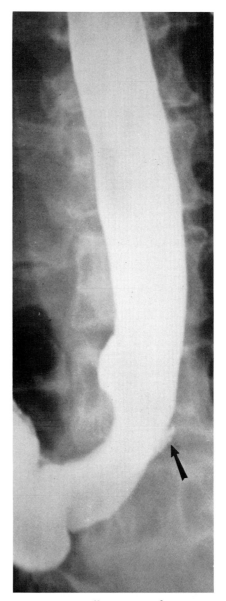

Fig. 13-13 Mallory-Weiss laceration (arrow) at the esophagogastric junction following forcible vomiting. Demonstration of these superficial mucosal tears is unusual.

affected lymph nodes heal and become fibrotic, they exert traction on a small area of the esophageal wall. As a result of intraesophageal pressure phenomena, these areas respond by becoming diverticula (Fig. 13-14). They are generally not

(Text continues on page 170.)

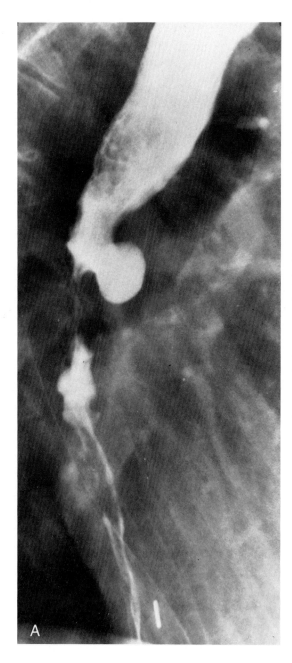

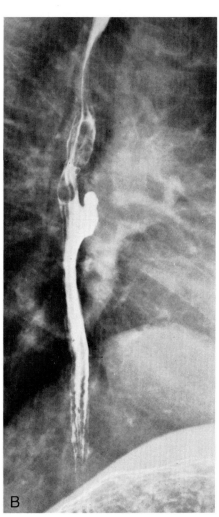

Fig. 13-14 (A & B) Two examples of midesophageal diverticula of the traction-pulsion type. In Fig. B, esophageal varices are also visible.

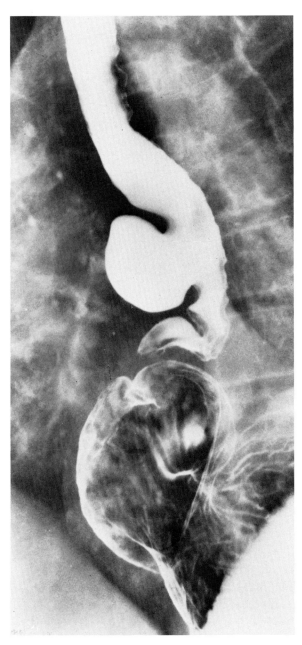

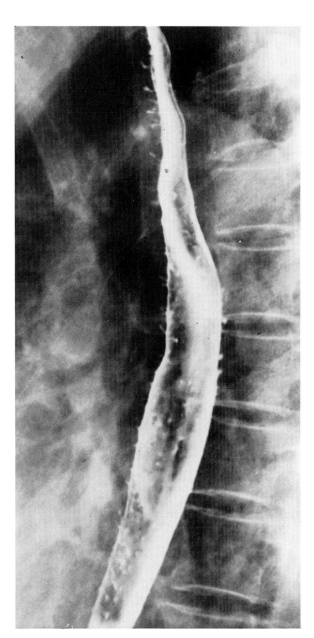

Fig. 13-15 Example of an epiphrenic diverticulum. Most epiphrenic diverticula are associated with hiatus hernia.

Fig. 13-16 Numerous intramural diverticula extending almost the full length of the esophagus. These are dilated glandular structures, and their presence has been associated with chronic inflammation.

larger than 2 or 3 cm and are seldom the cause of symptoms.

Epiphrenic Diverticula

Epiphrenic diverticula occur in the distal third of the esophagus, just above the diaphragm, and are often associated with hiatus hernia (Figs. 13-12C and 13-15). They may become considerably larger than the typical traction-pulsion diverticula seen at the carina, and may retain food and/or cause dysphagia. As with a Zenker's diverticulum, it is important to evaluate these patients for esophageal stricture, hiatus hernia, or gastroesophageal reflux, since these may produce an elevated intraesophageal pressure that will interfere with successful surgical correction.

Intramural Diverticula

Intramural diverticula are rare, and may occur individually or in large numbers along varying lengths of the esophagus (Fig. 13-16). The "diverticula" are in actuality dilated glandular structures. Although their exact cause is uncertain, they have been variously associated with moniliasis, chronic inflammation due to reflux esophagitis, and distal strictures. Their most common radiographic presentation is that of numerous, tiny flask-shaped protrusions of barium, usually located in the distal esophagus, and generally no larger than 1 to 2 mm.

FUNCTIONAL DISORDERS

Unlike the more distal segments of the gastrointestinal tract, the esophagus is the site of a wide variety of well-defined functional disorders. Several of these are seen with great regularity and are capable of causing significant symptoms. A summary of pathologic conditions known to alter esophageal motility in a manner detectable radiologically is presented in Table 13-1.

Table 13-1. Entities Capable of Causing Abnormal or Absent Esophageal Motility

Achalasia
Diffuse esophageal spasm
Presbyesophagus
Connective tissue disorder
  Scleroderma
  Dermatomyositis
  Rheumatoid arthritis
  Polyarteritis nodosa
Neuropathic state
  Diabetic neuropathy
  Alcoholic neuropathy
  Cerebral lesion
  Poliomyelitis
  Multiple sclerosis
Anticholinergic drugs
Esophagitis
  Reflux esophagitis
  Moniliasis
  Caustic ingestion
  Radiation
Primary disease of striated muscle
  Muscular dystrophy
  Myasthenia gravis
  Myotonic dystrophy
Chaga's disease
Thyrotoxicosis
Myxedema

Achalasia

Achalasia is manifested by an inability of the lower esophageal sphincter to relax for the passage of food. The disease is associated with degeneration of the mysenteric plexus of the esophagus and is progressive in its severity. Its onset is usually noted in the young adult years, and its presence causes dysphagia and aspiration of retained esophageal contents. Nourishment of the patient is often adversely affected.

Radiologically, an air-fluid level may be visible in the upper esophagus on plain films or fluoroscopically even before barium is administered. The barium then enters a dilated, fluid- and food-filled esophagus (Fig. 13-17A). At the esophagogastric junction a long, narrow segment is encountered with an appearance often described as resembling a "rat's tail" (Figs. 13-17B). Proximal to the narrowed segment, peristalsis may be entirely lacking or it may be present but disorganized. In the latter case, the entity is termed "vigorous achalasia" (Fig. 13-17C).

Although the tapered narrowing of the distal

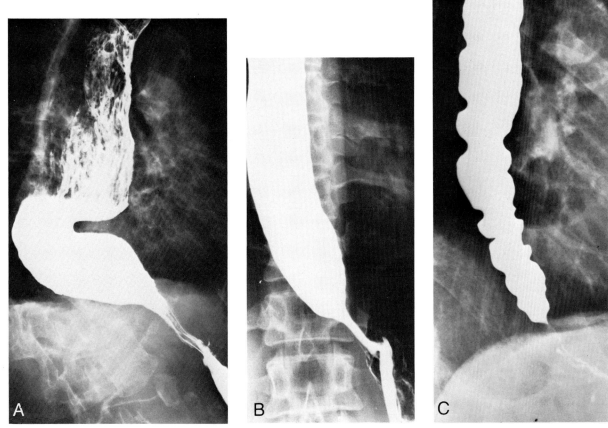

Fig. 13-17 (A) Achalasia with a fluid-filled, dilated esophagus, and an elongated esophagogastric junction. Slight irregularity of the esophagogastric junction is due to previous dilatations. (B) Typical rat-tail configuration with esophageal dilatation in a patient with newly discovered achalasia. (C) Example of "vigorous" achalasia with indentation of the barium column by uncoordinated esophageal contractions.

esophagus in achalasia is quite characteristic, an adenocarcinoma of the esophagogastric junction may mimic this appearance by infiltrating the distal esophagus submucosally. Thus, endoscopy should be performed in all newly discovered cases, particulary in patients over 30 years old. A further precaution is that the incidence of primary carcinoma of the esophagus is increased in patients with longstanding achalasia, and the esophagus should therefore be carefully examined in such patients to rule out this possibility.

Chaga's Disease

Chaga's disease mimicks the radiographic appearances of achalasia, with a dilated esophagus and an elongated, narrowed esophagogastric junction. The parasite *Trypanosoma cruzi* is the causative organism, and it provokes a degeneration of the myenteric plexus of the esophagus that is essentially indistinguishable from that of achalasia. The definitive diagnosis of Chaga's disease is made on the basis of the complement fixation test for *T cruzi*. The distribution of the parasite and the disease is limited to parts of South America.

Scleroderma

Scleroderma of the esophagus causes degeneration of the smooth muscle components of the esophageal wall. The eventual manifestation is esophageal dilatation and lack of a primary wave in the distal two-thirds of the esophagus. The proximal third of the esophagus remains contractile because of its striated musculature. The malfunction is accompanied by gastroesophageal reflux, and after a period of time the resulting esophagitis causes ulceration and stricture of the distal esophagus, almost invariably accompanied by hiatus hernia.

Radiologically, the most common presentation of scleroderma of the esophagus is that of a dilated distal esophagus lacking normal peristalsis (Fig. 13-18). The loss of peristalsis in the distal two-thirds of the esophagus as observed radiologically may be one of the first clinical signs of scleroderma, and it may precede definitive skin changes. Hiatal hernia is a common associated finding, as are the radiologic signs of reflux esophagitis. In longstanding cases, esophageal stricture may also be present. Advanced scleroderma of the esophagus may thus present radiologically as a dilated, immobile esophagus with hiatus hernia, reflux esophagitis, and stricture. *Dermatomyositis, rheumatoid arthritis,* and *periarteritis nodosa* infrequently cause esophageal manifestations virtually identical to scleroderma.

Diffuse Esophageal Spasm

Diffuse esophageal spasm is characterized by forcible, nonperistaltic contractions of the distal esophagus. The esophageal contraction resembles severe tertiary contractions and may produce transient pseudodiverticula (Fig. 13-19). The characteristic of diffuse esophageal spasm that differentiates it from marked tertiary contractions is that it is accompanied by intense chest pain. The radiologic diagnosis is made difficult because it is both difficult and unusual to provoke the symptomatic spasms while the patient is being examined. Apart from detecting diffuse esophageal spasm directly, the purpose of the radiologic examination in these patients is to rule out the possibility of hiatal hernia and reflux esophagitis as contributing factors.

Presbyesophagus

Presbyesophagus is an occasional cause of dysphagia in the elderly. It is thought to be due to

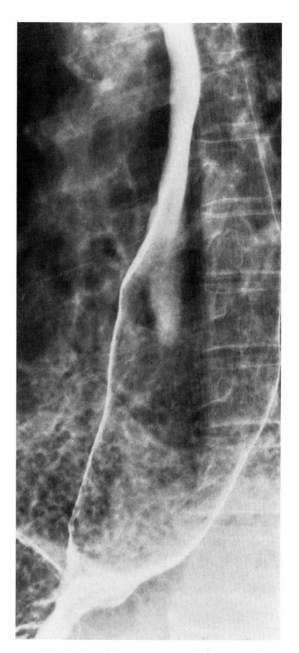

Fig. 13-18 Scleroderma causing dilatation of the esophagus. Severe pulmonary fibrosis, in the form of honeycombing of the base of the lung, is visible through the shadow of the esophagus.

neuromuscular degenerative changes related to the aging process.

Radiologically, one sees one or more of the following abnormalities of motor function. Primary waves may be infrequent and incomplete or they

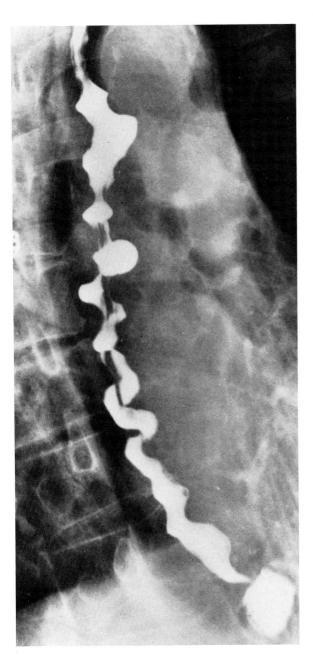

Fig. 13-19 Severe tertiary contractions in a patient with esophagospasm. These uncoordinated contractions may segment the esophagus into barium-containing pseudodiverticula.

may be totally absent. Tertiary contractions are usually present to a variable degree, ranging from mild segmental contractions to diffuse spasm. In occasional cases, the lower esophageal sphincter may fail to open, producing a radiologic picture similar to that of mild achalasia.

Diabetic and Alcoholic Neuropathy

Diabetic and alcoholic neuropathy are also manifest in the esophagus radiologically mainly as a decrease or absence of the primary peristaltic wave. Tertiary contractions may be seen as well. These two varieties of esophageal dysmotility are radiologically virtually indistinguishable from presbyesophagus and are only occasionally the cause of dysphagia.

A summary of conditions known to alter esophageal motility is presented in Table 13-1.

INFLAMMATORY DISEASES

These are among the most common of gastrointestinal disorders, particulary reflux esophagitis and its complications. A broad variety of other diseases is also capable of causing esophageal inflammatory changes, although less frequently, and are listed in Table 13-2.

Table 13-2. Inflammatory Diseases of the Esophagus in Approximate Order of Prevalence

Reflux esophagitis
Candidiasis
Herpes zoster
Chemical injury
Columnar-lined esophagus
Zollinger-Ellison disease
Cytomegalic inclusion disease
Radiation therapy
Crohn's disease
Tuberculosis
Syphilis
Histoplasmosis
Actinomycosis
Sporotricosis
Blastomycosis
Echinococcosis
Cysticercosis
Trichinosis
Filariasis

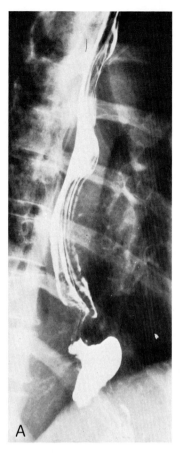

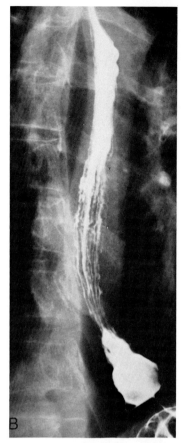

Fig. 13-20 (A & B) Examples of thickening and irregularity of esophageal folds in reflux esophagitis, as seen by mucosal relief technique. (C & D) Reflux esophagitis as demonstrated by double-contrast technique. The earliest manifestations of this disease on double-contrast films are granularity and a "tree bark" appearance. (Fig. D from Gelfand DW, Ott DJ: Anatomy and techniques in evaluating the esophagus. Semin Roentgenol 16:168, 1981.)

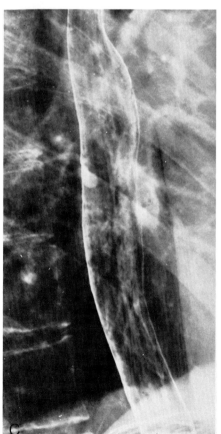

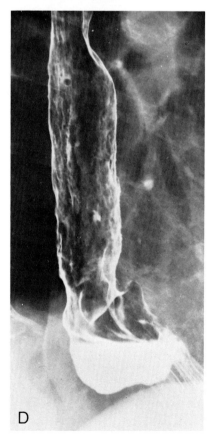

Reflux Esophagitis

Reflux esophagitis is at least as common as peptic ulcer disease and is intimately associated with the presence of hiatal hernia, which appears to play a permissive role. In its mildest form reflux esophagitis consists of mild mucosal erythema, and radiographic findings are usually absent. With slightly more advanced inflammation of the wall of the esophagus, radiographic findings may be present and consist of thickened, irregular folds on mucosal relief films (Figs. 13-20A and B) or a granular mucosa on double-contrast films (Figs. 13-20C and D).

With more severe esophagitis, ulceration and stricture occur and are usually located just proxi-

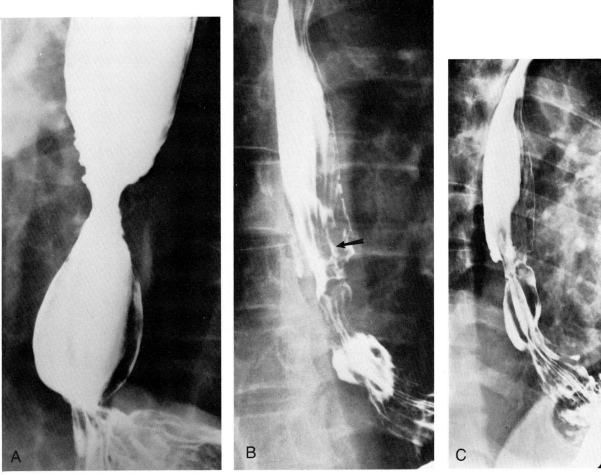

Fig. 13-21 (A) Ulcerations of the distal esophagus due to reflux esophagitis, seen on a barium-filled film as marginal irregularities and out-pouchings of the barium suspension. The patient also has a marked stricture. (Ott DJ, Gelfand DW, Wu WC: Sensitivity of single contrast radiology in esophageal disease. Gastrointest Radiol 8:105, 1983.) (B) Ulcerations of the distal esophagus in reflux esophagitis as seen on mucosal relief films. The ulcers are visible as linear collections between swollen folds (arrow). (C) Ulcer of the distal esophagus as shown by double-contrast technique in a patient with reflux esophagitis. A linear, longitudinally oriented ulcer surrounded by edema is visible just above the stricture that has formed at the esophagogastric junction. (Fig. C from Ott DJ, Gelfand DW, Lane TG, Wu WC: Radiologic detection and spectrum of appearances of peptic esophageal strictures. J Clin Gastroenterol 4:11, 1982.)

mal to the esophagogastric junction. Radiologically, the ulcers are visible on full column films at the margins of the barium column as a fine irregularity (Figs. 13-21A and 13-22). On mucosal relief films, a combination of thickened folds and crevices retaining barium may be seen (Fig. 13-21B). When double-contrast technique is employed, the ulcers are mainly perceived en face (Fig. 13-21C).

Stricture may finally result from persistent, severe esophagitis and may be detected as a lack of distensibility on both full column and double-contrast films (Fig. 13-22). Strictures will not be apparent if only mucosal relief films are taken since distention is required for their demonstration. During periods of exacerbation, almost all cases

with stricture will demonstrate radiologic evidence of the presence of ulceration.

Scarring of the esophagus due to reflux esophagitis may take at least two additional forms. Transverse or converging folds may be found in the distal esophagus (Fig. 13-23A), often in association with obvious stricture, and pseudodiverticula may be formed due to local cicatrization (Fig. 13-23B).

Peptic Ulcers

Discrete peptic ulcers of the distal esophagus are usually associated with reflux esophagitis, but may occasionally be seen without other evidences of

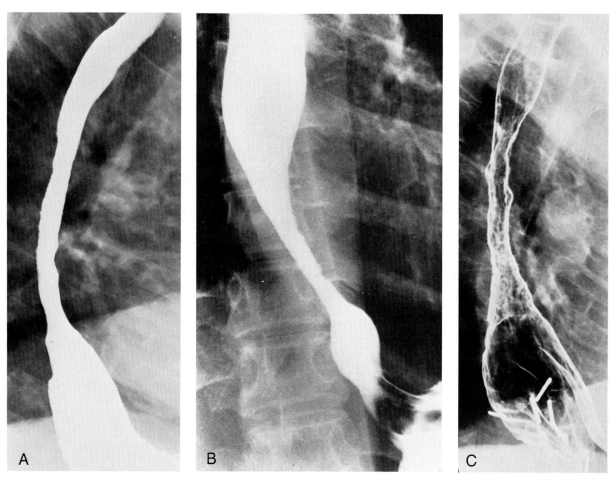

Fig. 13-22 (A–C) Examples of strictures of the distal esophagus caused by reflux esophagitis. Marginal irregularity and irregularity of the mucosal surface reflect continued inflammatory activity; (Fig. B from Ott DJ, Gelfand DW, Wu WC: Reflux esophagitis: Radiographic and endoscopic correlation. Radiology 130:583, 1979.)

Fig. 13-23 (A) Scarring due to reflux esophagitis, resulting in transverse and converging folds at the esophagogastric junction (arrow). Ulcers are visible more proximally as marginal irregularities on the posterior wall of the esophagus. (Ott DJ, Wu WC, Gelfand DW: Reflux esophagitis revisited: Prospective analysis of radiologic accuracy. Gastrointest Radiol 6:1, 1981.) (B) Pseudodiverticulum (arrow) caused by scarring in a patient with reflux esophagitis. A marked stricture is seen immediately distal to the pseudodiverticulum. (Ott DJ, Gelfand DW, Lane TG, Wu WC: Radiologic detection and spectrum of appearances of peptic esophageal strictures. J Clin Gastroenterol 4:11, 1982.)

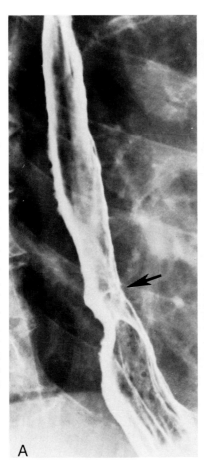

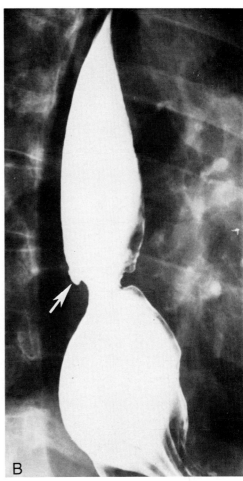

esophagitis. However, they are virtually always associated with hiatus hernia. Esophageal peptic ulcers tend to be deeper and more clearly defined than the typical erosions and small ulcerations more commonly seen with reflux esophagitis. This entity has also been described in older literature as marginal ulcer with short esophagus.

Radiologically, peptic ulcer of the esophagus is seen as a well-defined collection of barium lying at or just above the esophagogastric junction (Fig. 13-24). The lesion is usually several millimeters in diameter and almost as deep. It requires differentiation from the pseudodiverticula that may form in a distal esophagus badly scarred by esophagitis. In general, esophageal peptic ulcers are rigid and unchangeable and may be surrounded by a ring of visible edema, while pseudodiverticula usually change shape and size during the examination.

Zollinger-Ellison Syndrome

Zollinger-Ellison syndrome may occasionally present radiologically as severe reflux esophagitis with ulcers and stricture. These are the consequences of the gastric hypersecretion stimulated by the gastrin-producing pancreatic islet cell tumor that is the root cause of the syndrome. Other radiologic signs of Zollinger-Ellison disease will also be present, such as multiple gastric and duodenal ulcers, gastric hyper-rugosity, and thickened folds in the proximal small bowel.

Columnar-Lined Esophagus

Columnar-lined esophagus, also known as *Barrett's esophagus* and the *Allison-Johnstone anomaly*, may closely mimic the appearances of reflux esophagitis, similarly producing a stricture above a hiatal hernia. In most cases, the esophagus below the stricture is lined with columnar epithelium. Rarely, an isolated island of columnar epithelium may be present at the stricture, with squamous esophageal mucosa above and below.

The radiographic appearance of this entity has several consistent features. Hiatus hernia is almost always present, and at a variable distance above the esophageal hiatus, a distinct constriction may be visible marking the squamocolumnar junction (Fig. 13-25). In about half of cases, this is further above the esophagogastric junction than the strictures commonly seen in association with reflux esophagitis, and the esophagus below the constriction is slightly dilated. Thus, the presence of hiatus hernia plus a stricture located more proximally than would be expected with reflux esophagitis should suggest columnar-lined esophagus. In addition, a discrete Barrett's ulcer may be detected in the region of the stricture. A further sign of Barrett's esophagus is the occasional presence on double-contrast films of a distinct reticular pattern in the columnar-lined distal esophagus.

Recent data suggest that Barrett's esophagus is not as uncommon as previously thought. Furthermore, there may be a significant incidence of adenocarcinoma arising from the junctional columnar epithelium. This suggests that these patients must be carefully examined and closely followed.

Infectious Esophagitis

Infectious esophagitis is most frequently caused by *Candida albicans*, the resulting inflammatory process being commonly referred to as *candidiasis* or *moniliasis*. The advent of steroids and the increasing use of cancer chemotherapy has greatly increased the incidence of this entity in recent years. Esophageal candidiasis also occurs with increased frequency in patients with diabetes mellitus.

The earliest radiologic signs of esophageal can-

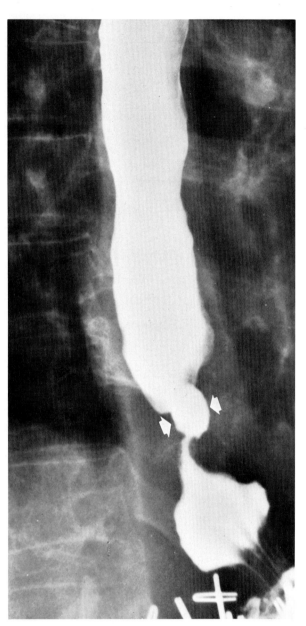

Fig. 13-24 Distal esophageal peptic ulcer associated with hiatus hernia and stricture. (Gelfand DW, Ott DJ: Anatomy and techniques in evaluating the esophagus. Semin Roentgenol 16:168, 1981.)

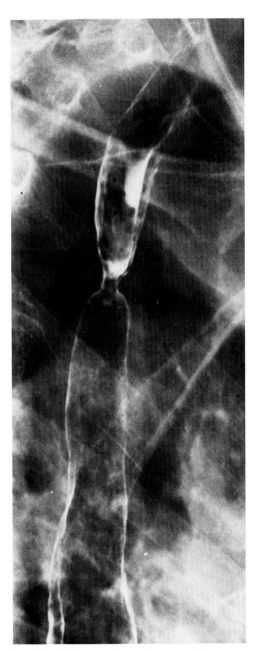

Fig. 13-25 Barrett's esophagus, visible as a stricture of the proximal esophagus with a flaccid and slightly dilated esophagus distal to the constriction.

didiasis are isolated mucosal plaques and/or a granular mucosal surface (Fig. 13-26A). With more severe disease, a cobblestone appearance becomes apparent as shallow ulcerations and a pseudomembrane form (Fig. 13-26B). Candidiasis rarely progresses to transmural ulceration and/or stricture (Fig. 13-26C). Patients predisposed to esophageal candidiasis by virtue of steroid or chemotherapeutic treatment and complaining of dysphasia should have a careful examination of the esophagus that includes both double-contrast and mucosal relief films. Visual inspection of the pharynx by the radiologist is also warranted, since almost all patients with esophageal candidiasis will have monilial lesions in the pharynx.

Several other specific infections of the esophagus also occur. *Herpes zoster* causes superficial ulcerations of the esophagus, usually discrete and similar to aphthoid ulcers. In more severe cases, however, there is more extensive ulceration and the radiologic picture may resemble candidiasis (Fig. 13-26D). *Tuberculous* esophagitis is increasingly uncommon, but takes several forms: single or multiple ulcers capable of penetrating the wall of the esophagus and most often located at or above the carina, fibrotic stricture due to tuberculous mediastinitis, or fine nodular changes due to granulomata in the submucosal layer of the esophagus. *Syphilis* of the esophagus is now quite rare, and takes the form of either an inflammatory stricture or extrinsic pressure caused by a gummatous mass. Other infectious agents reported to involve the esophagus include *histoplasmosis, actinomycosis, sporotricosis, blastomycosis, cytomegalic inclusion disease, echinococcosis, cysticerosis, trichinosis* and *filariasis*.

Chemical Esophagitis

Chemical esophagitis is most frequently caused by ingestion of alkaline caustics such as the lye used in drain cleaners. Other corrosive agents include household ammonia and bleaches, strong acids, phenols, various oral medications, silver nitrate, and iodine compounds.

Roentgenograms taken immediately after corrosive ingestion may be normal. If the esophageal mucosa has sloughed, intramural contrast material

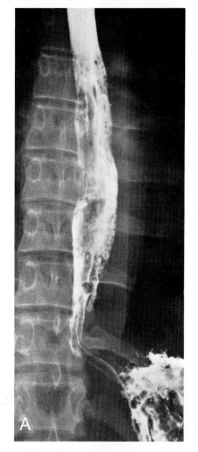

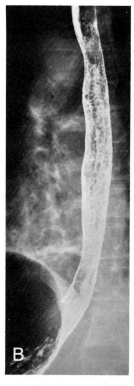

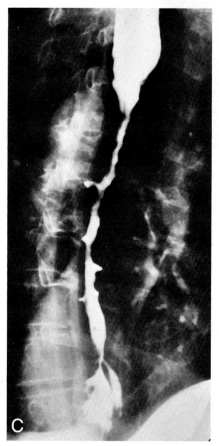

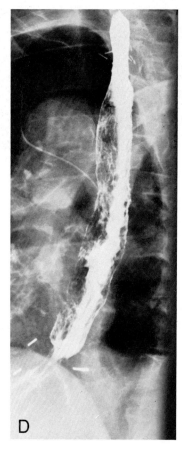

Fig. 13-26 (A) Isolated plaques, small ulcers, and granularity in a patient with mixed candidiasis and herpetic esophagitis. The patient had been receiving chemotherapy. (B) Diffuse granularity and ulcerations in a patient with total esophageal involvement by candidiasis. The patient was receiving anticancer therapy. (C) Candidiasis causing a lengthy esophageal stricture and transmural ulcerations. The patient was receiving steroids and antimetabolites for treatment of leukemia. (Fig. C from Ott DJ, Gelfand DW: Esophageal stricture secondary to candidiasis. Gastrointest Radiol 2:323, 1978.) (D) Severe herpetic esophagitis essentially indistinguishable from candidiasis.

may be detected beneath necrotic superficial layers. Use of a water-soluble contrast material is recommended during the acute phase due to possible transmural necrosis and perforation.

After 2 or 3 weeks, there is progressive stricture of the areas of injury. Stricture formation is usually well developed after 2 or 3 months, and after severe injury the lumen of the esophagus may become almost totally occluded (Fig. 13-27). Strictures due to corrosive ingestion are rarely perfectly smooth, and if there has been repeated therapeutic dilatation of the stricture, considerable irregularity may be present.

Crohn's Disease

Crohn's disease of the esophagus is very rare and is almost always accompanied by Crohn's disease

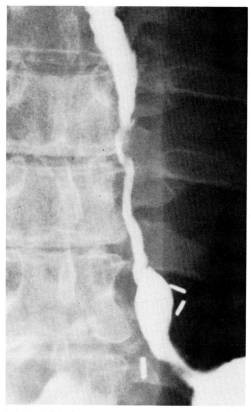

Fig. 13-27 A severe, irregular stricture of the distal esophagus following ingestion of drain cleaner and repeated attempts at dilatation.

elsewhere in the gastrointestinal tract. The radiologic appearance most often reported is that of erosions or ulceration, but reported cases are sufficiently rare that a definite pattern has not become discernible. Perforation of the esophagus due to Crohn's disease has been reported, with formation of sinus tracts and esophagobronchial fistulae.

Differential Diagnosis

Differential diagnosis may be necessary in cases of esophagitis or stricture where a specific cause is not identifiable by history. This usually involves differentiating between reflux esophagitis, columnar-lined esophagus, and monilial or herpetic esophagitis, and the following points are helpful. In reflux esophagitis, the esophageal irregularities and possible stricture are usually concentrated immediately proximal to a visible hiatus hernia. With columnar-lined esophagus, hiatus hernia is similarly present, but the stricture is often at some distance above the hiatal hernia, and the distinctive reticular pattern of the junctional columnar epithelium may be seen. In moniliasis or herpetic esophagitis, involvement of the esophagus is usually widespread by the time the patient has been referred for radiologic evaluation, and hiatus hernia is not a necessary component. A more complete list of causes of inflammatory lesions of the esophagus is presented in Table 13-2.

BENIGN NEOPLASMS

Benign neoplasms are uncommon in the esophagus and occasionally are of unusual or bizarre nature. Benign tumors of epithelial origin are particularly rare, in contrast to their frequency in the remainder of the gastrointestinal tract. Tumors of mesenchymal origin typically take the forms displayed by these neoplasms throughout the gut.

Leiomyoma

Leiomyoma is the most common benign neoplasm of the esophagus. It usually presents as an intramural mass, with sharply defined margins. In

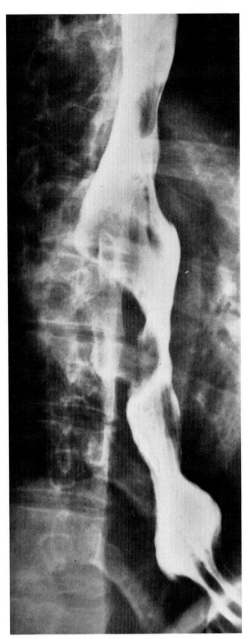

Fig. 13-28 Large leiomyoma of the esophagus causing a smooth, lobulated mass within the esophageal wall.

the esophagus, in contrast to elsewhere in the gut, the lesion seldom ulcerates. Since the overlying mucosa is usually intact, the round or elliptical defect seen radiographically is smooth (Fig. 13-28). When a potential leiomyoma is larger than 5 cm, however, the possibility of leiomyosarcoma

should also be raised. Other tumors of mesothelial origin, such as lipoma and fibroma, may duplicate the appearance of a leiomyoma.

Polypoid Lesions

Polypoid lesions of the esophagus of mucosal or submucosal origin are usually papillomatous, of mixed cellularity, or lipomatous. These extremely rare tumors are usually small and may be single or multiple. Tumors of mixed cellularity occasionally grow to considerable size, however, and may present as elliptical or sausage-shaped filling defects within the lumen of the esophagus.

Cysts

Cysts of the esophageal wall are radiologically similar in appearance to benign tumors and may cause intramural or extrinsic defects. Although usually termed *duplication cysts,* the epithelium within these cysts may be of either gastrointestinal or respiratory origin. Retention cysts, with origin in the glandular structures of the submucosa, have also been reported.

Table 13-3. Potential Intramural Lesions of the Esophagus

Benign tumors
  Leiomyoma
  Lipoma
  Fibroma
  Angioma
  Papilloma
  Tumor of mixed cellularity
  Granular cell tumor
Polypoid primary malignancy
  Carcinoma
  Leiomyosarcoma
  Carcinosarcoma
  Lymphoma
Extrinsic invading malignancy
  From primary in lung
  From mediastinal node metastases or lymphoma
  From stomach invading submucosally
Metastatic tumor
  Breast
  Melanoma
Varices
Duplication cyst
Retention cyst
Primary melanoma
Abscess
Foreign body

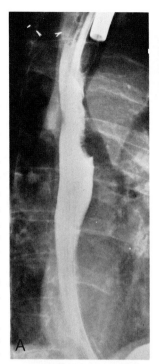

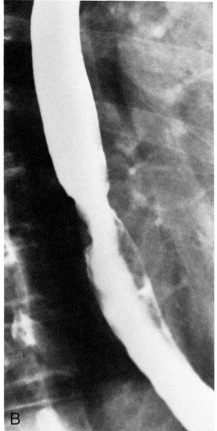

Fig. 13-29 (A) Plaque-like carcinoma of the mid-esophagus found incidentally during an upper gastrointestinal series performed for unrelated reasons. Discovery of such small, asymptomatic lesions at this early stage is unusual. (B) Small carcinoma of the esophagus that is beginning to assume a circumferential configuration. (Fig. B from Gelfand DW, Ott DJ: Anatomy and techniques in evaluating the esophagus. Semin Roentgenol 16:168, 1981.) (C) Carcinoma circumferentially involving several centimeters of the esophagus. An ulceration within the tumor is visible posteriorly. (Fig. C reprinted by permission of the publisher from Ott DJ: Radiologic evaluation of the esophagus. In Castell DO, Johnson LF, eds: Esophageal Function in Health and Disease. New York, copyright 1983 by Elsevier Science Publishing Co., Inc., pp 211–235.) (D) Carcinoma of the esophagus with development of an esophagobronchial fistula. Barium is visible (arrow) within the left mainstem bronchus.

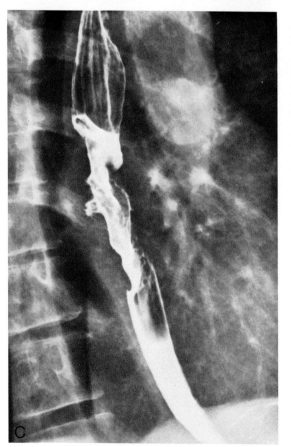

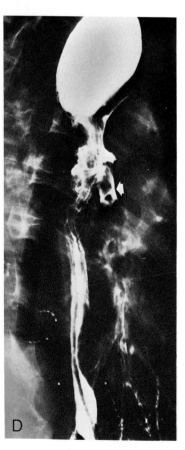

Differential diagnosis of the above entities usually involves distinguishing between a benign intramural tumor or cyst and an extrinsic tumor that has partially invaded the wall of the esophagus. A helpful point is that the center of a mass of intramural origin usually projects in line with the wall of the esophagus while the center of an extrinsic mass is usually projected outside the wall of the esophagus. Specific radiologic differentiation between the various mesenchymal tumors and similar appearing cysts is usually possible only for the lipoma, which may be detectably deformable and radiolucent. A more extensive list of potential intramural lesions of the esophagus is presented in Table 13-3.

MALIGNANT NEOPLASMS

The variety of malignant lesions encountered in the esophagus is smaller than in the more distal segments of the gastrointestinal tract. For practical purposes, the overwhelming majority will be either squamous cell carcinoma of the esophagus proper or adenocarcinoma of gastric or junctional origin involving the esophagogastric region.

Squamous Cell Carcinoma

Squamous cell carcinoma may occur anywhere in the esophagus, and its radiographic appearance depends on the stage at which it is discovered (Fig. 13-29). The earliest lesion is usually manifest as a small plaque on the side of the esophagus. The tumor is only rarely discovered in this form, however, possibly because symptoms at this point are seldom severe enough to bring the patient to evaluation. More commonly, the lesion is first detected when it has become more extensive and has ulcerated. At this stage it usually involves several centimeters of esophageal wall. Carcinoma of the esophagus eventually involves the entire circum-

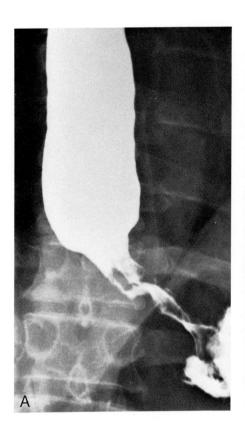
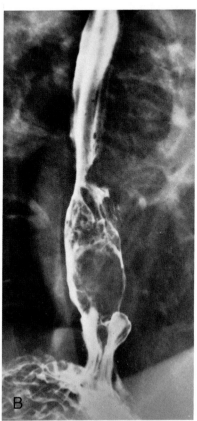

Fig. 13-30 (A & B) Adenocarcinomas of the esophagogastric junction presenting with a typically malignant appearance.

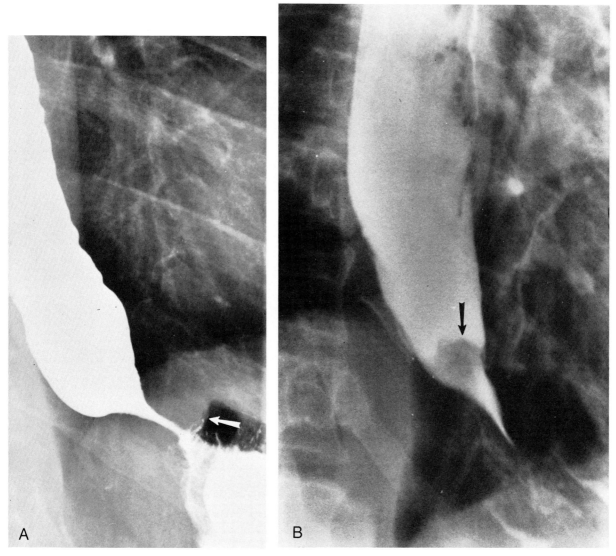

Fig. 13-31 (A) Adenocarcinoma of the esophagogastric junction submucosally infiltrating the distal esophagus, causing an appearance similar to achalasia. However, a mass of tumor was visible on the gastric side of the esophagogastric junction (arrow), suggesting the nature of the lesion. (B) Adenocarcinoma of the esophagogastric junction with an appearance partially simulating achalasia. In this case, a tumor mass has begun to form, (arrow) strongly suggesting the presence of malignancy. (Fig. B from Ott DJ, Gelfand DW, Wu WC, Kerr RM: Secondary achalasia in esophagogastric carcinoma: Re-emphasis of a difficult differential problem. Rev Interam Radiol 4:135, 1979.)

ference of the esophagus, producing stricture, abrupt margins, and other signs of advanced malignancy.

Esophageal carcinoma undergoes a characteristic sequence of changes during and after radiotherapy. Shortly after radiotherapy is completed, the radiologic appearance of the esophagus returns almost to normal, usually with a slight stricture remaining. However, the tumor invariably recurs, and eventually the typically malignant, irregular configuration again becomes apparent. In its terminal phase, the recurrent carcinoma almost always produces complete obstruction. Tracheoesophageal or bronchoesophageal fistula is a further complication often occurring in the final stages of the disease (Fig. 13-29D).

Adenocarcinoma

Adenocarcinoma originating in gastric or junctional columnar epithelium is the malignancy most commonly occurring at the esophagogastric junction. It generally presents appearances similar to squamous cell carcinoma, except that tumor may also be visible on the wall of adjacent areas of the proximal stomach. Within the esophagus, the tumor most often produces the typical signs of malignancy, with a sharp demarcation and an irregular surface (Fig. 13-30). In a fairly common and more subtle form, however, adenocarcinoma may invade the distal esophagus submucosally, causing a benign-appearing stricture or an appearance closely mimicking achalasia (Fig. 13-31). Because of this possibility, all strictures of the distal esophagus warrant endoscopic examination and biopsy.

Varicoid Carcinoma

Varicoid carcinoma is a rare presentation of carcinoma of the esophagus in which the tumor infiltrates the distal esophageal folds without totally obliterating them. The resulting irregular thickening of folds resembles esophageal varices (Fig. 13-32).

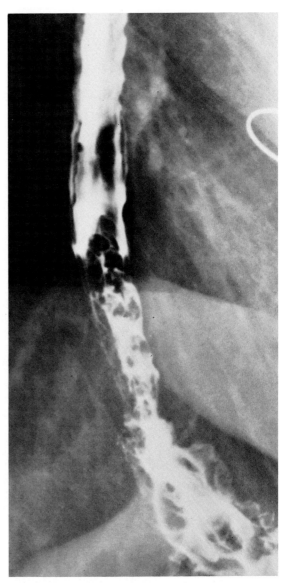

Fig. 13-32 Varicoid carcinoma of the distal esophagus causing nodular swelling of the distal esophageal folds. The similarity of this type of lesion to ordinary esophageal varices should be noted.

Carcinosarcoma

Carcinosarcoma is a rare malignancy of mixed cellularity and a low order of malignancy. Most lesions present as large, lobulated filling defects. These tumors may be relatively smooth in appearance due to an intact overlying mucosa.

Carcinoma of the Lung

Carcinoma of the lung invading the esophagus characteristically occurs in the region of the carinal lymph nodes. Although metastatic tumor enlarging a lymph node usually causes an extrinsic impression on the esophagus (Fig. 13-33A), when invasion occurs, the tumor may disrupt the mucosal surface of the esophagus and assume the appearances of a primary malignancy. It should also be noted that invasion of the esophagus by carcinoma of the lung is one of the more common causes of tracheoesophageal and esophagobronchial fistulae in adults (Fig. 13-33B).

Malignant Lymphoma and Metastases

Malignant lymphoma only rarely invades the esophagus from adjacent lymph nodes. Similarly, primary malignant lymphoma of the esophagus is extremely rare. Metastatic malignancy of the esophagus from a distant site is also extremely rare.

Differential Diagnosis

Differential diagnosis is at times required between malignant lesions of the esophagus and potentially malignant-appearing benign processes,

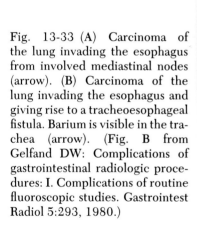

Fig. 13-33 (A) Carcinoma of the lung invading the esophagus from involved mediastinal nodes (arrow). (B) Carcinoma of the lung invading the esophagus and giving rise to a tracheoesophageal fistula. Barium is visible in the trachea (arrow). (Fig. B from Gelfand DW: Complications of gastrointestinal radiologic procedures: I. Complications of routine fluoroscopic studies. Gastrointest Radiol 5:293, 1980.)

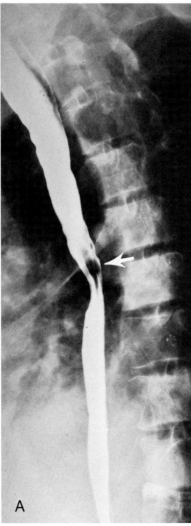

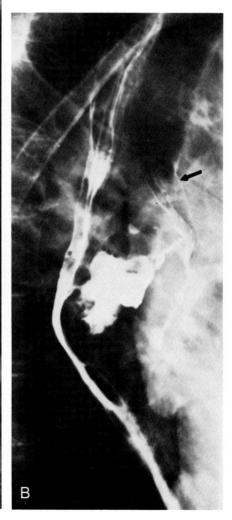

A

B

188   *Gastrointestinal Radiology*

Table 13-4. Potentially Malignant-Appearing Lesions of the Esophagus

Primary carcinoma
Invading carcinoma
    From stomach
    From primary in lung
    From mediastinum
Metastatic malignancy
    Breast carcinoma
    Melanoma
Carcinosarcoma
Lymphoma
Primary melanoma
Kaposi's sarcoma
Reflux esophagitis with stricture
Columnar-lined esophagus
Peptic ulcer
Varices

such as an irregular stricture due to reflux esophagitis. Conversely, a moderate number of carcinomas of the esophagus cause submucosal infiltration with a relatively benign appearance. As a consequence of these uncertainties, all lesions of the esophagus causing a fixed narrowing, with the exception of an obvious Schatzki ring, should at first presentation be subjected to endoscopic inspection and biopsy to rule out or establish the presence of malignancy. A list of those entities capable of causing malignant-appearing lesions of the esophagus is presented in Table 13-4.

EXTRINSIC MASSES

The proximity of the esophagus to the heart, great vessels and mediastinal lymph nodes ensures that enlargement of these structures of any significant degree may be manifest as deviation of the esophagus from its normal course within the mediastinum.

Enlargement of the Heart

Enlargement of the heart is the most common cause of extrinsic compression of the esophagus. Its usual effect is displacement of the distal third of the esophagus posteriorly. If the enlargement is primarily left atrial, the arcuate displacement may be characteristic in that it ends above the dia-

phragm (Fig. 13-34A). Except for left atrial enlargement, esophageal displacement due to cardiac enlargement is seldom specific for a particular chamber enlargement.

Tortuosity of the Aorta

Tortuosity or ectasia of the aorta causes the normal indentation on the left side of the esophagus at the aortic arch to be broader and/or deeper than usual. Also, if the descending thoracic aorta be-

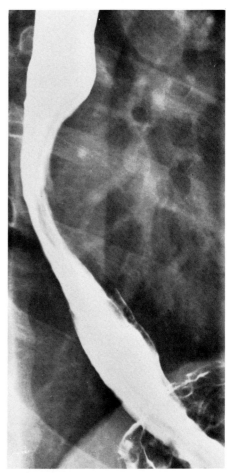

Fig. 13-34 Typical impression upon the distal esophagus in a patient with an enlarged left atrium due to mitral valvular disease. Left atrial involvement is the only specific chamber enlargement reliably discernible on the esophagogram.

comes elongated and tortuous, the loosely adherent esophagus may be pulled posteriorly and to the left with the aorta. If the distal thoracic aorta becomes tortuous and dilated, the distal esophagus may be displaced further to the right than normal. It may then angle sharply to the left as it courses around the aorta just proximal to the esophageal hiatus (Fig. 13-35). This acute angulation and stretching has been reported as causing dysphasia in the elderly.

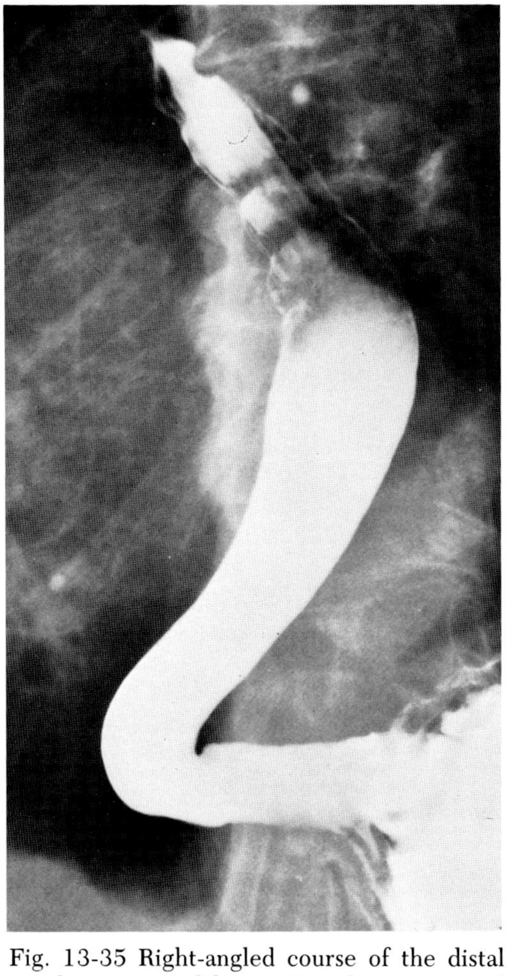

Imprints of Anomalous Vessels

Imprints of anomalous vessels also occur, primarily near the aortic arch. The most common of these is the *anomalous right subclavian artery*, or *Arteria lusoria*, which causes a posterior imprint just above the aortic arch with a characteristic angulation upward and to the right (Fig. 13-36). It

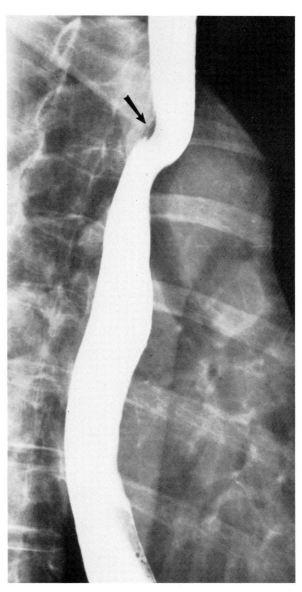

Fig. 13-35 Right-angled course of the distal esophagus caused by aortic enlargement and tortuosity. This elderly individual was experiencing dysphagia, presumably on this basis. (Gelfand DW, Ott DJ: Anatomy and techniques in evaluating the esophagus. Semin Roentgenol 16:168, 1981.)

Fig. 13-36 Impression upon the posterior aspect of the esophagus caused by an anomalous right subclavian artery (arrow), also known as arteria lusoria.

may be the cause of a rare swallowing difficulty known as dysphagia lusoria. A less common anomalous vascular imprint on the esophagus is the *right aortic arch*, which deviates the esophagus at the crossing of the aortic arch to the left instead of to the right.

Table 13-5. Abnormal Extrinsic Impression on the Esophagus

Aortic arch (ectasia, aneurysm, tortuosity)
Cardiac enlargement
Mediastinal lymph node enlargement
Mediastinal neoplasm
Anomalous vessel
   Aberrant right subclavian
   Right aortic arch
   Anomalous innominate artery
   Aortic diverticulum
   Double aortic arch
   Anomalous left pulmonary artery
Duplication cyst

Mediastinal Tumors and Cysts

Mediastinal tumors and cysts may also cause extrinsic compression or deviation of the course of the esophagus. The direction in which the esophagus is deviated depends on the location of the mass and to a certain extent suggests its potential origin. Masses of lymph node origin are the most commonly encountered mediastinal masses likely to press upon the wall of the esophagus or deviate its course. They arise in the middle mediastinum, most often anterior to the esophagus, and thus tend to deviate the esophagus in a posterior or lateral direction (Fig. 13-37). Thyroid and thymic masses originate in the anterior mediastinum and typically deviate the thoracic esophagus posteriorly. Masses of neurogenic origin arise posteriorly and usually deviate the esophagus anteriorly. A summary of entities capable of causing extrinsic compression or deformity of the esophagus is presented in Table 13-5.

SUGGESTED READINGS

Structural Abnormalities: Hiatus Hernia

Berridge FR, Friedland GW, Tagart REB: Radiological landmarks at the oesophagogastric junction. Thorax 21:499, 1966.

Dodds WJ: Current concepts of esophageal motor function: Clinical implications for radiology. Am J Roentgenol 128:549, 1977.

Friedland GW: Historical review of changing concepts of lower esophageal anatomy: 430 BC–1977. AJR 131:373, 1978.

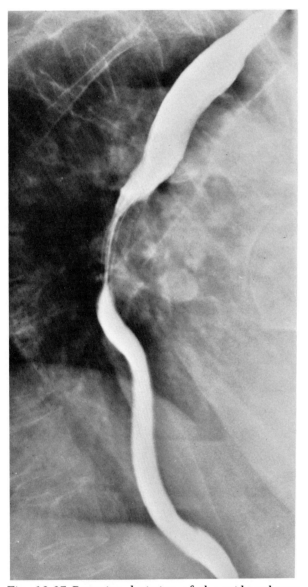

Fig. 13-37 Posterior deviation of the midesophagus produced by mediastinal lymph node enlargement in a patient with metastatic carcinoma.

Gelfand DW, Ott DJ: Areae gastricae traversing the esophageal hiatus: A sign of hiatus hernia. Gastrointest Radiol 4:127, 1979.

Schatzki R, Gary JE: Dysphagis due to a diaphragm-like localized narrowing in the lower esophagus ("lower esophageal ring"). Am J Roentgenol 70:911, 1953.

Wolf BS: The roentgen diagnosis of minimal hiatus hernia. J Mount Sinai Hosp NY 23:738, 1956.

Structural Abnormalities: Varices

Cockerill EM, Miller RE, Chernish SM, et al: Optimum visualization of esophageal varices. Am J Roentgenol 126:512, 1976.

Kirsch IE, Blackwell CC, Bennett HD: Roentgen diagnosis of oesophageal varices: Comparison of roentgen and oesophagoscopic findings in 502 cases. Am J Roentgenol 74:477, 1955.

Otto DL, Kurtzman RS: Esophageal varices in superior vena caval obstruction. Am J Roentgenol 92:1000, 1964.

Waldram R, Nunnerly WR, Davis M, et al: Detection and grading of esophageal varices by fibre-optic endoscopy and barium swallow with and without Buscopan. Clin Radiol 28:137, 1977.

Structural Abnormalities: Webs

Friedland GW, Filly R: The postcricoid impression masquerading as an esophageal tumor. Am J Dig Dis 20:287, 1975.

Goyal RK, Bauer L, Spiro HM: The nature and location of the lower esophageal ring. N Engl J Med 284:1175, 1971.

Kelley ML, Frazer JP: Symptomatic mid-esophageal webs. JAMA 197:143, 1966.

Pitman RG, Fraser GM: The post-cricoid impression on the esophagus. Clin Radiol 16:34, 1965.

Schatzki R, Gary JE: Dysphagia due to diaphragm-like localized narrowing in the lower esophagus ("lower esophageal ring"). Am J Roentgenol 70:911, 1953.

Seaman WB: The significance of webs in the hypopharynx or upper esophagus. Radiology 89:32, 1967.

Shifflett DW, Gilliam JH, Wu WC, et al: Multiple esophageal webs. Gastroenterology 77:556, 1979.

Structural Abnormalities: Diverticula

Cho SR, Sanders MM, Turner MA, et al: Esophageal intramural pseudodiverticulosis. Gastrointest Radiol 6:9, 1981.

Hodes PJ, Atkins JP, Hodes BL: Esophageal intramural diverticulosis. Am J Roentgenol 96:411, 1966.

Localio SA, Stahl WM: Diverticular disease of the alimentary tract. Curr Probl Surg: 3–47, Jan 1968.

Troupin R: Intramural esophageal diverticulosis and moniliasis—a possible association. Am J Roentgenol 104:613, 1968.

Functional Disorders

Atkinson M, Summerling MD: Oesophageal changes in systemic sclerosis. Gut 7:402, 1966.

Bennett JR, Hendrix TR: Diffuse esophageal spasm: A disorder with more than one cause. Gastroenterology 59:273, 1970.

Carter R, Brewer LA: Achalasia and esophageal carcinoma. Am J Surg 130:114, 1975.

Hale CH, Schatzki R: Roentgenological appearance of the gastrointestinal tract in scleroderma. Am J Roentgenol 51:407, 1944.

Herrera AF, Colon J, Valdes-Dapena A, Roth JLA: Achalasia or carcinoma? The significance of the Mecholyl test. Am J Dig Dis 15:1073, 1970.

Schroder JS, Hatcher CR: Achalasia of the esophagus. JAMA 202:620, 1967.

Soergel KH, Zboralske FF, Amberg JR: Presbyesophagus: Esophageal mobility in nonagenarians. J Clin Invest 43:1472, 1964.

Stevens MB, Hookman P, Siegal CI, et al: Aperistalsis of the esophagus in patients with connective-tissue disorders and Raynaud's phenomenon. N Engl J Med 270:1218, 1964.

Zboralske FF, Dodds WJ: Roentgenographic diagnosis of primary disorders of esophageal mobility. Radiol Clin North Am 7:147:1969.

Inflammatory Diseases: Reflux Esophagitis, Stricture, Ulcer

Allison PR, Johnstone AS, Royce GB: Short esophagus with simple peptic ulceration. J Thorac Surg 12:432, 1943.

Dodds WJ, Dehn TG, Hogan WJ, et al: Severe peptic esophagitis in a patient with Zollinger-Ellison syndrome. Am J Roentgenol 113:237, 1971.

Koehler RE, Weyman PJ, Oakley HF: Single- and double-contrast techniques in esophagitis. AJR 135:15, 1980.

Ott DJ, Dodds WJ, Wu WC, et al: Current status of radiology in evaluating for gastroesophageal reflux disease. J Clin Gastroenterol 4:365, 1982.

Ott, DJ, Gelfand DW, Wu WC: Reflux esophagitis: Radiologic and endoscopic correlation. Radiology 130:583, 1979.

Ott DJ, Wu WC, Gelfand DW: Reflux esophagitis revisited. Gastrointest Radiol 6:1, 1981.

Rabin MS, Schmaman IB: Radiological changes of reflux esophagitis. Clin Radiol 30:187, 1979.

Wolf BS, Som ML, Marshak RH: Short esophagus with esophagogastric or marginal ulceration. Radiology 61:473, 1953.

Inflammatory Diseases: Columnar-Lined Esophagus

Allison PR, Johnstone AS: The lower esophagus lined by columnar epithelium. Thorax 8:87, 1953.

Barrett NR: The lower esophagus lined by columnar epithelium. Surgery 41:881, 1957.

Robbins AH, Vincent ME, Saini M, Schimmel EM: Revised radiologic concepts of the Barrett's esophagus. Gastrointest Radiol 3:377, 1978.

Inflammatory Diseases: Infectious Esophagitis

Berg JW: Esophageal herpes: A complication of cancer therapy. Cancer 8:731, 1955.

Goldstein HM, Dodd GD: Radiologic spectrum of opportunistic infections of the upper gastrointestinal tract. Am J Roentgenol 129:419, 1977.

Levine MS, Laufer I, Kressel HY, Friedman HM: Herpes esophagitis. AJR 136:863, 1981.

Lewicki AM, Moore JP: Esophageal moniliasis. Am J Roentgenol 125:218, 1975.

Ott DJ, Gelfand DW: Esophageal stricture due to candidiasis. Gastrointest Radiol 2:323, 1978.

Schneider R: Tuberculous esophagitis. Gastrointest Radiol 1:143, 1976.

Thoeni R, Margulis AR: Gastrointestinal tuberculosis. Semin Roentgenol 14:283, 1979.

Inflammatory Diseases: Chemical Esophagitis

Boal DKB, Newburger PE, Teele RL: Esophagitis induced by combined radiation and Adriamycin. AJR 132:567, 1979.

Goldstein HM, Rogers LF, Fletcher GH, Dodd GD: Radiological manifestations of radiation induced injury to the normal upper gastrointestinal tract. Radiology 117:135, 1975.

Martel WM: Radiologic features of esophagogastritis secondary to extremely caustic agents. Radiology 103:31, 1972.

Muhletaler CA, Gerlock AJ, deSoto L, Halter SA: Acid corrosive esophagitis: Radiographic findings. AJR 134:1137, 1980.

Teplick JG, Teplick SK, Ominsky SH, Haskin ME: Esophagitis caused by oral medication. Radiology 134:23, 1980.

Inflammatory Diseases: Crohn's Disease

Dyer NH, Cook PL, Kemp Harper RA: Oesophageal stricture associated with Crohn's disease. Gut 10:549, 1969.

Frohlich H, Huchzermeyer H, St. Stender H: Roentgenologische Befunde bei der Osophagitis regionalis Crohn. Fortschr Röntgenstr 125:497, 1976 (in German with English abstract).

Gelfand MD, Krone CL: Dysphagia and ulceration in Crohn's disease. Gastroenterol 55:510, 1968.

Ghahremani GG, Gore RM, Breuer RI, Larson RH: Esophageal manifestations of Crohn's disease. Gastrointest Radiol 7:199, 1982.

Benign Neoplasms

Barlow D: Enterogenous cyst of the esophagus. Br J Surg 45: 100, 1957.

Bruneton JN, Drouillard J, Roux P, et al: Leiomyoma and leiomyosarcoma of the digestive tract — a report of 45 cases and review of the literature. Eur J Radiol 1:291, 1981.

Farman J, Rosen Y, Dallemand S, et al: Esophagitis cystica: Lower esophageal retention cysts. Am J Roentgenol 128:495, 1977.

Jang GC, Clouse ME, Fleischner FG: Fibrovascular polyps — a benign intraluminal tumor of the esophagus. Radiology 92:1196, 1969.

Parnell SAC, Peppercorn MA, Antoniolle DA, et al: Squamous cell papilloma of the esophagus. Gastroenterology 74:910, 1978.

Plachta A: Benign tumors of the esophagus. Review of the literature and report of 99 cases. Am J Gastroenterol 38:639, 1962.

Schatzki R, Hawes LE: The roentgenologic appearance

of extramucosal tumors of the esophagus. Am J Roentgenol 48:1, 1942.

Vithespongse V, Blank S: Ciliated epithelial esophageal cyst. Am J Gastroenterol 56:436, 1971.

Whitaker JA, Deffenbaugh LD, Cooke AR: Esophageal duplication cyst. Am J Gastroenterol 73:329, 1980.

Malignant Neoplasms

Anderson MF, Harell GS: Secondary esophageal tumors. AJR 135:1243, 1980.

Carnovale RL, Goldstein HM, Zornoza J, Dodd GD: Radiologic manifestations of esophageal lymphoma. Am J Roentgenol 128:751, 1977.

Gloyna RE, Zornoza J, Goldstein HM: Primary ulcerative carcinoma of the esophagus. Am J Roentgenol 129:599, 1977.

Goldstein HM: Esophagus. In Steckel RJ, Kagan AR, eds: Diagnosis and Staging of Cancer: A Radiologic Approach. Philadelphia, WB Saunders, 1976, pp 110–128.

Itai Y, Kogure T, Okuyama Y, Akiyama H: Superficial esophageal carcinoma. Radiologic findings in double-contrast studies. Radiology 126:597, 1978.

Kormano MJ, Yrjana J: Radiology of uncommon esophageal neoplasms. Eur J Radiol 1:51, 1981.

Libshitz IL, Lindell MM, Dodd GD: Metastases to the hollow viscera. Radiol Clin North Am 20:487, 1982.

McCort JJ: Esophageal carcinosarcoma and pseudosarcoma. Radiology 102:519, 1972.

Nussbaum M, Grossman M: Metastases to the esophagus causing gastrointestinal bleeding. Am J Gastroenterol 66:467, 1976.

Sostman HD, Keohane MF, Lee CH, et al: Primary esophageal melanocarcinoma. Br J Radiol 53:589, 1980.

Turnbull, ADM, Goodner JT: Primary adenocarcinoma of the esophagus. Cancer 22:915, 1968.

Wiot JW, Felsen B: Current concepts in cancer. Esophagus: Radiologic differential diagnosis. JAMA 226:1548, 1973.

Yates CW, Le Vine MA, Jensen KM: Varicoid carcinoma of the esophagus. Radiology 122:605, 1977.

Zornoza J, Lindell MM: Radiologic evaluation of small esophageal carcinoma. Gastrointest Radiol 5:107, 1980.

14

Abnormalities of the Stomach

STRUCTURAL DISORDERS

Structural disorders of the stomach may be either congenital or developmental in origin and are characterized by abnormality of the structure of the stomach unaccompanied by inflammation or neoplasm.

Diverticula

Diverticula of the stomach occur in two locations. The most common form is the *true gastric diverticulum* containing muscularis propria, which occurs just below the esophagogastric junction on the posterior aspect of the lesser curvature (Fig. 14-1). These diverticula are generally not larger than 3 or 4 cm and are thought to be without symptoms. Food almost never collects in this type of diverticulum and diagnosis is seldom a problem, since the stream of barium leaving the esophagus tends to flow across the entrance of the diverticulum filling it with barium. Since they are extremely rare in children, this form of gastric diverticulum is thought to be of developmental origin.

The less common *intramural gastric diverticulum* occurs on the greater curvature proximal to the pyloric canal. They are rarely more than a few millimeters in diameter and are lenticular in shape, following the contour of the wall of the stomach. Being intramural, they do not protrude appreciably from the normal contour of the stomach. Like the larger diverticula seen in the proximal stomach, they are thought to be asymptomatic. Intramural gastric diverticula, because of their location and small size, are occasionally confused with small greater curvature ulcers or with the central indentation found in cases of aberrant pancreas, which occur in the same region.

Intramucosal gastric diverticulum is extremely rare. This form of diverticulum consists of an invagination of the mucosa into the submucosal layer. A sac is formed, the walls of which are mucosa and areolar tissue. The sac fills with barium during the course of an examination and often can be seen protruding into the lumen of the stomach.

Antral Web

In rare individuals, a distinct web may be found in the gastric antrum just proximal to the pylorus, creating a small third chamber between the stomach and duodenal bulb. Partial gastric outlet obstruction may occur if the opening through the

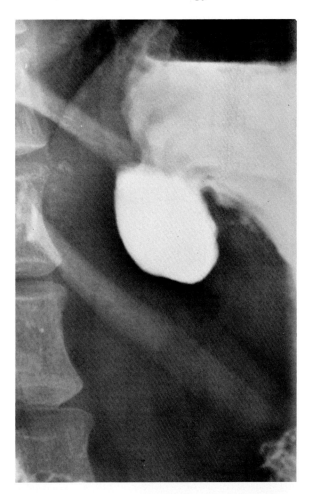

Fig. 14-1 Gastric diverticulum in the most common location, high on the posterior aspect of the lesser curvature.

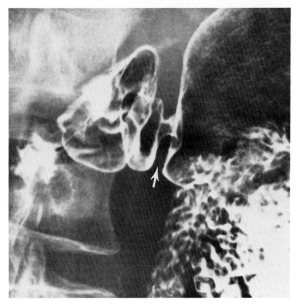

Fig. 14-2 Antral web (arrow) demarcating a third small chamber between itself and the pyloric canal.

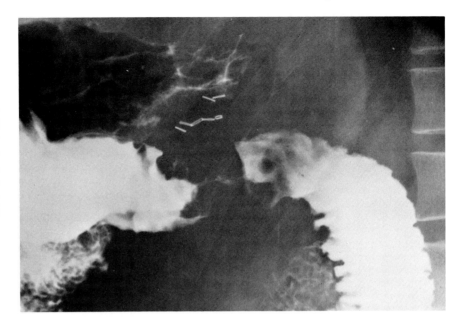

Fig. 14-3 Adult type of hypertrophic pyloric stenosis with an irregular funnel-shaped narrowing of the distal antrum and pyloric canal. Irregular projections of barium associated with this condition must be differentiated from ulcerations.

web is sufficiently narrow. The radiologic diagnosis is established by demonstration of the web and the small preduodenal chamber (Fig. 14-2).

Pyloric Hypertrophy

Pyloric hypertrophy presents in several forms in the adult patient. Least common is the infantile type of hypertrophic pyloric stenosis encountered in an adult. In these patients, the abnormality has probably been present since infancy and has the radiologic characteristics of the infantile disease. A large knot of pyloric muscle tissue is present that bulges in retrograde fashion into the lumen of the antrum, causing the typical "shoulders" used to identify the disease in infants. Also, the pyloric channel lumen is long and narrow, often with a small star-shaped chamber in its midst, which should not be misinterpreted as a peptic ulcer.

A second form of adult pyloric hypertrophy is more commonly encountered and consists of diffuse hypertrophy of both the pyloric muscle and the adjacent musculature of the antrum. In these instances, there is a funnel-shaped entrance to the pyloric canal, which is narrowed and elongated (Fig. 14-3). The shoulder-like configuration of the distal antrum seen in the infantile variety of pyloric hypertrophy is absent. The contour of the entrance

to the hypertrophied area may be somewhat irregular, and during certain phases of peristaltic contraction, small irregularly shaped chambers, which require differentiation from peptic ulcer, may form as the muscle contracts. The adult type of pyloric hypertrophy is frequently associated with inflammatory changes in the antrum, and may be a response to chronic antral gastritis or peptic ulcer.

The mildest form of pyloric hypertrophy in adults is known as *torus hypertrophy.* In this entity, the circular muscles of the pyloric canal hypertrophy in a manner that elongates the pyloric canal slightly and characteristically produces a small ulcer-like niche in the superior aspect of the pyloric canal where the circular muscle bundles diverge slightly. Its importance is that the barium collection within the canal can mimic peptic ulcer.

Gastric Varices

In patients with esophageal varices, gastric varices are almost always present as well. The most common cause of both esophageal and gastric varices in clinical practice is alcoholic hepatic cirrhosis. Because alcoholism is reasonably common, and optimum demonstration of gastric varices requires special effort at fluoroscopy, one should always try to determine beforehand if the patient has poten-

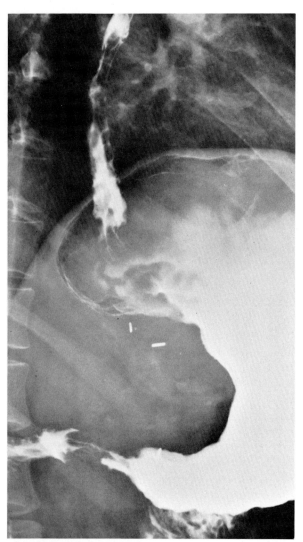

Fig. 14-4 Gastric varices appearing as large irregular folds at the esophagogastric junction. Esophageal varices are also visible.

tial alcoholism and/or hepatic cirrhosis.

Radiologically gastric varices take the form of widened, tortuous, irregularly enlarged folds in the esophagogastric region, the gastric fundus, and the proximal body of the stomach (Fig. 14-4). Often, the varices will appear as rounded enlargements of gastric folds that have been described as being "grape-like." To best demonstrate gastric varices, a double-contrast view of the proximal stomach in moderate distension is required.

Volvulus

Volvulus of the stomach is a rare but serious occurrence that may take any combination of two basic forms. The first form is *organoaxial volvulus*, in which the stomach rotates around its own long axis. The second type is known as *mesenteric-axial volvulus*, in which the axis of the volvulus is perpendicular to the long axis of the stomach.

The radiographic appearances produced by combinations of these two types of volvulus, complete and incomplete as well as obstructing and nonobstructing, are quite varied. Furthermore, because of the considerable variation in the normal position of the stomach, the radiologic diagnosis of gastric volvulus is not always as obvious as might be imagined. Usually, the radiologic diagnosis of volvulus is made on the basis of seeing a large, fluid-filled viscus in the upper abdomen on plain films, inability to demonstrate the lumen of the stomach in its normal position, partial or complete obstruction of the flow of barium somewhere between the esophagus and pyloris, or demonstration with barium of the actual twist (Fig. 14-5).

The clinical importance of gastric volvulus is twofold in that the twist may obstruct the lumen of the stomach or it may compromise the stomach's blood supply. Many cases of gastric volvulus are associated with eventration or traumatic rupture of the left leaf of the diaphragm, in which the subsequent migration of the stomach into the thorax is accompanied by partial or complete volvulus. Symptoms do not usually occur unless the stomach has twisted 180° or more. The stomach may then obstruct and become filled with fluid. The classic clinical triad in gastric volvulus is epigastric pain, wretching with little or no regurgitation of gastric contents, and inability to intubate the stomach.

Isolated Heterotaxy

Isolated heterotaxy of the stomach is a rare congenital anomaly in which the stomach is on the right side of the abdomen, located behind the liver. The entity is primarily a problem to the radiologist and the endoscopist but not to the patient who is usually asymptomatic. The radiologic difficulty presented is that the air and fluid within the pa-

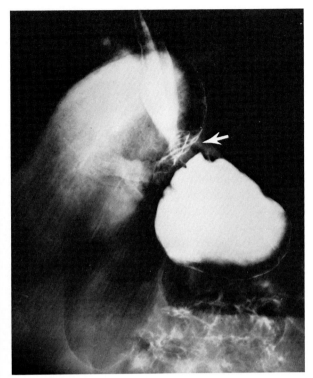

Fig. 14-5 Gastric volvulus associated with rupture of the left diaphragm. Much of the stomach has wrapped itself around the esophagogastric junction, with the area of twist being clearly visible (arrow).

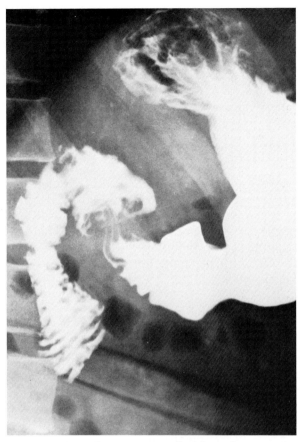

Fig. 14-6 Typical appearance of prolapsed gastric mucosa in the base of the duodenal bulb.

tient's stomach may simulate a large abscess cavity in the posterior regions of the liver on abdominal plain films, and the liver itself may appear as a large, abnormal mass in the upper abdomen.

Prolapse of Gastric Mucosa

Prolapse of gastric mucosa is a frequent radiographic finding of questionable clinical significance. The gastric mucosa is not firmly attached to the underlying muscularis, the intervening areolar tissue allowing considerable independent movement of the mucosa. In response to propulsion by peristalsis, the antral mucosa may prolapse into the base of the duodenal bulb. This can be an intermittent or fixed finding. At surgery or endoscopy, the prolapsed folds are occasionally erythematous and swollen, very rarely showing small bleeding points.

Whether prolapse of gastric mucosa is capable of causing epigastric pain or bleeding in any significant number of patients remains open to question.

The radiographic appearances of prolapsed gastric mucosa are those of an umbrella-like or mushroom-shaped mass of folds in the base of the duodenal bulb (Fig. 14-6). Most often, the caliber of the folds does not differ from those of the gastric mucosa within the stomach. Occasionally, however, the folds are swollen and slightly irregular. Whether this appearance is significant for indicating inflammation of the prolapsed folds has not been firmly established.

A more important radiographic consequence of prolapse of gastric mucosa is that it complicates the search for peptic ulcer in the gastric antrum and duodenal bulb. Barium caught between the adjacent, tortuous folds often forms collections that mimic the presence of peptic ulcer. Occasionally, distension, compression, or passage of a peristaltic wave will cause the folds to return to the stomach, allowing more careful evaluation of both the duodenal bulb and the previously prolapsed region of gastric mucosa.

FUNCTIONAL DISORDERS

With normal gastric peristalsis, propulsive waves begin in the body of the stomach and progress distally in an orderly fashion. Disorders of gastric peristalsis are relatively simple in their expression in that they decrease or eliminate the normal gastric peristalsis and may progress to gastric dilatation.

Gastroparesis Diabeticorum

Gastroparesis diabeticorum is the most common significant disorder of gastric peristalsis in the intact stomach. Many diabetics exhibit gastric peristalsis that is decreased but still present, without associated symptoms. However, in patients with severe or prolonged diabetes, particularly during periods of acute illness, gastroparesis may become complete. This results in functional obstruction and progressive dilatation of the stomach. The patients may then experience upper abdominal pain, nausea, electrolyte disturbances, and occasionally shock.

Radiologically, fully developed diabetic gastroparesis often presents as a series of plain films of the abdomen showing a consistently dilated stomach over several days. An examination with barium suspension or water-soluble contrast materials confirms the lack of gastric peristalsis and that the dilated viscus is in fact the stomach. Although the presence of fluid or food in the stomach often precludes thorough evaluation, one can usually demonstrate that obstruction is not causing the gastric dilatation.

Scleroderma

Scleroderma is a rare cause of gastroparesis. Smooth muscle of the stomach wall may be destroyed in a manner similar to that occurring elsewhere in the gastrointestinal tract. The overall result is decreased peristalsis, delayed emptying, and dilatation. The incidence of significant gastric involvement in scleroderma is only a small fraction of those cases of scleroderma exhibiting changes elsewhere in the gastrointestinal tract.

Gastric Outlet Obstruction

Gastric outlet obstruction at or beyond the pylorus is a frequent cause of gastric dilatation with decreased or absent gastric peristalsis. It is most commonly the result of a pyloric channel ulcer with edema and obstruction of the pylorus. However, obstructing carcinomas of the distal gastric antrum, duodenum, pancreas, and proximal small bowel may also cause gastric dilatation (Fig. 14-7). Gastroparesis in this circumstance results from decompensation of smooth muscle.

Barium sulfate suspension is the best contrast medium for the investigation of an obstructed stomach, since the density of the barium allows it to be maneuvered by gravity into the region of the pylorus and duodenum, often outlining the lesion causing the obstruction. Water-soluble contrast materials are of lesser density and are more quickly diluted by retained gastric secretions. In addition, most of these patients are nauseous and intermittently vomiting, and water-soluble contrast agents in this circumstance may be potentially dangerous in that they cause pulmonary edema if vomited and aspirated.

INFLAMMATORY DISEASES

Inflammatory diseases of the stomach encompass both the most commonly encountered and widely varied gastric pathology of importance to the radiologist. They can be subdivided into the two broad categories of (1) peptic ulcer and related entities and (2) granulomatous, infectious, and other diffuse diseases.

PEPTIC ULCER AND RELATED ENTITIES

Gastric ulcer is the most common disease of the stomach amenable to reliable radiologic diagnosis. It is estimated that 25 percent of all individuals

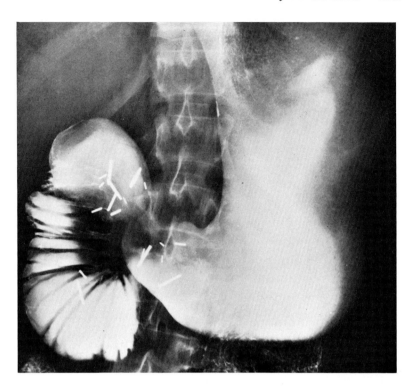

Fig. 14-7 Gastric dilatation and atony due to postsurgical obstruction of the third portion of the duodenum.

develop peptic ulcer, gastric or duodenal, during their lifetime. Only a fraction, however, seek medical care and have a definitive diagnosis established on the basis of radiologic or endoscopic findings.

Gastric ulcers are unusual in children and are most often found in young and middle-aged adults. They also occur in the aged, albeit less commonly, despite the onset of achlorhydria. Gastric ulcers are frequent among alcoholics, and large gastric ulcers of more than 1 cm in size are more common in alcoholics and the economically disadvantaged, the latter seeking care only when the ulcer has become unbearably painful or complicated by perforation, bleeding, or obstruction. Gastric ulcers are frequent in patients routinely taking aspirin or other anti-inflammatory drugs, particularly in patients with rheumatoid arthritis. Although disputed, ulcers may also be more common in patients receiving corticosteroids or cancer chemotherapy.

The distribution of gastric ulcers within the stomach follows a distinct pattern, with ulcers being most common on or near the lesser curvature and distal to the angularis. The location of gastric ulcers may also be specific for certain causative factors. Patients taking aspirin tend to develop ulcers along the distal greater curvature. This is

thought to be due to the ingested aspirin coming to rest in the most dependent area of the stomach, which in an upright individual is the distal greater curvature. The distribution of gastric ulcers and erosions in alcoholics is more diffuse, but mainly in the distal stomach. Elderly patients have a more random distribution of gastric ulcers, which tend to be larger and more resistant to medical therapy. Gastric ulcers in the aged require particularly careful evaluation because of the increased incidence of carcinoma in this age group.

The radiologic diagnosis of gastric ulcer is one of the most completely investigated areas of gastrointestinal radiology, and an entire terminology has developed describing the various radiologic signs found in association with gastric ulcer.

En Face Signs of Benign Gastric Ulcer

Most gastric ulcers will be radiographically demonstrated en face, particularly on compression and double-contrast views. The basic en face sign of gastric ulcer is that of a round or oval collection of barium within the ulcer itself (Figs. 14-8A and B). While most gastric ulcers have a round or oval

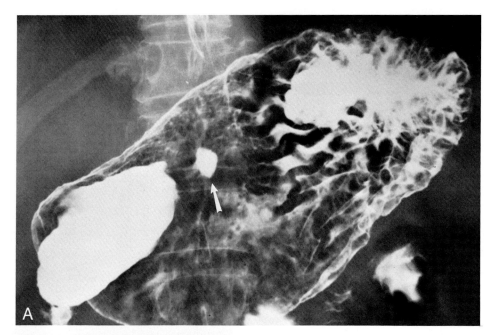

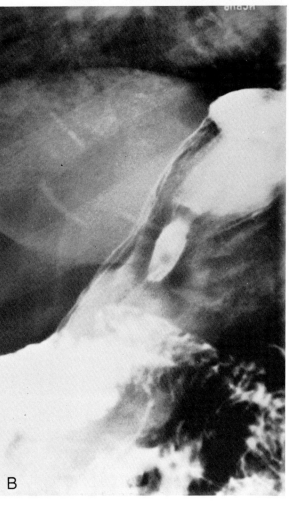

Fig. 14-8 En face signs of benign gastric ulcer. (A) An ovoid collection of barium lying in a benign gastric ulcer (arrow) located on the posterior aspect of the lesser curvature. (B) Large ovoid ulcer situated high on the lesser curvature of the stomach. Note the smooth radiolucent mound of edema surrounding the lesion.

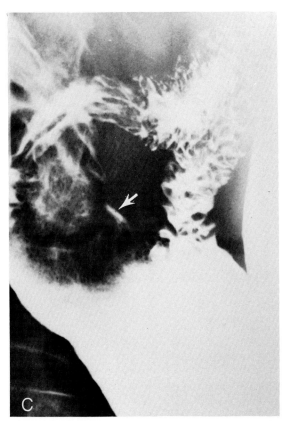

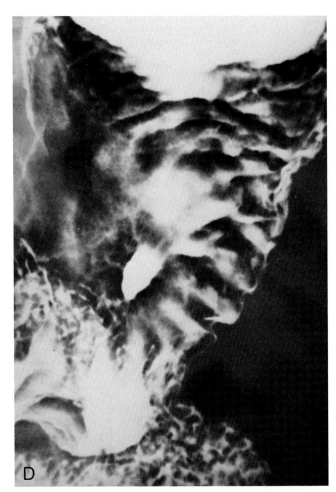

Fig. 14-8 *(continued)* (C) Benign antral ulcer of linear configuration (arrow) as demonstrated with compression filming. (D) Large benign gastric ulcer situated on the posterior wall of the body of the stomach, and surrounded by converging folds and a smooth mound of edema.

contour, a smaller number will have a linear, teardrop, or serpiginous contour (Fig. 14-8C). Some indication of the depth of the ulcer can be obtained on the basis of the density or amount of barium within the ulcer.

With chronicity, an ulcer may be accompanied by a converging fold pattern. This is due to the production of collagenous tissue at the base of the ulcer, which then contracts as it matures. The resulting area of lessened distensibility causes a converging fold pattern to appear when the wall of the stomach is put under tension by distension or compression. The folds entering the region of a benign gastric ulcer usually are smooth in character, without nodular enlargements in the region of the ulcer.

Since peptic ulcers often produce edema of the immediately adjacent region of the wall of the stomach, an edematous "ulcer mound" may be found surrounding the ulcer. This elevated surround is characterized by being rather uniform and smooth (Figs. 14-8B and D). If considerable edema surrounds the ulcer, the mucosal pattern around the ulcer may be effaced, and folds entering the region of the ulcer may disappear or fade before they reach the margin of the ulcer.

Profile Signs of Benign Gastric Ulcer

When the stomach is distended by barium, an ulcer may be clearly visible only when viewed in

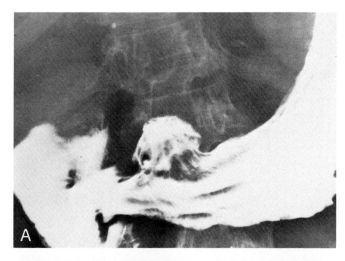

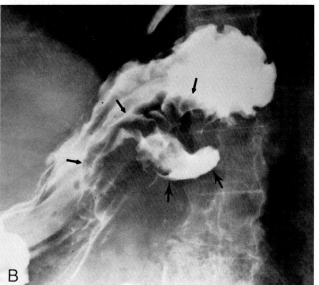

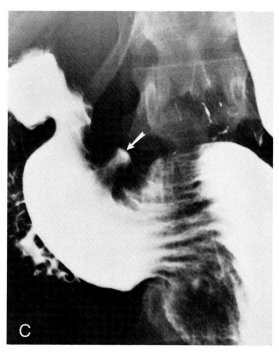

Fig. 14-9 Profile signs of benign gastric ulcer. (A) Large, deep penetrating ulcer situated on the distal lesser curvature. (B) Large penetrating benign gastric ulcer (lower arrows) located high on the posterior wall of the stomach. The ulcer is surrounded by a huge mound of edema (smaller upper arrows). (C) Lesser curvature antral ulcer (arrow) surrounded by its symmetrical mound of edema.

profile. The barium protruding into the ulcer presents a cross-sectional view of both the ulcer and the surrounding mucosal surface. A discussion of the terminology associated with the profile view of a benign gastric ulcer demonstrates the more pertinent characteristics.

The "ulcer niche" was described by Haudek and represents the barium filling the depression or crater constituting the ulcer proper. The contour of the niche clearly indicates the size and depth of

the ulcer, which may vary from 2 or 3 mm to several centimeters. Because the depth of a lesion has considerable diagnostic and prognostic importance, an attempt always should be made to obtain at least one radiograph demonstrating a gastric ulcer in profile. A very deep lesion (Figs. 14-9A and B) suggests possible penetration of the gastric wall and indicates that healing under medical therapy might be prolonged. Also, a relatively deep ulcer is almost always benign.

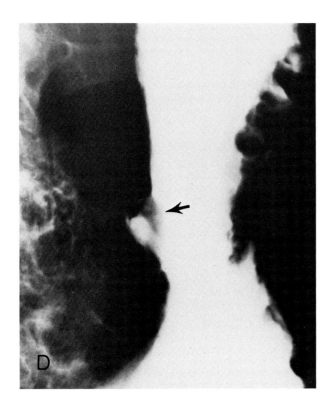

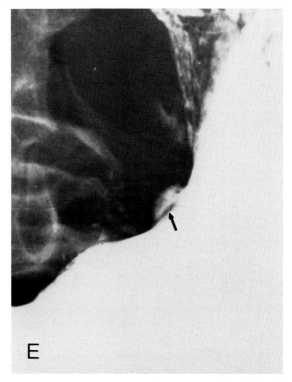

Fig. 14-9 *(continued)* (D) Lesser curvature ulcer of moderate size accompanied by a marked ulcer collar (arrow). (E) Lesser curvature benign gastric ulcer with an easily visible Hampton's line (arrow). (F) Large, deep lesser curvature ulcer accompanied by a prominent incisura (arrow).

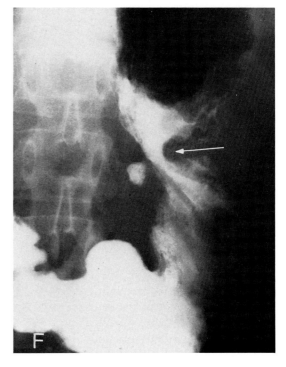

The "ulcer mound," as mentioned above, is an area of edema surrounding the ulcer, and it causes the ulcer to appear as if it is resting on a gently sloped mass (Figs. 14-9B and C). Generally, the inflammation surrounding an ulcer is evenly distributed. On profile views of the ulcer mound, therefore, the raised area on each side of an ulcer tends to be symmetrical.

The "ulcer collar" is seen with ulcers of considerable depth and is a thick rim of radiolucency present at the neck of the ulcer (Fig. 14-9D). It represents inflamed, undermined gastric wall and inflammatory thickening of the neck of the ulcer.

Hampton's line is a very thin radiolucency traversing the neck of a gastric ulcer (Fig. 14-9E). It represents intact, undermined gastric mucosa. Hampton's line is seen far less commonly than the ulcer mound or ulcer collar, but its visualization is considered a virtually 100 percent certain sign that the ulcer is benign.

The *incisura* is an indentation of the greater curvature of the stomach found in relation to a benign ulcer (Fig. 14-9F), but has also been described in relation to gastric carcinoma. Shortening of the lesser curvature is a further secondary sign of gastric ulcer, and usually is the result of fibrosis produced by a large healing or chronic lesser curvature ulcer.

Benign versus Malignant Ulcers

After detecting a gastric ulcer, the radiologist's next obligation is to categorize its radiographic characteristics as benign, malignant, or indeterminant in appearance. Before gastroscopy was widely available, this was of crucial importance, since it often determined whether surgery would be performed.

Radiologic signs of benign ulcers may be characterized as follows:

1. The benign ulcer protrudes beyond the expected contour of the stomach.
2. The benign ulcer has considerable depth in relation to its size at the mucosal surface.
3. The ulcer mound surrounding a benign ulcer is smooth and symmetrical.
4. A smooth ulcer collar across the opening of an ulcer suggests a benign lesion.

5. A Hampton's line is an almost certain sign that an ulcer is benign.
6. An ulcer that is exquisitely round, oval, or linear in contour is usually benign.
7. The folds entering the margin of a benign ulcer or fading into its ulcer mound will be smooth.
8. There are no nodules or masses, other than a symmetrical ulcer mound, in the region of a benign ulcer.
9. Benign ulcers will usually show considerable healing after 2 to 3 weeks of medical therapy and will usually heal completely within 6 to 8 weeks.

Radiologic signs of malignant ulcer tend to be the converse of the above and are as follows:

1. A malignant ulcer is often irregular in contour as seen en face or in profile.
2. The malignant ulcer tends to be shallow in relation to its overall size.
3. The malignant ulcer will generally not protrude beyond the normal contour of the stomach.
4. The margin of the malignant ulcer is usually nodular or otherwise irregular, in contrast to the typically smooth ulcer collar.
5. The malignant ulcer may sit upon a mass that is irregular or asymmetrical, differing from the typical benign ulcer mound.
6. Hampton's line is never seen in conjunction with a malignant ulcer.
7. Folds entering the region of a malignant ulcer may be thickened, irregular, club-shaped, or may

Table 14-1. Gastric Ulcers and Similar Lesions

Developmental
  Aberrant pancreas
  Intramural diverticulum
  Pyloric chamber in pyloric hypertrophy
Inflammatory
  Peptic ulcer
  Crohn's disease
  Tuberculosis
  Syphilis
  Eosinophilic gastritis
  Pseudolymphoma
Neoplastic
  Ulcerated leiomyoma or leiomyosarcoma
  Ulcerated carcinoma
  Ulcerated lymphoma
  Metastatic melanoma

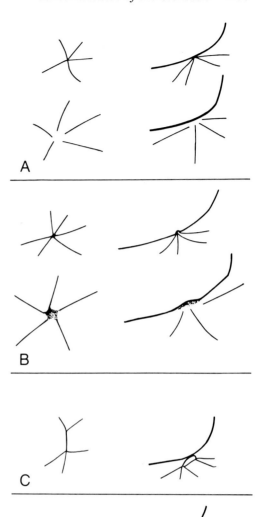

Fig. 14-10 Diagrammatic representation of various forms of gastric ulcer scar. (A) Converging folds. (B) Converging folds with small pit or depression. (C) Linear ulcer scar accompanied by converging folds. (D) Small depression or pit without converging folds (Figs. A–D from Gelfand DW, Ott DJ: Gastric ulcer scars. Radiology 140:37, 1981).

merge prior to reaching the margin of the ulcer.

8. The region surrounding a malignant ulcer is usually rigid and lacking in normal peristalsis due to infiltration of the adjacent wall of the stomach by tumor.

9. Malignant ulcers fail to heal completely with medical therapy, there being very rare exceptions to this rule.

Using the above criteria, it is possible to make a distinction between benign and malignant ulcer in the majority of cases. A very small percentage of ulcers with typically benign macroscopic characteristics will be found on biopsy or at surgery to have histologic evidence of malignancy. However, these covert malignant ulcers virtually always fail to heal completely with medical therapy, thus indicating their potential malignancy. In another small percentage of gastric ulcers, the radiologic appearances will be indeterminate. The nature of these ulcers can be determined by endoscopy with biopsy or by a test of therapy with careful radiologic follow-up.

Although the major differentiation in gastric ulcers is usually between benign peptic ulcer and malignant ulcer, a variety of other entities may present predominantly as ulceration. These are reviewed in Table 14-1.

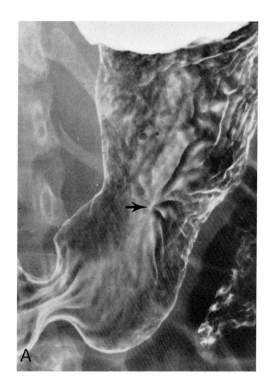

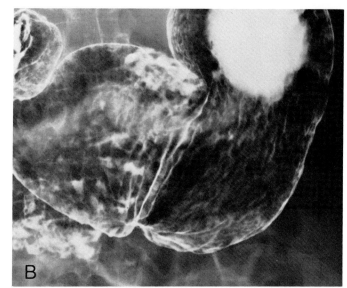

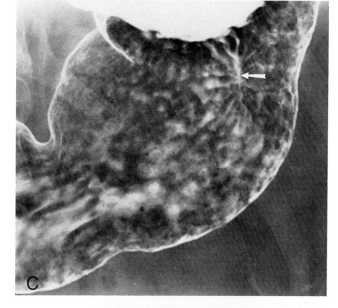

Fig. 14-11 Representative radiographic examples of gastric ulcer scars. (Gelfand DW, Ott DJ: Gastric ulcer scars. Radiology 140:37, 1981.) (A) Ulcer scar visible as converging folds on the posterior wall of the body of the stomach (arrow). (B) Converging folds and an incisura due to an ulcer scar on the greater curvature. (C) Ulcer scar visible as converging folds with a linear center (arrow), the residue of a large, healed gastric ulcer. (D) Gastric ulcer scar visible as nodular converging folds on the posterior wall of the distal antrum. A small central depression is visible. The irregularity of folds in this ulcer scar makes it almost indistinguishable from early gastric cancer.

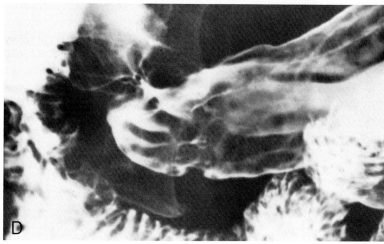

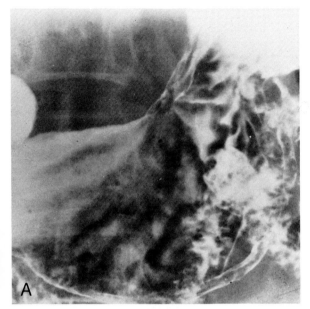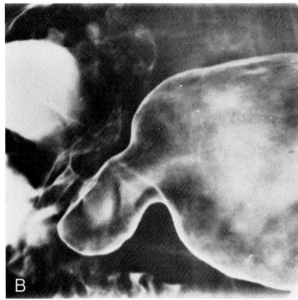

Fig. 14-12 Gross distortions of the stomach produced by healing of gastric ulcers. (A) Shortening of the lesser curvature accompanied by converging folds. (Gelfand DW: The double-contrast upper gastrointestinal series in the Japanese style. Am J Gastroenterol 63:216, 1975.) (B) Antral narrowing following healing of a lesser curvature ulcer. (Gelfand DW, Ott DJ: Gastric ulcer scars. Radiology 140:37, 1981.)

Gastric Ulcer Scars

Gastric ulcers are often accompanied by converging folds, and when the ulcer itself has finally healed, the converging fold pattern usually remains visible. These ulcer scars may be seen as the residue of approximately 50 percent of gastric ulcers, with the larger ulcers more likely to result in a visible scar. As with gastric ulcers, gastric ulcer scars are more common in the distal half of the stomach and at or near the lesser curvature. Radiologic demonstration of gastric ulcer scars is best accomplished with double-contrast technique.

The several appearances of gastric ulcer scar are summarized diagrammatically in Figure 14-10. The most typical presentation is that of a converging fold pattern unaccompanied by obvious ulceration (Figs. 14-11A and B and 14-12A), but at times having a small pit at its center. A gastric ulcer scar also may contain a linear depression in its center (Fig. 14-11C), usually the result of healing of a very large gastric ulcer. The converging folds of a gastric ulcer scar are usually uniform, but irregularity or nodularity of folds accompanying a gastric ulcer scar require differentiation from gastric cancer (Fig. 14-11D). Scarring may also produce deformity of the stomach, usually shortening of the lesser curve or antral narrowing (Fig. 14-12).

Zollinger-Ellison Syndrome

A severe form of peptic ulcer disease is found in the presence of a gastrin-producing pancreatic islet cell tumor, the complex of findings being known as the Zollinger-Ellison syndrome. The presence of the gastrin-producing islet cell tumor causes immense gastric hypersecretion. The usual consequence is large or multiple peptic ulcerations, which may occur anywhere in the distal esophagus, stomach, duodenum, or proximal jejunum. There is also a diffuse and often severe inflammation of mucosal surfaces throughout the upper gastrointestinal tract.

Radiologically, Zollinger-Ellison syndrome presents several characteristic findings. The stomach is full of gastric secretions, which dilute the barium

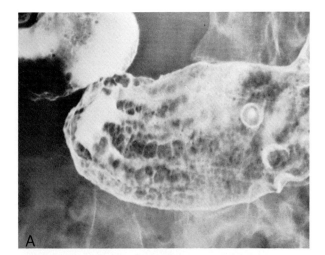

Fig. 14-13 Various manifestations of gastric erosions. (A) Multiple, complete gastric erosions. Some of the lesions contain visible central collections of barium. Others are visible as nodular swellings. Several polyps are also apparent. (B) Multiple gastric erosions seen during compression filming. At least three gastric erosions are demonstrated on this particular spot film (arrows). (C) Multiple gastric erosions demonstrated as nodular swellings of the rugae.

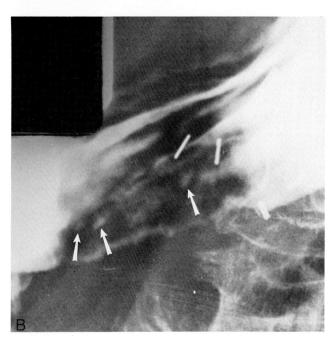

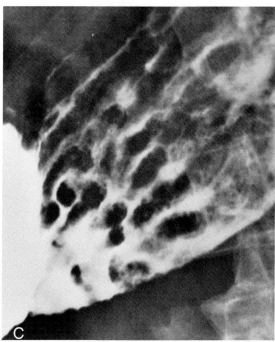

suspension and may render radiologic evaluation of the upper gastrointestinal tract difficult. The gastric rugae, duodenal folds, and proximal jejunal folds are thickened and irregular in contour. Multiple gastric ulcers, often of considerable size, are common. The pancreatic tumor itself is generally small and does not cause sufficient pancreatic enlargement to be detectable during the upper gastrointestinal study.

Gastric Erosions

These small superficial ulcerations exist in a gray area of nomenclature that lies between peptic ulcer disease and gastritis. By definition, gastric erosions are small ulcerations that do not penetrate the muscularis mucosa. They are found with considerable frequency in patients with large intakes of alcohol or aspirin. They are also seen as a result of stress and in patients with severe trauma, particularly following massive head injuries or burns.

Gastric erosions may be demonstrated by either double-contrast technique or careful compression filming. Double-contrast films show best those erosions lying on the posterior wall of the distal half of the stomach (Fig. 14-13A). Careful compression films show erosions on both the anterior and posterior wall of the distal half of the stomach (Fig. 14-13B), but may be difficult to obtain in muscular patients or in those with stomachs lying transversely high in the abdomen. Although it is best to identify the small collection of barium within an erosion, very often only the elevated, nodular edematous region underlying the erosion can be demonstrated (Fig. 14-13C).

Gastric erosions appear radiographically as small, shallow collections of barium generally no more than 1 to 2 mm in diameter and 1 mm in depth. "Complete," "numular," or "variolar" erosions are those surrounded by edema, which raises the adjacent mucosa and produces a slight radiolucent halo around the lesion (Figs. 14-13A and 14-14A). When the edema is absent, the erosions may be termed *incomplete*. The radiologic diagnosis of gastric erosions is most easily made in the presence of multiple complete erosions. Although single erosions and incomplete erosions are often seen endoscopically, their radiologic diagnosis is unreliable, even with excellent technique. Although reported figures are sparse, it is probable that fewer than 50 percent of patients with gastric erosions have their erosions identified radiologically.

GASTRITIS

In its several forms, gastritis is one of the most puzzling areas of gastrointestinal radiology. Part of the difficulty exists because gastritis is often manifested as little more than a change of the mucosal surface from pink to red. Within the limits of physics, it is simply not possible to make such a color-dependent diagnosis radiologically. A second problem is that the various forms of gastritis have never been definitively classified, either pathologically or endoscopically. It is thus difficult to make a precise radiologic diagnosis of gastritis in a situation where the endoscopists and pathologists have not yet agreed on strict criteria for the diagnosis and classification of the entity.

Despite the above difficulties, several distinct and relatively common forms of gastritis are amenable to radiologic diagnosis. There are also several forms of gastritis due to specific infectious agents or associated with known system illnesses, and these may produce distinctive radiologic changes.

The following is a description of those forms of gastritis that are amenable to radiologic diagnosis. It will be recognized that there is considerable overlap in the radiographic findings presented by the several forms of gastritis described. Therefore, all attempts at the radiologic diagnosis of gastritis based on the following descriptions should be made in correlation with available clinical information.

Erosive Gastritis

Multiple gastric erosions are often accompanied by diffuse gastritis, particularly in the gastric antrum. As mentioned earlier, many of these cases are associated with alcohol or aspirin intake. The radiographic findings of gastric erosions have been described above (Fig. 14-13). Radiographically, the diagnosis of erosive gastritis is made on the basis of detection of the erosions since there is little that is radiologically distinctive about the gastritis found in association with the erosions.

Antral Gastritis

Diffuse or patchy inflammation of the antral mucosa, particularly in the prepyloric area, is a common endoscopic finding. Radiologically, more emphasis has been placed upon the diagnosis of antral gastritis in the European literature than in publications emanating from North America. Empirically, there is some association of antral gastritis with peptic ulcer disease and gastric erosions and with the intake of alcohol. On biopsy, antral gastritis may prove to be acute, superficial, atrophic, or erosive in nature.

Radiologically, antral gastritis may be diagnosed on the basis of the following findings (Fig. 14-14).

(Text continues on page 214.)

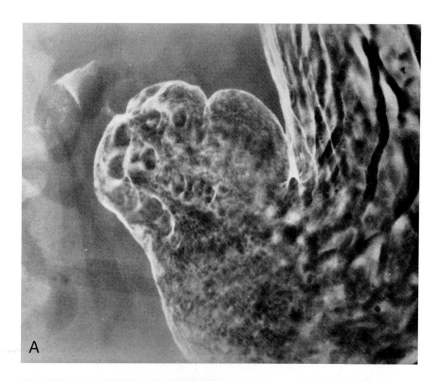

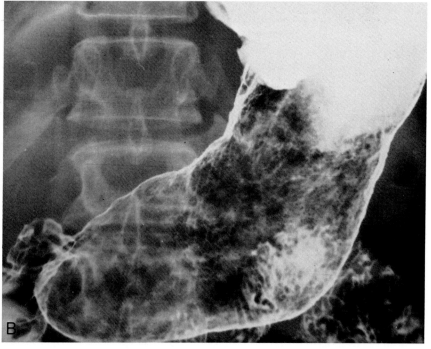

Fig. 14-14 Examples of antral gastritis of differing etiology. (A) Erosive antral gastritis visible mainly as nodular swellings of the mucosa, many of which are arranged in rows. (B) Atrophic antral gastritis with loss of the areae gastricae in the distal stomach.

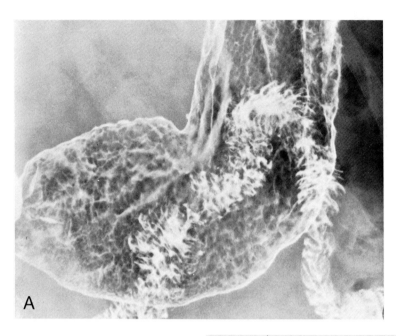

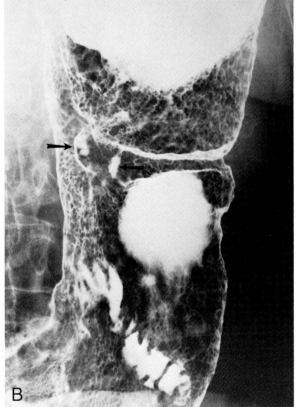

Fig. 14-15 Examples of hypertrophic gastritis. (A) En-larged, irregular areae gastricae associated with a small lesser curvature ulcer. (B) Enlarged, very prominent areae gastricae surrounding two active gastric ulcers (arrows).

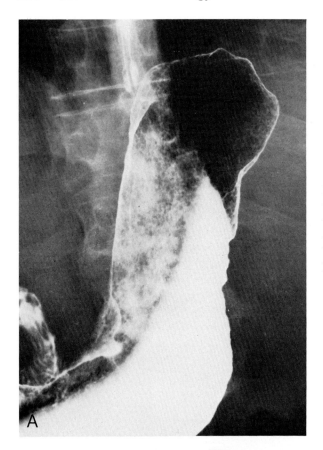

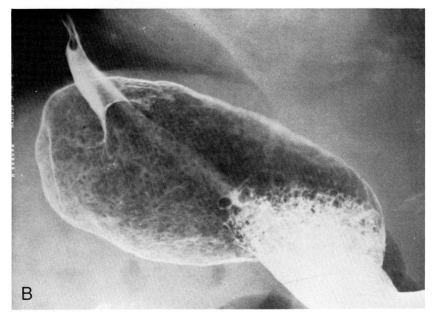

Fig. 14-16 Radiographic manifestations of atrophic gastritis. (A) The proximal stomach is tubular in configuration and completely lacking in folds. Small, prominent areae gastricae are visible. (B) Total absence of rugae in the fundus of the stomach. The areae gastricae are small, prominent, and abnormally separated from each other.

The distal antrum is often less distensible than the remaining portions of the stomach and may be narrow in caliber. There may be an abrupt change in surface pattern from the body of the stomach to the antrum. Folds in the distal antrum may be thickened, nodular, and/or spiculated. On double-contrast examinations, there may be a peculiar transverse orientation of the areae gastricae, which are more prominent in the distal antrum than in the remaining portions of the stomach.

Hypertrophic Gastritis (Hypersecretory Gastropathy)

Hypertrophic gastritis appears endoscopically as erythema and thickening of the gastric rugae, usually throughout the stomach. It is in many cases clinically associated with gastric hypersecretion and with peptic ulcer disease. Hypertrophic gastritis may not be a true gastritis, since inflammatory cells are not a prominent element histologically.

The radiologic appearance of hypertrophic gastritis is that of thickened folds, with prominent areae gastricae visible throughout the stomach (Fig. 14-15). The stomach is often filled with secretions at the onset of the examination. The areae gastricae will often be far larger than the normal 1 or 2 mm size, occasionally reaching 4 or 5 mm in diameter. They also become increasingly angular or polygonal, rather than round or oval. An association between prominence and enlargement of the areae gastricae and the presence of peptic ulcer disease has recently been demonstrated. Thus, when this form of hypertrophic change is seen radiologically, it should be regarded as the signal for a thorough investigation of the stomach and duodenum for peptic ulcer.

Atrophic Gastritis and Gastric Atrophy

Atrophic gastritis and gastric atrophy are common findings in elderly patients and occur with somewhat lesser frequency in younger individuals. By the time a patient has reached 80 years of age, there is an approximately 75 percent chance that the patient will have achlorhydria and the radio-logic signs of atrophic gastritis. Atrophic gastritis and gastric atrophy are capable of causing epigastric pain and early satiety, and they are associated with an increased frequency of gastric polyps and gastric carcinoma. Although the existence of gastric atrophy does not rule out the presence of gastric ulcers, duodenal ulcers are virtually never found in these patients.

The radiologic findings of gastric atrophy and atrophic gastritis are as follows:

1. Almost total lack of normal folds in the proximal two-thirds of the stomach; a few folds may be visible in the antrum (Fig. 14-16).
2. A tubular appearance of the overall shape of the stomach, particularly on upright films (Fig. 14-16A).
3. Small, prominent areae gastricae separated by widened grooves (Fig. 14-16B).
4. In many cases, virtual absence of the areae gastricae.

Menetrier's Disease

In the rare case of Menetrier's disease, the gastric mucosa appears to be wildly hypertrophic, with greatly thickened mucosal folds resembling the surface of the cerebral cortex. These changes are most marked in the proximal stomach and along the greater curvature, with the gastric antrum being free of disease. Histologically, there is inflammation, atrophy, metaplasia, and cystic glandular degeneration. Clinically, the patients present with epigastric pain, achlorhydria, and gastrointestinal protein loss, all of these symptoms being inconstant features of the disease.

Radiologically, the disease is characterized by thick, nodular, or mass-like folds located primarily in the proximal stomach and along the greater curvature. Unlike tumor infiltration causing similar hyper-rugosity, the gastric wall is not rigid. Nevertheless, radiographic differentiation of Menetrier's disease from gastric carcinoma or lymphoma may be difficult, and endoscopy is usually performed to establish the diagnosis histologically and to rule out malignancy. A listing of potential causes of thickened gastric folds is presented in Table 14-2.

Table 14-2. Thick Gastric Folds

Noninflammatory
  Normal
  Varices
  Hypersecretory state°
  Amyloidosis
Inflammatory
  Hypertrophic gastritis°
  Peptic ulcer
  Zollinger-Ellison syndrome
  Crohn's disease
  Menetrier's disease
  Eosinophilic gastritis
  Tuberculosis
  Postirradiation gastritis
  Corrosive gastritis
  Pancreatitis
  Strongyloidiasis
  Phlegmonous gastritis
  Pseudolymphoma
Neoplastic
  Carcinoma
  Metastatic neoplasm
  Invasive pancreatic carcinoma
  Lymphoma
  Gastric polyposis

°May be the same entity.

Crohn's Disease

In a substantial minority of patients with well-developed Crohn's disease elsewhere in the gastrointestinal tract, endoscopic and histologic evidence of at least minimal Crohn's disease in the stomach will be present. Radiologically, however, gastric involvement will be detected less frequently because of the minimal involvement. Nevertheless, because of the reasonable incidence of Crohn's disease in the stomach, a careful radiologic assessment of the stomach should be performed in conjunction with any small bowel series intended to evaluate known small bowel involvement.

The radiologic findings in Crohn's disease of the stomach in its early stages are minimal and nonspecific (Fig. 14-17). One early finding is a subtle rearrangement of the fold pattern of the stomach, with prominent folds coursing downward from the body of the stomach toward the greater curvature and absence of the normal rugae paralleling the curvatures in the gastric antrum. Another early finding is the presence of aphthoid ulcers, which are small erosions surrounded by a halo of edema. However, their discovery in the stomach of a patient with Crohn's disease elsewhere does not incontrovertibly establish the diagnosis of gastric

Crohn's disease, since coexistent gastritis, gastric erosions, or peptic ulcer disease is as likely in these patients as in the general population.

With more severe involvement by Crohn's disease, the gastric folds become more obviously thickened and more extensive ulcerations may be seen, particularly in the region of the pylorus (Fig. 14-18A). With severe involvement, ulceration and fibrosis may obliterate the demarcation between the distal antrum, pyloric channel, and duodenal bulb, changing the pyloroduodenal area into an irregular region without well-defined landmarks (Fig. 14-18B). Obliteration of the pyloric canal, characteristic of advanced Crohn's disease of the stomach and duodenum, may also be seen in gastroduodenal tuberculosis and eosinophilic gastritis.

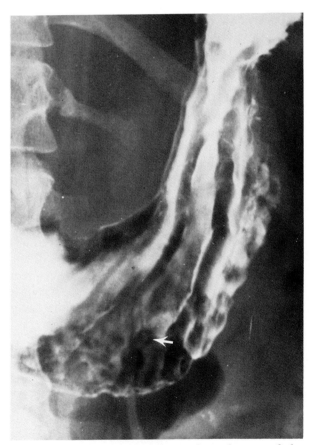

Fig. 14-17 Example of early Crohn's disease of the stomach showing thickened folds coursing down to the greater curvature, as well as the presence of one or more aphthoid ulcers (arrow).

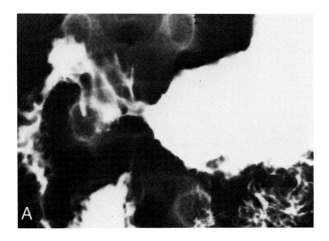

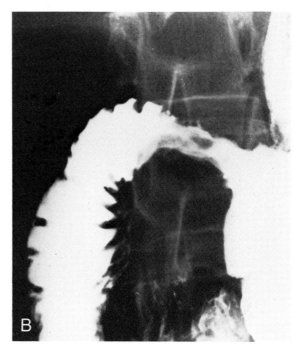

Fig. 14-18 Two cases of advanced Crohn's disease of the stomach, with the most severe changes typically located distally. (A) Ulceration, contraction, and deformity of the distal antrum, pyloric canal, and duodenal bulb. (B) Destruction of the normal landmarks of the pyloric region.

Eosinophilic Gastritis

Gastritis presenting with an abundance of eosinophils histologically may take two general forms and may represent more than a single disease process. The first type of eosinophilic gastritis is that of a diffuse, ulcerating lesion in large measure duplicating the various radiographic findings of Crohn's disease or tuberculosis. This diffuse form of eosinophilic gastritis is often associated with eosinophilic lesions elsewhere in the gastrointestinal tract. Many of these patients have a history of allergy, and there is speculation that certain cases are the result of occult parasitic infestation.

The second variety of eosinophilic gastric disease is that of a polypoid lesion. On histologic investigation there is a dense fibrous stroma with heavy inflammatory infiltration by eosinophils.

Pseudolymphoma

Pseudolymphoma (lymphoreticular hyperplasia of the stomach) is an inflammatory state with the ability to mimic both true lymphoma and carcinoma in its gross pathologic and radiographic appearances. The usual presentation is that of an ulcerating and/or infiltrating lesion, often involving an extensive portion of the stomach. Differentiation from malignancy may be impossible on the basis of the radiologic examination and may be difficult histologically as well. Clinically, most patients present with some combination of epigastric pain, nausea, vomiting, and weight loss. The disease occurs predominantly in males and is relatively rare.

Tuberculosis

Tuberculosis of the stomach is unusual, being far less common than tuberculosis of the small bowel or colon. Gastric tuberculosis may occur as a large, localized ulceration simulating peptic ulcer or as an infiltrating lesion producing more typical granulomatous and hyperplastic changes. This latter type may destroy the landmarks of the pyloric canal. Since gastric tuberculosis may closely mimic other ulcerative, granulomatous, and neoplastic diseases, biopsy is generally required to establish

218 Gastrointestinal Radiology

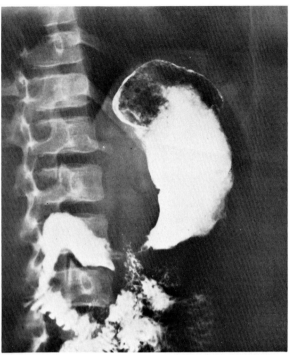

Fig. 14-19 Gastric syphilis causing a funnel-shaped contraction of the gastric antrum. (Willeford G, Childers JH, Hepner WR: Gumma of the stomach in congenital syphilis. Pediatrics 10:162, 1952. Copyright American Academy of Pediatrics 1952.)

the diagnosis by demonstration of the tubercle bacilli.

Histoplasmosis

Gastric histoplasmosis is usually found in association with severe involvement of other organs by this disease. Cases of gastric histoplasmosis are extremely rare and radiographic findings are variable, ranging from large, discrete ulcers to infiltrating disease simulating tuberculosis, carcinoma, and lymphoma.

Candidiasis

Candidiasis very rarely involves the stomach, usually occurring as an opportunistic infection in patients with suppressed immunity. Discrete polypoid lesions, multiple nodules, and aphthoid ulcers have been described.

Gastric Syphilis

Gastric syphilis may present in at least three varieties. The most common, and not at all unusual prior to the advent of antibiotics, was that of an infiltrating lesion causing diffuse constriction of the distal stomach similar to that of linitis plastica (Fig. 14-19). Two other presentations of gastric syphilis are also mentioned in the literature but are less common: masses caused by gummas, and constricting lesions of the body or angularis of the stomach.

Amyloidosis of the Stomach

Amyloidosis of the stomach is another rare entity and is even less frequently seen than eosinophilic gastritis. Amyloidosis of the stomach usually occurs as a manifestation of the primary form of amyloidosis. It causes irregular thickening of the wall, with rigidity and narrowing of the lumen, usually affecting the distal stomach. It is one of the several rarely encountered causes of thickened gastric folds listed in Table 14-2.

Corrosive Gastritis

Ingestion of corrosives may produce a severe gastritis, occasionally resulting in gastric necrosis and death. In general, acidic agents are more injurious to the stomach than alkaline chemicals. The normally acid gastric secretions have the ability to neutralize moderate amounts of ingested alkaline substances, such as the lye used in drain cleaners. On the other hand, gastric secretions, being acid, have no ability to neutralize ingested acids. Probably the most common cause of severe corrosive gastritis is the suicidal ingestion of household bleach, which is an acidic solution of sodium hypochlorite.

The initial consequence of ingesting a corrosive agent is a rapid necrosis of the gastric mucosa. In severe cases the full thickness of the gastric wall may become necrotic, leading to perforation. In less severe cases, the denuded gastric wall becomes progressively fibrotic. The result is a deformed, contracted, and occasionally obstructed stomach. The final outcome is often total gastrectomy.

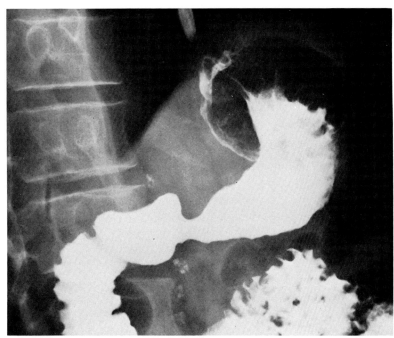

Fig. 14-20 Late manifestation of corrosive gastritis showing severe fibrotic contraction of the entire stomach.

The radiographic findings in corrosive gastritis depend on the severity of the chemical insult and the time interval after ingestion. Initially, one sees swelling and irregularity of the gastric rugae. As the mucosa sloughs, barium may flow between it and the remaining gastric wall. After a week or two, fibrotic contraction of the stomach begins to occur, quickly producing a shrunken appearance without visible folds similar to that of linitis plastica or syphilis (Fig. 14-20).

Emphysematous Gastritis and Intramural Gastric Emphysema

The presence of air within the wall of the stomach may be the result of any of several causative factors, ranging in severity from almost totally benign to life threatening. Because of the potential severity of certain of the associated disease processes, visualization of air within the wall of the stomach should be regarded as an alarming radiographic finding. The causes of emphysematous gastritis and intramural gastric emphysema include the following:

1. *Infection by gas-producing organisms* may cause localized accumulation of gas within the wall of the stomach. This is a rare but extremely serious disease process that may be amenable to treatment by antibiotics.

2. In *corrosive gastritis,* air is infrequently seen within the wall of the stomach. Usually, this is a sign of necrosis of the gastric wall and impending perforation.

3. *Gastric infarction,* usually the result of compromise of the gastric blood supply by volvulus or surgery, may cause necrosis of the stomach, allowing air to dissect within the gastric wall.

4. *Violent vomiting* may cause tears of the gastric mucosa, allowing gas to dissect within the wall of the stomach.

5. *Dissection of air in the mediastinum and retroperitoneal tissues,* often originating in a ruptured pulmonary bleb, may lead to dissection of air into the wall of the stomach in a process similar to the benign form of pneumatosis intestinalis.

Radiologic findings in emphysematous gastritis or intramural gastric emphysema are those of thin, arcuate collections of gas following the contour of the gastric wall. These are most easily seen on plain films of the upper abdomen. Careful inspection of films taken during barium studies is required to detect the intramural gas collections, since the greater radiographic penetrance used during bar-

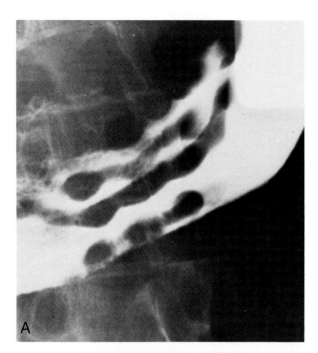

Fig. 14-21 Examples of gastric polyps. (A) Hyperplastic polyps oriented along the rugae. (B) Multiple adenomatous polyps.

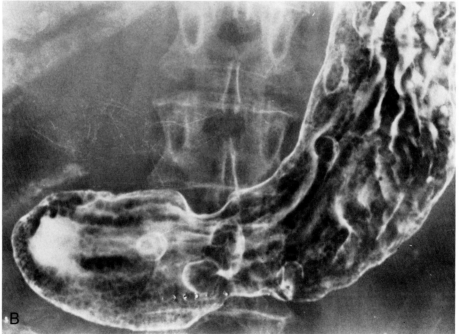

ium examinations frequently overexposes the soft tissues adjacent to the barium.

BENIGN NEOPLASMS AND NEOPLASTIC-LIKE DISEASES

Benign neoplasms and neoplastic-like diseases fall into several categories: tumors of mucosal origin, tumors of mesenchymal origin, cysts and duplications, and aberrant pancreatic tissue. While there can be considerable resemblance among these radiologically, the majority of cases will present with findings leading either to a specific diagnosis or to a short list of likely possibilities. The important considerations are the size and contour of the lesion, its location, its numbers, and its association with other disease entities.

Gastric Polyps

Gastric polyps occur in two major varieties: the more numerous hyperplastic polyps and the larger but less common adenomatous polyps. They are frequently found in association with gastric achlorhydria and atrophic gastritis and are most often seen in the elderly. Polyps may be single or multiple and both types may occur in the same patient. Hyperplastic polyps have no malignant potential, but there is a very small chance that an individual adenomatous polyp may degenerate into gastric carcinoma. Thus, patients with gastric polyps, particularly those with large lesions or large numbers of lesions, should be carefully evaluated radiologically and endoscopically. If technically possible, adenomatous polyps should be removed endoscopically as a prophylactic measure.

Hyperplastic polyps are smooth or ovoid lesions generally smaller than 1 cm (Fig. 14-21A), although they may occasionally be larger. Adenomatous polyps are often larger than 1 cm (Fig. 14-21B), but clear differentiation between them and hyperplastic polyps is not always possible. Many polyps appear to sit on a broad base on top of the gastric folds themselves. Less frequently, polyps may develop a stalk. Polyps in the distal antrum, particularly, have a tendency to develop a long stalk and they may then prolapse through the

Table 14-3. Small Gastric-Filling Defects
Noninflammatory
Aberrant pancreas
Duplication cyst
Varix
Enlarged fold
Inflammatory
Gastric erosion
Peptic ulcer
Eosinophilic polypoid lesion
Polypoid pseudolymphoma
Neoplastic
Adenomatous polyp
Peutz-Jehgers disease
Cronkhite-Canada syndrome
Benign mesenchymal tumor
Leiomyoma
Lipoma
Angioma
Fibroma
Neurilemmoma
Villous adenoma
Carcinoid
Lymphoma
Metastatic lesion

pyloric canal into the duodenal bulb where they can be mistaken for duodenal tumors.

The radiologic criteria for establishing the benign nature of a gastric polyp are similar to those used in evaluating polyps of the colon. Benign polyps, most of which will be hyperplastic, tend to be small, usually less than 1 cm in diameter, and clearly round or oval. Their surface should be smooth, rather than crenelated or irregular. Although many benign polyps in the stomach will be on a broad base, they are more certain to be benign if a stalk can be identified. A particular hazard exists where polyps are numerous, since it is difficult to thoroughly evaluate all of the polyps present in the stomach under this circumstance. This is complicated by the fact that the likelihood of eventual malignant change is significant when many adenomatous polyps are present. In the presence of numerous polypoid lesions, endoscopic inspection with biopsy and/or removal of any suspicious lesions should be performed.

Other lesions may simulate the appearance of a small, hyperplastic or round adenomatous polyp (Table 14-3). Virtually any of the mesenchymal, intramural tumors can present as a small, round lesion in the early stages of growth. In occasional cases of Menetrier's disease, the enlargement of

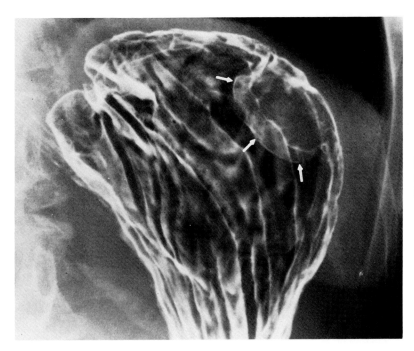

Fig. 14-22 Leiomyoma of smooth spherical appearance (arrows) located in the fundus of the stomach.

folds may assume a polypoid appearance, presenting in a manner similar to that of multiple adenomatous polyps. Occasionally, blood-borne intramural metastases may present as small, spherical lesions if the overlying mucosa has not yet been destroyed. Also, an occasional carcinoid tumor or villous adenoma may present in the stomach as a small, polypoid lesion.

Villous Adenoma

Villous adenoma occur very infrequently in the stomach and generally present as polypoid lesions somewhat larger and more irregular in contour than the typical adenomatous polyp. On histologic inspection, a considerable fraction of gastric villous adenomas will be found to be malignant. Radiologically they are difficult to differentiate from an adenoma or polypoid carcinoma.

Carcinoid Tumors

The incidence of carcinoid tumors in the stomach is far less than in the ileum. The majority of reported gastric carcinoid tumors have presented as polypoid, well-defined lesions on a broad base, usually slightly larger than the typical adenomatous polyp. Most carcinoid tumors are malignant, and it is difficult to predict the natural history of a carcinoid tumor on the basis of its macroscopic or radiologic appearance. Indeed, a substantial minority of benign-appearing gastric carcinoids will be found to have metastasized by the time of discovery.

Tumors of Mesenchymal Origin

The broad category of tumors of mesenchymal origin occurs in the stomach with approximately the same frequency as seen elsewhere in the gastrointestinal tract. As elsewhere, the most common lesion is the *leiomyoma*. Additional types in this category include *lipoma*, *fibroma*, *angioma*, *neurilemmoma*, and *neurofibroma*. When first seen radiographically, these lesions usually present as spherical tumors smoothly covered by mucosa and sharply demarcated at their junction with the normal surrounding stomach wall (Fig. 14-22).

Several of the above mesenchymal tumors may present with individual characteristics allowing a specific diagnosis. Leiomyomas tend to outgrow

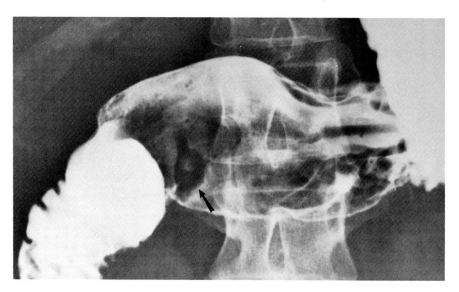

Fig. 14-23 Pancreatic rest visible in the distal stomach near the greater curvature. A small ulcer-like dimple is visible and is typical of these lesions.

their blood supply and ulcerate, the resulting ulceration often being visible radiologically. Their clinical presentation is often that of gastrointestinal bleeding. Lipomas are usually deformable, which may be demonstrable during compression filming. Also, their relative radiolucency may be detectable, especially if the lesion is large. Angiomas, although taking origin from mesenchymal elements, may protrude into the gastric lumen, with an appearance similar to that of adenomatous polyps. Furthermore, angiomas may be deformable, and more than one lesion may be present.

Duplication Cysts

Duplication cysts are congenital abnormalities consisting of cyst-like lesions containing fluid and lined by gastric mucosa. They may present as either extrinsic or intramural lesions and tend to be located in the distal stomach. When intramural in location, a gastric duplication of modest size may present an appearance identical to a benign mesenchymal tumor.

Aberrant Pancreas

Pancreatic tissue of rather normal architecture may develop in the wall of the distal stomach or duodenal loop. Generally, there are no symptoms associated with the presence of aberrant pancreatic tissue in these locations. Their importance is their ability to mimic the presence of a small ulcer or neoplasm. Radiographically, aberrant pancreatic tissue takes the form of a polypoid or plaque-like mass in the distal stomach, usually on the distal greater curvature (Fig. 14-23). The lesion is always broad based, and frequently there is a small ulcer-like dimple on the surface of the lesion caused by the presence of an incompletely formed pancreatic duct.

MALIGNANT NEOPLASMS

Malignant neoplasms of the stomach consist mainly of carcinomas and lymphomas, the former being more common. Malignancies of spindle cell origin are rare. Among the gastric malignancies, the varied presentations of gastric carcinoma have been most extensively described.

CARCINOMA OF THE STOMACH

Although extremely prevalent in Japan, carcinoma of the stomach is a decreasing problem in Western countries. However, the considerable incidence of carcinoma of the stomach in Japan has stimulated development of sophisticated diagnostic techniques for the diagnosis and classification of

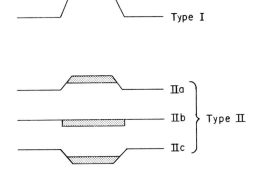

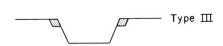

Fig. 14-24 Diagrammatic representation of the Japanese classification of early gastric cancer. Type I is a protruding lesion. Type III is a malignant ulceration. Type II lesions involve minimal protrusion or depression and are the most subtle and difficult to detect.

carcinoma of the stomach, particularly in its early stages.

Early Gastric Cancer

Early gastric cancer is defined as a lesion that has not invaded the muscularis propria and is in effect still confined to the mucosa. The Japanese morphologic classification of these early gastric lesions, now almost universally accepted, is presented in Figure 14-24.

While there is considerable variation in the presentation of early gastric cancer, the most common form is that of a slightly depressed, irregular lesion accompanied by clubbed or irregular converging folds (Figs. 14-25A and B). The association of converging folds with early gastric cancer is due to the scirrhotic reaction induced in the gastric wall by many of these malignancies. Within the more central portions of the lesion, an element of nodularity can usually be discerned. Often, the folds at the margin of the lesion are slightly widened or club-shaped or may merge in a plaque-like fashion as they enter the region of the depressed area. This presentation of early gastric cancer conforms to the Japanese classification IIc. Early lesions presenting as classification type I take the form of a plaque-like or polypoid elevation of the gastric mucosa (Fig. 14-25C).

Malignant Ulcer

One of the early, classic descriptions in gastrointestinal radiology is that of the malignant ulcer, a carcinoma of the stomach that has ulcerated. In its earliest form, the malignant ulcer is simply an early gastric cancer that has ulcerated within its central region. For early gastric cancer, this conforms to the Japanese classification type IIc plus III. Where most of the malignancy has been eroded by ulceration, differentiation from benign gastric ulcer may be quite difficult.

In its more advanced stages, a malignant ulcer can be conceived of as a carcinomatous mass that has ulcerated, with much of the remaining mass being obvious radiologically (Fig. 14-26A). Carman's meniscus sign was an early attempt to describe the radiologic findings in this type of lesion. In the original publication, Carman's meniscus was an ulcer excavating a mass (Fig. 14-26B).

Advanced Gastric Cancers

At some point in their development, most gastric carcinomas will assume the typical appearances of a large gastrointestinal carcinoma. At this stage, an obvious, irregularly contoured mass will be visible. A large ulceration may or may not be present within the mass, and the mass-like element domi-

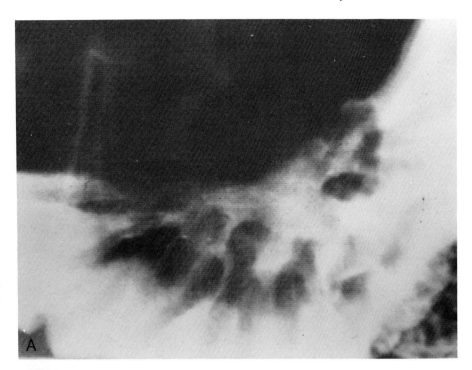

Fig. 14-25 Examples of early gastric cancer. (A) Type IIc lesion with depressed center and nodular, club-shaped converging folds as demonstrated by compression. (Gelfand DW, Ott DJ: Gastric ulcer scars. Radiology 140:37, 1981). (B) Type IIc lesion demonstrated on double-contrast view. (Gelfand DW: The double-contrast upper gastrointestinal series in the Japanese style. Am J Gastroenterol 63: 216, 1975.) (C) Type IIa lesion of plaque-like configuration (arrow).

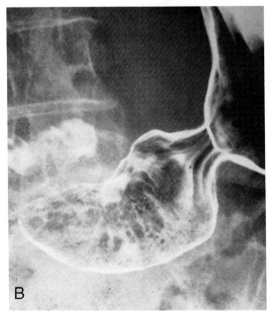

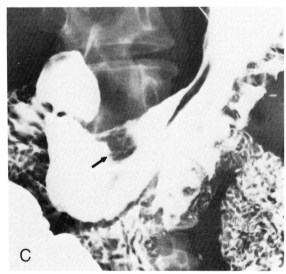

nates the lesion. The radiographic diagnosis of this sort of advanced cancer is a challenge only in the sense of having to differentiate between gastric cancer and lymphoma.

The radiographic appearances of a well-developed carcinoma are usually those of an irregularly contoured mass of considerable size (Figs. 14-27A and B). Eventually, the tumor may completely en-

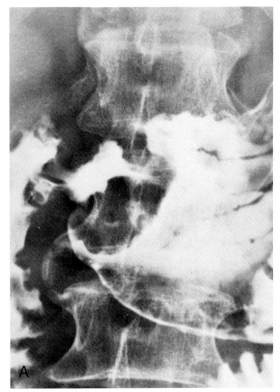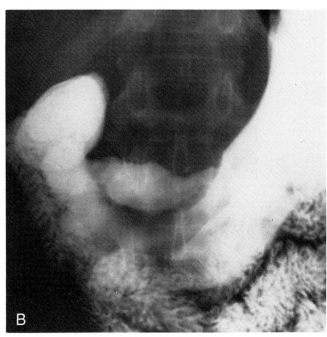

Fig. 14-26 Examples of advanced ulcerating gastric carcinoma. (A) Large ulcerating mass situated at the entrance of the pyloric canal. (B) Large lesser curvature malignant ulcer demonstrating a Carman's meniscus sign.

circle the stomach (Fig. 14-27C) and attain considerable size, involving most of the stomach (Fig. 14-27D). At the margins of the lesion, there may be a "shelf" or angular demarcation. The irregular surface of the lesion often has the appearance of the surface of a cauliflower (Figs. 14-27A and B), and one or more large ulcerations may be present. If located in the antral region, a large encircling carcinoma may partially or completely obstruct the outlet of the stomach (Fig. 14-27C).

A subtle sign of gastric cancer is stiffening of a segment of the gastric wall. This may be noted as straightening of the wall and/or lessened distensibility (Fig. 14-28A). The rigid area may fail to flex with peristalsis, and this finding has been described as a "board floating on the waves" (Fig. 14-28B).

Most frankly malignant-appearing gastric lesions are carcinomas, with a minority being lymphomas. However, a variety of other malignant and nonma-lignant diseases may suggest the presence of carcinoma or lymphoma (Table 14-4) and must be considered in the differential diagnosis under the appropriate circumstances.

Linitis Plastica

Carcinoma of the stomach not infrequently presents as diffuse infiltration and thickening of a considerable portion of the stomach, occasionally the entire stomach. The latter is the "leather bottle" stomach described in pathology texts. Histologically, the tumor differs from other carcinomas of the stomach in the extent of fibrosis and infiltration of carcinomatous cells. The overlying mucosa is often largely intact, although infiltrated by carcinoma, and large ulcers are not a dominant aspect.

Radiologically, linitis plastica is seen as a stomach decreased in size and lacking the normal rugal

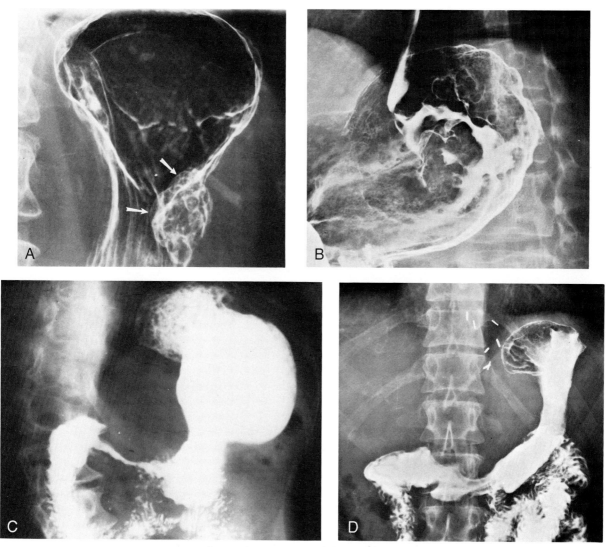

Fig. 14-27 Large gastric carcinomas of typical appearance. (A) Irregular polypoid lesion in the proximal stomach (arrows). (B) Large lesion of cauliflower configuration at the esophagogastric junction. (C) Large carcinoma encircling and partially obstructing the distal antrum. (D) Linitis plastica involving most of the stomach.

pattern (Fig. 14-27D). The mucosal surface often has a smooth or finely granular appearance atypical of other forms of malignancy. The diameter of the lumen of the stomach is usually decreased in the involved areas, with an obvious rigidity, lack of distensibility, and absence of peristalsis. Although the radiologic diagnosis is seldom difficult, other lesions may produce a similar appearance and should be considered in the differential diagnosis when clinically appropriate (Table 14-5).

Gastric Lymphoma

Lymphoma of the stomach is less common than gastric carcinoma. The majority of gastric lymphomas are of the non-Hodgkin's variety, although Hodgkin's disease of the stomach occasionally occurs. Lymphoma most often involves the stomach primarily or may less commonly be invasive from adjacent sites, particularly the periaortic lymph nodes.

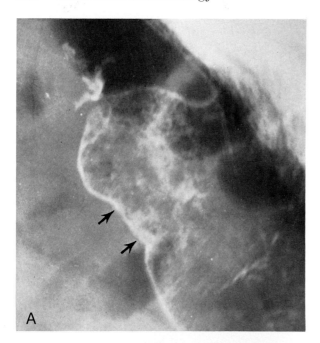

Fig. 14-28 Subtle gastric carcinomas causing stiffening of a segment of the gastric wall. (A) Retraction and stiffening of the distal greater curvature due to a small gastric carcinoma (arrows). The lesion was not initially detected on this study. (Gelfand DW, Ott DJ, Tritico R: Causes of error in gastrointestinal radiology: I. Upper gastrointestinal examination. Gastrointest Radiol 5:91, 1980.) (B) Plaque-like carcinoma causing stiffness of a segment of the greater curvature and demonstrating the phenomenon of "a board floating on the waves."

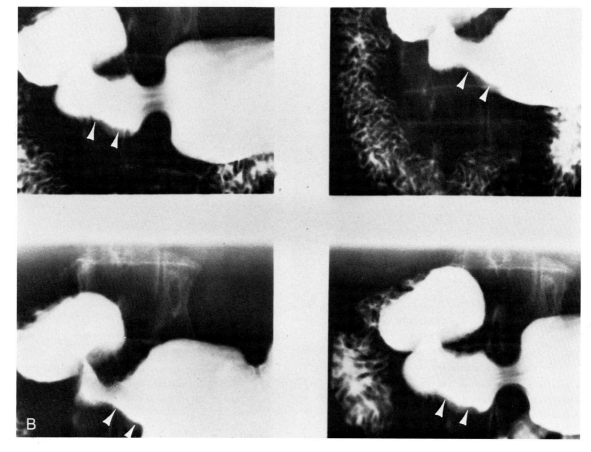

**Table 14-4. Localized
Malignant-Appearing
Gastric Lesions**

Nonmalignant
  Peptic ulcer
  Ulcer scar
  Gastric varices
  Confluent adenomatous polyps
  Menetrier's disease
  Crohn's disease
  Pseudolymphoma
  Tuberculosis
  Eosinophilic gastritis
  Syphilis
  Amyloidosis
  Prolapsing hiatal hernia
Malignant
  Carcinoma
  Lymphoma — primary
  Lymphoma — invasive
  Invasive pancreatic carcinoma
  Metastatic lesion

**Table 14-5. Gastric Lesions
Presenting as Linitis Plastica**

Carcinoma
Corrosive gastritis
Crohn's disease
Syphilis
Tuberculosis
Eosinophilic gastritis
Metastatic carcinoma
Lymphoma
Pseudolymphoma

Primary lymphoma may mimic any of the forms of gastric carcinoma. Most commonly, a primary lymphoma takes the form of an infiltrating lesion involving large areas of the stomach. It is one of the more frequent causes of thickening of the gastric folds (Table 14-2). In this presentation, the gastric wall is rigid, with considerable nodularity or thickening of the rugae (Figs. 14-29A and B). Ulcerations may be scattered over the involved area. A second presentation is that of a bulky, more localized mass, often ulcerated and quite similar to that seen in advanced gastric carcinoma. Rarely, lymphoma will present as a malignant ulcer.

Secondary involvement by lymphoma may occur when a large lymphomatous mass originating in the periaortic lymph nodes infiltrates the posterior wall of the stomach. The stomach is displaced anteriorly in a broad curve, and distorted folds and/or ulceration occasionally may be detected on the posterior wall due to invasion of the gastric wall by the lymphoma.

Metastatic lymphoma of the blood-born type occurs but is rare. This form occasionally presents as target lesions with dimpled or ulcerated centers.

MALIGNANT MESENCHYMAL TUMORS

Infrequently, malignant degeneration of a mesenchymal tumor, usually a leiomyosarcoma, will be encountered in the stomach. Leiomyosarcomas differ radiologically from benign leiomyomas primarily on the basis of size.

METASTATIC MALIGNANCIES

Occasionally, malignancies originating in distant organs will send blood-borne metastases to the wall of the stomach (Fig. 14-30). The most common are carcinoma of the breast, malignant melanoma, carcinoma of the lung, choriocarcinoma, and thyroid carcinoma in roughly that order. In their earliest stages, before destroying overlying mucosa, blood-born metastatic malignancies may present as intramural or submucosal nodules (Fig. 14-30A). As the lesions progress, however, they may assume any of the more obviously malignant forms described for carcinoma or lymphoma of the stomach. Two of the above types of metastatic lesions have propensities that should be noted. Malignant melanoma has a tendency to produce target or bulls-eye lesions, with central dimpling. Carcinoma of the breast may infiltrate the stomach wall without disrupting the overlying mucosa, causing lack of distensibility, rigidity, and a nodular or otherwise irregular mucosal surface in the involved area (Fig. 14-30B).

EXTRINSIC MASSES

The stomach is a very mobile structure, and large masses adjacent to it often cause readily discernible displacement. Extrinsic masses capable of displacing the stomach fall into three general categories: retrogastric masses, liver enlargement and splenic enlargement.

Retrogastric masses displace the stomach anteri-

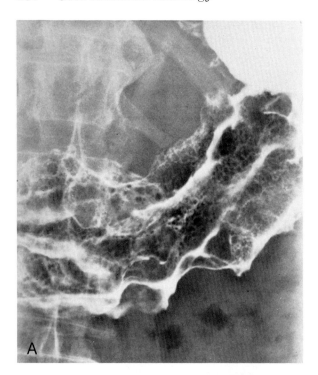

Fig. 14-29 Examples of widely infiltrating primary lymphoma of the stomach. (A) Diffuse thickening and irregularity of the gastric folds. (B) Nodular irregularity of the mucosal surface of almost the entire stomach.

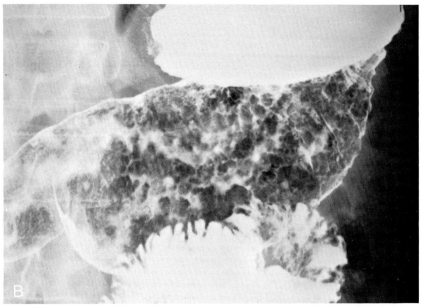

orly. In approximate order of frequency, these retrogastric masses are pancreatic tumors and cysts; generalized pancreatic enlargement secondary to pancreatitis; periaortic lymph node enlargement by metastatic malignancy or lymphoma; left renal masses; and lesser sac abscesses. Retrogastric masses of the above origins generally cause anterior displacement of the stomach, with a broad impression on the posterior wall. However, the exact size, shape, and location of the posterior wall

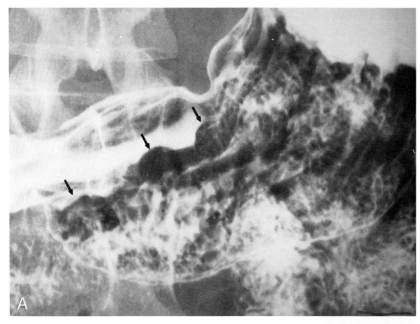

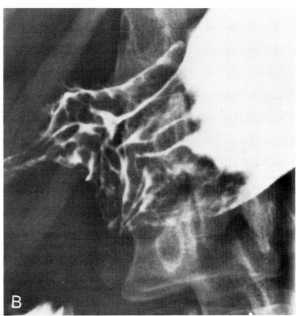

Fig. 14-30 Differing types of metastatic carcinoma involving the stomach. (A) Multiple well-defined nodules representing metastatic Kaposi's sarcoma in a patient with acquired immune deficiency syndrome (AIDS). (B) Nodularity and distortion of the gastric rugae due to metastatic scirrhous carcinoma of the breast.

impression is dependent on the size and location of the retrogastric mass and its exact relation to the stomach.

Liver enlargement generally displaces the stomach posteriorly, inferiorly, and to the left.

Splenic enlargement displaces the stomach inferiorly and toward the midline.

THE POSTOPERATIVE STOMACH

Until recently, most operative procedures were performed on the stomach for amelioration of peptic ulcer disease and could be classified into three general categories: partial gastrectomy with gastroenterostomy, partial gastrectomy with gastro-

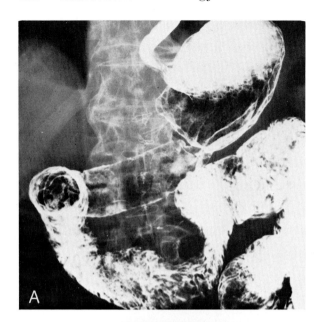

Fig. 14-31 Commonly encountered examples of gastric surgery. (**A**) Billroth I procedure with resection of most of the stomach. (**B**) Antrectomy with vagotomy.

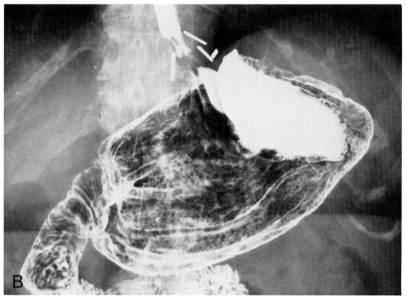

duodenostomy, and pyloroplasty. Recently, however, much gastric surgery has been performed to ameliorate gastroesophageal reflux and for the purposes of weight reduction, the latter taking the form of gastric plication or gastric bypass. The more commonly encountered varieties of gastric surgery are as follows:

1. *Billroth I procedure* consists of resection of most of the stomach, with gastroduodenostomy (Figs. 14-31A and 14-32C).

2. *Antrectomy* is a less radical version of the Billroth I procedure in which only the gastric antrum is resected and a gastroduodenostomy is performed (Fig. 14-31B).

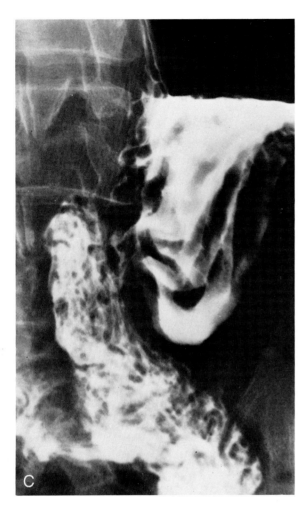

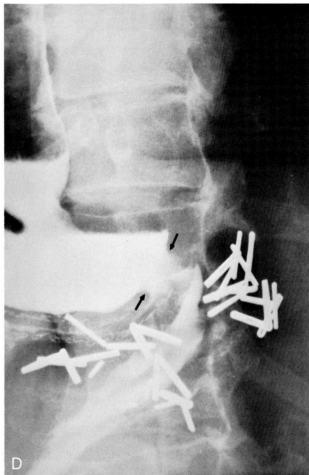

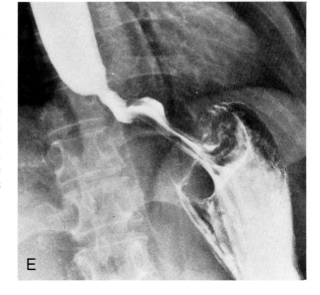

Fig. 14-31 *(continued)* (C) Billroth II type procedure. On this film, the afferent and efferent loops are superimposed at the anastomosis. (D) Horizontal type of gastric plication for weight reduction as seen several months after surgery. The passage through the plication (between the arrows) is larger than desirable. (E) Nissen fundoplication with its typical mass in the fundus of the stomach. A pre-existing distal esophageal stricture is also visible.

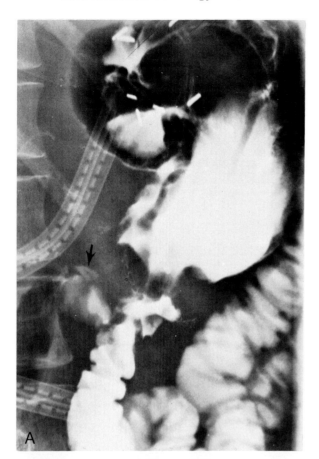

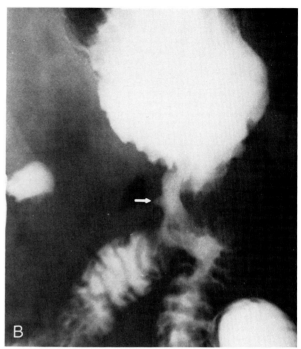

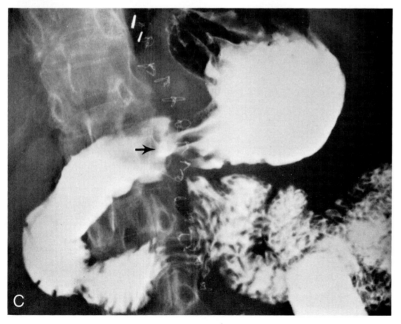

Fig. 14-32 Example of postoperative complications and sequelae following gastric surgery. (A) Anastomotic leak following partial gastrectomy and gastroenterostomy. Contrast material escaping at the anastomosis is visible (arrow). (B) Anastomotic ulcer (arrow) following a Billroth II type procedure. (C) Anastomotic ulcer (arrow) following a Billroth I type partial gastric resection.

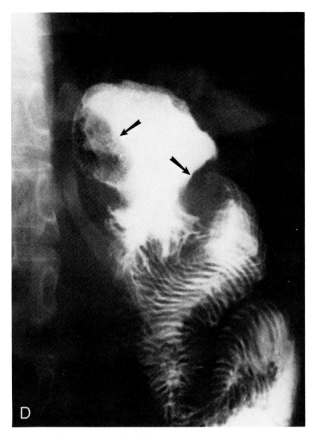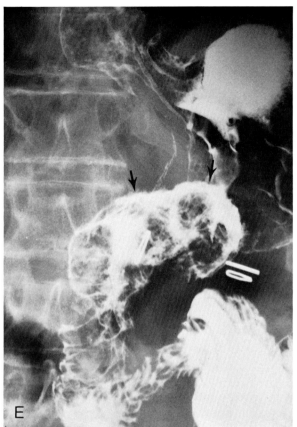

Fig. 14-32 (*continued*) (D) Recurrent gastric carcinoma (arrow) following partial gastric resection of a Billroth II variety. (E) Recurrent gastric carcinoma at the anastomosis manifested mainly as a giant ulceration (arrows).

3. *The Billroth II procedure* and its variants consist of subtotal gastric resection with a gastroenterostomy linking the gastric pouch to the small bowel distal to the ligament of Treitz (Figs. 14-31C and 14-32B and D). The several variations of this procedure primarily differ in the construction of the gastroenterostomy and the manner in which the small bowel is brought up to the anastamosis.

4. *Pyloroplasty* is the term applied to any of several operations designed to widen the lumen of the pyloric channel for purposes of promoting gastric drainage. The procedure is usually combined with vagotomy. Pyloroplasty destroys the normal contours of the pyloric canal, widening and deforming it.

5. *Gastric plication* consists of stapling a closure across the stomach just below the esophagogastric junction, leaving a very small lumen between the two gastric chambers thus created (Fig. 14-31D). This is a recent and relatively successful form of gastric surgery for weight reduction, and it has largely replaced the more complex procedure known as *gastric bypass.*

6. *Nissen fundoplication* is an antireflux procedure in which the gastric fundus is wrapped around the esophagogastric region. The resulting mass at the esophagogastric region seen radiographically is characteristic of the procedure (Fig. 14-31E).

7. *Total gastrectomy* is the procedure of choice in Zollinger-Ellison syndrome, as well as for many gastric carcinomas. Usually, the distal esophagus is sutured to jejunum that has been brought up to the anastomosis as part of a roux-en-Y.

COMPLICATIONS OF GASTRIC SURGERY

Radiologic investigation of potential complications following gastric surgery is a frequent necessity. The types of complications that occur are legion, and if one can imagine a particular complication as being possible, it has probably been reported. For purposes of brevity, however, only the major and more common complications of gastric surgery are discussed.

Anastomotic Leaks

During the immediate postoperative period, a small fraction of cases are plagued by breakdown of a surgical anastomosis (Fig. 14-32A), which is best investigated with water-soluble contrast material. Breakdown of a suture line may occur at the anastomosis of stomach to small bowel, at any enteroenteric anastomosis accompanying gastric surgery, and at the oversown proximal end of the duodenal bulb following Billroth II type procedures. Common radiologic signs of an anastomotic leak are contrast material leaving the viscus and appearing within the peritoneal cavity, filling of an adjacent abscess cavity, or demonstration of a fistula.

Marginal Ulcers

The Billroth I and II varieties of partial gastric resection are often not curative of peptic ulcer disease and the recurrent peptic ulcers that occur in the region of the anastomosis are termed marginal or postanastomotic ulcers (Figs. 14-32B and C). These ulcers may be difficult to identify radiologically because of the often confused overlapping fold patterns produced by the surgical procedure in the region of an anastomosis. Although it is best to directly identify the recurrent ulcer crater, unusual stiffness at an anastomosis, an edematous-appearing mass, or unusually thickened folds are excellent secondary radiographic signs that should lead to suspicion of the presence of marginal ulcer. However, the uncertainty of the radiologic diagnosis of marginal ulcer, with a sensitivity of approx-

imately 50 percent, has placed this diagnosis largely within the realm of endoscopy.

Jejunogastric Intussusception

In occasional patients with a Billroth II type resection, retrograde prolapse of the small bowel adjacent to the gastroenterostomy into the gastric pouch may occur resulting in partial or complete obstruction. This phenomenon is associated with marginal ulcer and may obstruct the afferent or efferent loop.

Recurrent Carcinoma

In patients who have had partial gastrectomy for localized carcinoma of the stomach, a considerable possibility of recurrence exists for several years. Furthermore, the incidence of carcinoma in patients with partial gastric resection for peptic ulcer has been shown to be higher than in the general population. The radiographic signs of recurrent gastric carcinoma are basically those of an infiltrating, polypoid, or ulcerating gastric malignancy presenting in the remaining gastric pouch (Figs. 14-32D and E).

Afferent Loop Syndrome

In patients who have had a Billroth II type procedure, the loop of bowel leading from the duodenum to the anastomosis is termed the afferent loop, while that leading distally from the anastomosis is termed the efferent loop. In occasional patients, the afferent loop may become dilated, due to one of two circumstances, and may cause epigastric distress. In the first instance, the afferent loop may become dilated due to partial obstruction at the anastomosis, pancreatic and duodenal secretions accumulating within the partially obstructed segment. In the second instance, the anastomosis may be constructed such that food flows almost directly from the esophagus into the afferent loop, causing dilatation of the afferent loop. Radiographically, the diagnosis of afferent loop syndrome is made by demonstrating the obstructed or dilated afferent loop.

Zollinger-Ellison Syndrome

Large or multiple ulcerations recurring in a patient's gastric pouch following partial gastric resection for ulcer disease should alert one to the possibility of the Zollinger-Ellison syndrome. In the presence of this syndrome due to a gastrin-producing tumor, partial gastric resection is ineffective in reducing the massive gastric acid secretion, since the acid-secreting mucosa of the proximal stomach remains in place and responds to the continuing elevated blood-gastrin levels. Total gastrectomy is the usual procedure of choice in Zollinger-Ellison syndrome, since it completely eliminates the possibility of gastric hypersecretion.

Gastric Bezoar

Gastric bezoar may occur in the intact stomach, but is a specific complication of subtotal gastrectomy, particularly when combined with vagotomy and performed in an edentulous patient. Poorly chewed fibrous foods are retained and become a matted mass. The lack of peristalsis and absence of hydrochloric acid in these patients contribute to formation of the bezoar.

Radiologically, a bezoar should be suspected in any patient with a large, discrete mass of retained food in a partially resected stomach, particularly if one is certain the patient has not eaten prior to the examination. A further sign of the presence of a bezoar is the observation that none of the food mass leaves the stomach with the flow of barium, as would ordinary semisolid food.

SUGGESTED READINGS

Structural Disorders

Bateson EM, Talerman A, Walrond ER: Radiological and pathological observations in a series of seventeen cases of hypertrophic pyloric stenosis of adults. Br J Radiol 42:1, 1969.

Belgrad R, Carlson HC, Payne WS, Cain JC: Pseudotumoral gastric varices. Am J Roentgenol 91:751, 1964.

Chepey JJ, Kurtzman RS: Isolated heterotaxy of the stomach. Am J Roentgenol 91:770, 1964.

Cho KY: Gastric antral diaphragm. Radiology 1:37, 1976.

Clements JL, Jinkins JR, Torres W, et al: Antral mucosal diaphragm in adults. AJR 133:1105, 1979.

Felson B, Berkmen YM, Hoyumpa AM: Gastric mucosal diaphragm. Radiology 92:513, 1969.

Ghahremani GG: Non-obstructive mucosal diaphragms or rings of the gastric antrum in adults. Am J Roentgenol 121:236, 1974.

Larson LJ, Carson HC, Dockerty MB: Roentgenologic diagnosis of pyloric hypertrophy in adults. Am J Roentgenol 101:453, 1967.

Levin EJ, Felson B: Asymptomatic gastric mucosal prolapse. Radiology 57:514, 1951.

Palmer ED: Collective review: Gastric diverticula. Int Abst Surg 92:417, 1951.

Rabushka SE, Melamed M, Melamed JL: Unusual gastric diverticula. Radiology 90:1006, 1968.

Scott WG: The radiographic diagnosis of prolapsed redundant gastric mucosa into the duodenum. Radiology 46:547, 1946.

Seaman WB: Hypertrophy of the pyloric muscle in adults: Analysis of 27 cases. Radiology 80:753, 1963.

Seaman WB: Focal hypertrophy of the pyloric muscle — torus hyperplasia. Am J Roentgenol 96:388, 1966.

Semb BKH, Halvorsen JF, Fossdal JE: Acute gastric volvulus with necrosis of the stomach and left lower pulmonary lobe. Acta Chir Scand 143:256, 1977.

Tan K: Intraluminal diverticula of the stomach. AJR 132:461, 1979.

Twining EW: Chronic hypertrophic stenosis of the pylorus in adults. Br J Radiol 6:644, 1933.

Wastell C, Ellis H: Volvulus of the stomach. Br J Surg 58:39, 1971.

Functional Disorders

Hoeffel JC, Senot P, Champineulle B, Drouin P: Gastric retention and gastric ileus in diabetes mellitus. Radiologe 20:540, 1980.

Kassander P: Asymptomatic gastric retention in diabetics (gastroparesis diabeticarum). Ann Intern Med 48:797, 1958.

Zitomer BR, Gramm HF, Kozak GP: Gastric neuropathy in diabetes mellitus: Clinical and radiologic observations. Metabolism 17:199, 1968.

Inflammatory Diseases: Benign Gastric Ulcers and Erosions

Amberg JR, Zboralske FF: Gastric ulcers after 70. Am J Roentgenol 96:393, 1966.

Braver JM, Paul RE, Phillips E, Bloom S: Roentgen diagnosis of linear ulcers. Radiology 132:29, 1979.

Carman RD: Benign and malignant gastric ulcers from a roentgenologic viewpoint. Am J Roentgenol 8:695, 1921.

Catalano D, Pagliari U: Gastroduodenal erosions: Radiological findings. Gastrointest Radiol 7:235, 1982.

Gelfand DW, Ott DJ: Gastric ulcer scars. Radiology 140:37, 1981.

Green PHR, Gold RP, Marboe CC, et al: Chronic erosive gastritis: Clinical, diagnostic, and pathological features in nine patients. Am J Gastroenterol 77:543, 1982.

Haudek M: Zur röntgenologischen Diagnose der Ulcerationen in der pars media des Magens. München Med Wschr 57:1787, 1910.

Kemp Harper RA, Green B: Malignant gastric ulcer. Clin Radiol 12:95, 1961.

Laufer I, Hamilton J, Mullens JE: Demonstration of superficial gastric erosions by double-contrast radiography. Gastroenterology 68:387, 1975.

Nelson SW: The discovery of gastric ulcers and the differential diagnosis between benignancy and malignancy. Radiol Clin North Am 7:5, 1969.

Op den Orth JO, Dekker W: Gastric erosions: Radiologic and endoscopic aspects. Diagn Imaging 45:88, 1976.

Ott DJ, Gelfand DW, Wu WC: Detection of gastric ulcer: Comparison of single- and double-contrast examination. AJR 139:93, 1982.

Ott DJ, Gelfand DW, Wu SC, Kerr RM: Sensitivity of single- vs double-contrast radiology in erosive gastritis. AJR 138:263, 1982.

Schumacher EC, Hampton AO: Radiographic differentiation of benign and malignant ulcers. Clin Sympos 8:161, 1956.

Sommer AW, Dysart DN, Haines RD: Pyloric channel ulcer: Radiologic aspects. JAMA 174:126, 1960.

Walk I: Erosive gastritis. Digestion 84:87, 1955.

Wolf BS: Observations on roentgen features of benign and malignant gastric ulcers. Semin Roentgenol 6:140, 1971.

Zboralske FF, Amberg JR: Detection of Zollinger-Ellison syndrome: The radiologist's responsibility. Am J Roentgenol 104:529, 1968.

Zollinger RM, Ellison EH: Primary peptic ulcerations of the jejunum associated with islet cell tumors of the pancreas. Ann Surg 142:709, 1955.

Inflammatory Diseases: Gastritis

Abell MR, Limond RV, Blamey WE, Martel W: Allergic granulomatosis with massive gastric involvement. N Eng J Med 282:665, 1970.

Ackerman AJ: Roentgenological study of gastric tuberculosis. Am J Roentgenol 44:59, 1940.

Athey PA, Goldstein HM, Dodd GD: Radiologic spectrum of opportunistic infections of the upper gastrointestinal tract. Am J Roentgenol 129:419, 1977.

Balikian JR, Yenikomshian SM, Jidejian YD: Tuberculosis of the pyloroduodenal area. Am J Roentgenol 101:414, 1967.

Bockus HL: Syphilis and the stomach. In Bockus HL, ed: Gastroenterology. Philadelphia, WB Saunders, 1974, p 1047.

Burhenne HJ, Carbone JV: Eosinophilic (allergic) gastroenteritis. Am J Roentgenol 96:332, 1966.

Cohen WC: Gastric involvement in Crohn's disease. Am J Roentgenol 101:425, 1967.

Cooley R: Primary amyloidosis with involvement of the stomach. Am J Roentgenol 70:428, 1953.

Cronan J, Burrell M, Trepeta R: Aphthoid ulcerations in gastric candidiasis. Radiology 134:607, 1980.

Culver GJ, Person HS, Montez M, Palanker HK: Eosinophilic gastritis. JAMA 200:641, 1967.

Dastur KJ, Ward JF: Amyloidoma of the stomach. Gastrointest Radiol 5:17, 1980.

Edelman MJ, March TL: Eosinophilic gastroenteritis. Am J Roentgenol 91:773, 1964.

Gaines GW, Steinbach HL, Lowenkaupt E: Tuberculosis of the stomach. Radiology 58:808, 1952.

Joske RA, Vaughan MB: The radiologic findings in histologically verified atrophic gastritis and gastric atrophy. Gastroenterology 42:7, 1962.

Laufer I, Truman T, deSa D: Multiple superficial gastric erosions due to Crohn's disease of the stomach. Radiologic and endoscopic diagnosis. Br J Radiol 49:726, 1976.

Laws JW, Pitman RG: Radiological features of pernicious anemia. Br J Radiol 33:229, 1960.

Legge DA, Carlson HC, Judd ES: Roentgenologic features of regional enteritis of the upper gastrointestinal tract. Am J Roentgenol 110:355, 1970.

Lichtenstein JE: Case 3 (gastric syphilis). Selected cases from the film interpretation session of the Society of Gastrointestinal Radiologists, 1980, Maui, Hawaii. Gastrointest Radiol 6:371, 1981.

Mackintosh CE, Kreel L: Anatomy and radiology of the areae gastricae. Gut 18:85, 1977.

Marshak RH, Maklansky D, Kurzban JD, Lindner AE: Crohn's disease of the stomach and duodenum. Am J

Gastroenterol 77:340, 1982.

Martell W, Abell MR, Allan TNK: Lymphoreticular hyperplasia of the stomach (pseudolymphoma). Am J Roentgenol 127:261, 1976.

Muhletaler CA, Gerlock AJ, de Soto L, Halter SA: Gastroduodenal lesions of ingested acids: Radiographic findings. AJR 135:1247, 1980.

Perez CA, Dorfman RF: Benign lymphoid hyperplasia of the stomach and duodenum. Radiology 87:505, 1966.

Reese DF, Hodgson JR, Dockerty MD: Grant hypertrophy of the gastric mucosa (Menetriere's disease): A correlation of roentgenographic, pathologic, and clinical findings. Am J Roentgenol 88:619, 1962.

Rose C, Stevenson GW: Corrrelation between visualization and size of the areae gastricae and duodenal ulcer. Radiology 139:371, 1981.

Seaman WB, Fleming RJ: Intramural gastric emphysema. Am J Roentgenol 101:431, 1967.

Turner MA, Beachley MC, Stanley D: Phlegmonous gastritis. AJR 133:527, 1979.

Benign Neoplasms and Neoplasm-Like Diseases

Balthazar EJ, Megibow A, Bryk D, Cohen T: Gastric carcinoid tumors: Radiographic features in eight cases. AJR 139:1123, 1982.

Bartels RJ: Duplication of the stomach: Case report and review of the literature. Am Surg 33:747, 1967.

Bruneton JN, Drouillard J, Roux P, et al: Leiomyoma and leiomyosarcoma of the digestive tract—a report of 45 cases and review of the literature. Eur J Radiol 1:291, 1981.

Davies PM: Smooth muscle tumours of the upper gastrointestinal tract. Clin Radiol 29:407, 1978.

Eklof O: Benign tumors of the stomach and duodenum. Acta Radiol 57:177, 1962.

Freeny PC, Vimont TR: Villous tumors of the stomach and small bowel. Arch Surg 113:255, 1978.

Gordon R, Laufer I, Kressel HY: Gastric polyps found on routine double-contrast examination of the stomach. Radiology 134:27, 1980.

Marshak RH, Lindner AE: Polypoid lesions of the stomach. Semin Roentgenol 6:151, 1971.

Miller JH, Gisvold JJ, Weiland LH, McIlrath DC: Upper gastrointestinal tract: Villous tumors. AJR 134:933, 1980.

Ming SC: The adenoma-carcinoma sequence in the stomach and colon. II. Malignant potential of gastric polyps. Gastrointest Radiol 1:121, 1976.

Ming SC, Goldman H: Gastric polyps; a histogenetic

classification and its relation to carcinoma. Cancer 18:721, 1965.

Op den Orth JO, Dekker W: Gastric adenomas. Radiology 141:289, 1981.

Morson BC, Dawson IMP, Spriggs AI: Gastrointestinal Pathology. Oxford, Blackwell, 1979, pp 187–189.

Pochaczevsky R, Sherman RS: The roentgen appearance of gastric argentaffinoma. Radiology 72:330, 1959.

Rose C, Kesseram RA, Lind JF: Ectopic gastric pancreas: A review and report of 4 cases. Diagn Imaging 49:214, 1980.

Malignant Neoplasms

Balthazar EJ, Davidian MM: Hyperrugosity in gastric carcinoma: Radiographic, endoscopic and pathologic features. AJR 136:531, 1981.

Balthazar EJ, Rosenberg H, Davidian MM: Scirrhous carcinoma of the pyloric channel and distal antrum. AJR 134:669, 1980.

Dutta SK, Costa BS: Umbilicated gastric polyposis: An indicator of metastatic gastric tumor. Am J Gastroenterol 71:598, 1979.

Kawai K, Tanaka H: Differential Diagnosis of Gastric Diseases. Chicago, Year Book Medical Publishers, 1974.

Koga M, Nakata H, Kiyonari H, et al: Roentgen features of the superficial depressed type of early gastric carcinoma. Radiology 115:289, 1975.

Libshitz HI, Lindell MM, Dodd GD: Metastases to the hollow viscera. Radiol Clin North Am 20:487, 1982.

Menuck LS: Gastric lymphoma, a radiologic diagnosis. Gastrointest Radiol 1:157, 1976.

Meyer JE, Ostfeld D: Fibrosarcoma of breast metastatic to stomach. J Can Assoc Radiol 30:265, 1979.

Montesi A, Graziani L, Pesaresi A, et al: Radiologic diagnosis of early gastric cancer by routine double-contrast examination. Gastrointest Radiol 7:205, 1982.

Nauert TC, Zornoza J, Ordonez N: Gastric leiomyosarcomas. AJR 139:291, 1982.

Potchen EJ, Khung CL, Yatsuhashi M: X-ray diagnosis of gastric melanoma. N Engl J Med 271:133, 1964.

Privett JTJ, Davies ER, Roylance J: The radiological features of gastric lymphoma. Clin Radiol 28:547, 1977.

Sherrick DW, Hodgson JR, Dockerty MB: The roentgenologic diagnosis of primary gastric lymphoma. Radiology 84:925, 1965.

Shirakabe H, Nishizawa M, Maruyama M, et al: Atlas of X-Ray Diagnosis of Early Gastric Cancer. Tokyo,

Igaku-Shoin, 1982.

Smith FR, Barkin JS, Hensley G: Choriocarcinoma of the stomach. Am J Gastroenterol 73:45, 1980.

The Postoperative Stomach

Agha FP, Harris HH, Boustany MM: Gastroplasty for morbid obesity. Roentgen evaluation and spectrum of complications. Gastrointest Radiol 7:217, 1982.

Aleman S: Jejunogastric intussusception: A rare complication of the operated stomach. Acta Radiol 29:383, 1948.

Burhenne HJ: Roentgen anatomy and terminology of gastric surgery. Am J Roentgenol 91:731, 1964.

Burhenne JH: The retained gastric antrum. Preoperative diagnosis of an iatrogenic syndrome. Am J Roentgenol 101:459, 1967.

Burrell M, Touloukian JS, Curtis AM: Roentgen manifestations of carcinoma in the gastric remnant. Gastrointest Radiol 5:331, 1980.

DeBakey M, Ochsner A: Bezoars and concretions. Surgery 4:934, 1938; 5:132, 1939.

Feldman F, Seaman WB: Primary gastric stump cancer. Am J Roentgenol 115:257, 1972.

Ott DJ, Munitz HA, Gelfand DW, et al: The sensitivity of radiography of the postoperative stomach. Radiology 144:741, 1982.

Rogers LF, Davis EK, Harle TS: Phytobezoar formation and food boli following gastric surgery. Am J Roentgenol 119:280, 1973.

Scobie BA, McGill DB, Priestley JT, Rovelstad RA: Excluded gastric antrum simulating Zollinger-Ellison syndrome. Gastroenterology 47:184, 1964.

Szemes GC, Amberg JR: Gastric bezoars after partial gastrectomy. Radiology 90:675, 1968.

Toye DKM, Hutton JFK, Williams JA: Radiological anatomy after pyloroplasty. Gut 11:358, 1970.

Williams JA, Fielding JF: Recurrent acute retrograde intragastric intussusception. Gut 11:840, 1970.

15

Abnormalities of the Duodenum

STRUCTURAL ABNORMALITIES

Abnormalities of structure unrelated to inflammation or neoplasm occur in the adult duodenum, but are seldom a cause of clinical problems leading to a radiologic examination.

Diverticula

Diverticula are frequent in the duodenum and become more common with advanced age. Two types of diverticula are seen in the duodenum, the mechanism of their formation being unclear.

Most prevalent are those diverticula extending outside the confines of the duodenum itself. They occur with greatest frequency in the second portion of the duodenal loop, but may occur anywhere along its length. Very common is the diverticulum extending from the medial aspect of the second portion of the duodenum into the vicinity of the head of the pancreas (Fig. 15-1). The neck of a diverticulum in this specific location is usually found adjacent to the major papilla, or the papilla may be incorporated into the neck or cavity of the diverticulum. Occasionally, food residue will be seen in a duodenal diverticulum during an upper gastrointestinal series, but these diverticula are generally considered to be asymptomatic.

Differentiation of a small diverticulum from an ulcer occasionally may be necessary. Diverticula generally have a proportionally narrower neck than the usual peptic ulcer, and unlike a duodenal ulcer, folds often traverse the neck. Furthermore, a diverticulum will usually change size in response to peristalsis, while an ulcer remains of constant size.

A second uncommon form of duodenal diverticulum is that of the intraluminal duodenum diverticulum (Fig. 15-2). This type of diverticulum lies entirely within the mucosal and submucosal layers and presents macroscopically as a sac within the lumen of the duodenum. The radiographic findings are subtle and are those of a thin radiolucent line, convex distally, outlining the extent of the diverticulum. The radiolucent line is the wall of the diverticulum, demarcated inside and out by barium suspension. Most intraluminal diverticula are found incidentally during upper gastrointestinal studies, but they occasionally cause partial duodenal obstruction and upper gastrointestinal obstructive symptoms.

Duodenal Varices

The pancreatoduodenal veins constitute part of the anastomotic network between the portal and systemic venous systems. In hepatic cirrhosis with portal hypertension, these veins may become enlarged, serving as collateral channels and forming submucosal duodenal varices.

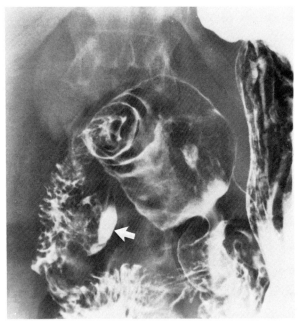

Fig. 15-1 Diverticulum of the medial aspect of the descending limb of the duodenum (arrow). An active ulcer is visible in the duodenal bulb.

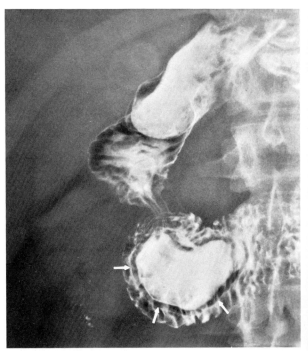

Fig. 15-2 Intraluminal diverticulum of the duodenum (arrows) visible as a radiolucent line in the distal duodenum.

The radiologic appearance of duodenal varices is similar to that of varices in the esophagus. They are seen as enlarged, irregular, occasionally nodular folds, most clearly visible in the first and second portions of the duodenum (Fig. 15-3). A point of differentiation from other large duodenal folds due to other causes (Table 15-1) is that duodenal varices may visibly change caliber in response to peristalsis and the application of compression. Folds thickened by inflammation or tumor infiltration are more consistent in appearance.

Annular Pancreas

A relatively rare anomaly, annular pancreas is a circular extension of the head of the pancreas around the second portion of the duodenum. Radiologically, it presents as a duodenal constriction with intact mucosal folds (Fig. 15-4A). It is an anomaly of the ventral anlage of the pancreas and contains its own pancreatic duct, which is demonstrable by endoscopic retrograde pancreatography (Fig. 15-4B). Annular pancreas must be differen-

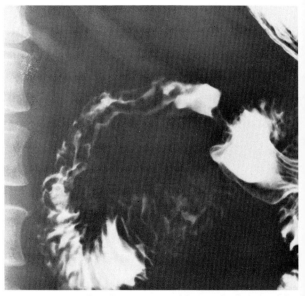

Fig. 15-3 Duodenal varices visible as thick, irregular folds coursing through the proximal portion of the duodenum.

Table 15-1. Thickened Duodenal Folds

Noninflammatory
  Normal
  Gastric hypersecretion
  Zollinger-Ellison Disease
  Edema
  Intestinal lymphangectasia
  Intramural hemorrhage
  Amyloidosis
  Varices
Inflammatory
  Nonspecific duodenitis
  Pancreatitis
  Giardiasis
  Hookworm
  Strongyloidiasis
  Eosinophilic enteritis
  Tuberculosis
  Crohn's disease
  Whipple's disease
Neoplastic
  Pancreatic cancer
  Lymphoma

tiated from duodenal stenoses due to peptic ulcer disease, pancreatitis, or pancreatic carcinoma. When it occurs in infants it also must be differentiated from duodenal atresia, duplication, and congenital bands.

Aberrant Pancreas

Although seen much more frequently in the distal stomach, aberrant pancreatic tissue may be found anywhere in the duodenum and in the proximal small bowel as well. Its appearance in the duodenum does not differ from that already described in the stomach. It forms a hemispheric or plaque-like benign-appearing tumor of approximately 1 to 2 cm in size, often with a central dimple representing an attempt at pancreatic duct formation. It is an asymptomatic condition, of importance only in its differentiation from true neoplasms.

Superior Mesenteric Artery Syndrome

Superior mesenteric artery syndrome refers to obstruction of the duodenal loop at the crossing of the superior mesenteric artery. It is usually seen in individuals who have lost significant weight, usually after trauma. It is common in patients suffering from severe burns and in patients who are in

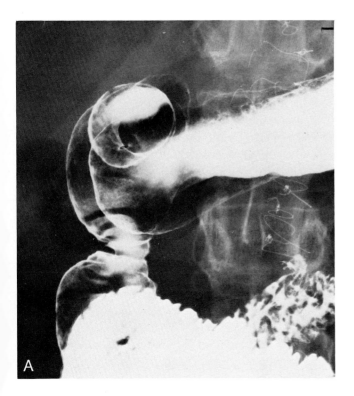
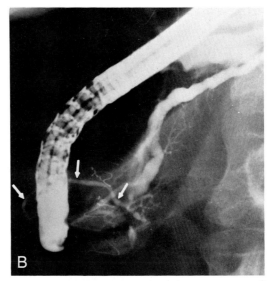

Fig. 15-4 Annular pancreas. **(A)** Constriction of the defending segment of the duodenum visible during an upper gastrointestinal examination. **(B)** Pancreatography showing the duct (arrows) within the pancreatic segment circling the duodenum.

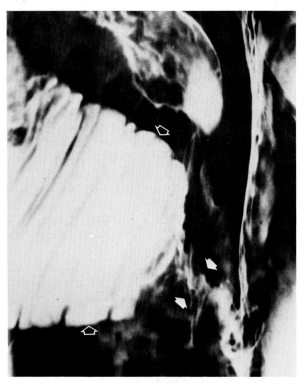

Fig. 15-5 Superior mesenteric artery obstruction with dilatation of the third portion of the duodenum (open arrows) and obstruction at the crossing of the superior mesenteric vessels (solid arrows).

body casts. The duodenal obstruction is thought to be due to trapping of the duodenal loop between the superior mesenteric artery and the aorta in a patient in whom the sparse retroperitoneal fat is insufficient to maintain space between the two vessels for the duodenum.

The radiologic diagnosis of superior mesenteric artery syndrome is made by demonstration of obstruction of the third segment of the duodenal loop at the crossing point of the superior mesenteric artery (Fig. 15-5). Duodenal dilation is always present proximal to the point of obstruction. A further diagnostic sign is the churning back and forth of the duodenal contents.

FUNCTIONAL DISORDERS

Several entities are capable of causing functional disturbances of duodenal motility. They may be manifest as either hyper- or hypomotility of the duodenal bulb or loop, hypomotility often being accompanied by duodenal dilatation.

Peptic ulcer and *duodenitis* most often cause hypermotility of the duodenal loop, presumably the result of an irritant stimulus. Thus, the presence of spasm or increased peristalsis is often used as a clue to the existence of these entities. When the associated inflammation is severe, however, peristalsis may cease almost totally, resulting in a flaccid duodenum. Duodenal *Crohn's disease* is an uncommon cause of the same effects on peristalsis.

Scleroderma (systemic sclerosis) affects the smooth muscle of the duodenum in a significant manner. The destruction of smooth muscle frequently accompanying scleroderma will often result in marked dilatation of the duodenal loop. Similar changes are seen in occasional cases of *dermatomyositis*.

INFLAMMATORY DISEASES

Inflammatory diseases are the most prevalent disorders leading to the radiologic examination of the duodenum. They may be divided into two basic groups by their relative incidence: (1) duodenal ulcer and duodenitis, which are of greatest incidence, and (2) all others.

DUODENAL ULCER

Duodenal ulcer is the most common form of peptic ulcer disease and is thought to be considerably more common than gastric ulcer. Duodenal ulcer bears many radiographic similarities to gastric ulcer, with almost identical radiologic signs of activity.

Profile signs of duodenal ulcer mimic those of gastric ulcer (Fig. 15-6). Barium fills the niche representing the ulcer proper. Surrounding most duodenal ulcers is an ulcer mound created by adjacent inflammatory edema. Unfortunately, the duodenal bulb is often tucked behind the gastic antrum and it may be difficult to turn the patient into a position in which an ulcer is clearly visible in profile.

En face signs of duodenal ulcer are more frequently employed than profile signs, since it is generally easier to obtain an en face view of a duodenal ulcer crater. The single most reliable

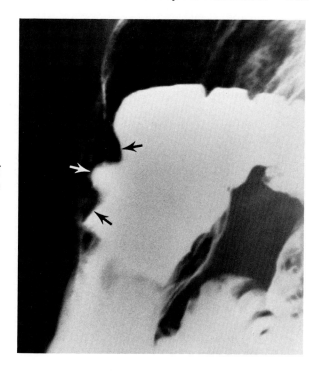

Fig. 15-6 Profile view of an ulcer on the anterior wall of the duodenal bulb. The ulcer niche (white arrow) is surrounded by a sloping mound of edema (black arrows).

method of demonstrating ulcers en face, in the author's opinion, is that of compression filming. Double-contrast views of the duodenum, most often obtained in the supine or supine oblique positions, readily demonstrate posterior wall duodenal ulcers, but often fail to show anterior wall lesions.

When seen en face, the ulcer crater usually appears round or oval, and it is often surrounded by a radiolucent halo, representing the ulcer mound (Figs. 15-7A and B). With chronicity or healing, converging folds may be plainly seen entering the region of the ulcer (Figs. 15-7C and D). Indeed, an efficient way to find a duodenal ulcer in a deformed duodenal bulb is to search carefully at the central point of any convergence of folds. Although most ulcers are rounded in contour, a minority present with linear or irregular shapes.

Multiple ulcers may be expected in a small percentage of patients with active duodenal ulcers. The identification of multiple duodenal ulcers is complicated because they usually occur in the patient with chronic peptic ulcer disease who has an extremely deformed duodenal bulb. It is my experience that in most patients with multiple duodenal ulcers, one or more of the ulcers may not be identified radiologically, as compared to endoscopic re-

sults, although active peptic ulcer disease of the duodenum will be correctly diagnosed. Zollinger-Ellison syndrome should be suspected whenever large or multiple ulcers are encountered, particularly if accompanied by gastric hypersecretion and greatly thickened gastric and duodenal folds.

Duodenal Deformity

Granulation tissue is produced in the base of a chronic or healing duodenal ulcer and is transformed eventually into collagenous tissue. Collagenous tissue shrinks as it matures, drawing adjacent areas of the duodenal wall toward the site of the ulcer. The result is a converging fold pattern (Figs. 15-7C, and D), a "cloverleaf" deformity or most commonly, some combination of the two (Figs. 15-8A – C).

With sufficient deformity, sac-like pseudodiverticula may form (Fig. 15-8C). These may collect barium and often require differentiation from an active ulcer. Pseudodiverticula may be differentiated from ulcer on two points. First, pseudodiverticula change size in response to peristalsis or application of compression while the size of an ulcer is constant. Second, pseudodiverticula

(Text continues on page 248)

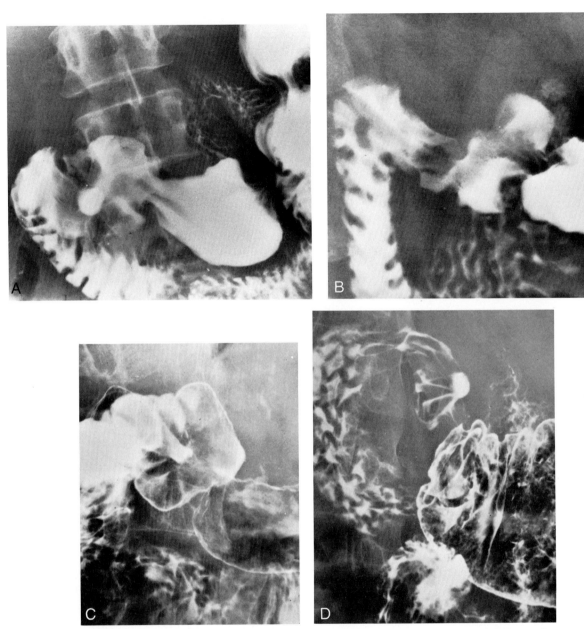

Fig. 15-7 En face views of duodenal ulcers illustrating various radiographic characteristics. (A) Large ulcer near the apex of the duodenal bulb accompanied by a radiolucent halo representing surrounding edema. (B) Compression spot film demonstrating a small ulcer accompanied by a large mound of edema. (C) Double-contrast view of folds converging towards a posterior wall bulbar ulcer. (D) Mucosal relief view of a duodenal ulcer illustrating folds converging into the site of the ulcer.

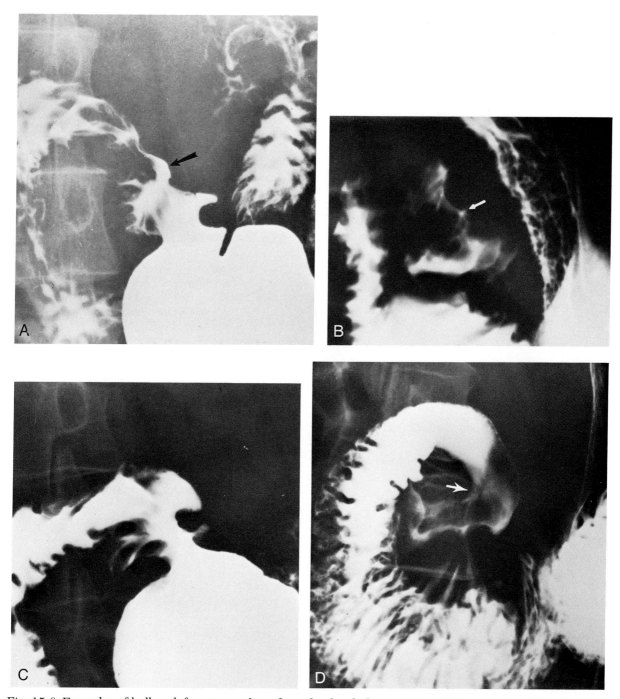

Fig. 15-8 Examples of bulbar deformity resulting from duodenal ulcer activity. (A) Constriction of the duodenal bulb near its apex due to an active ulcer (arrow). (B) Severe bulbar deformity associated with a small active ulcer (arrow). In this instance, much of the deformity is due to surrounding edema. (C) "Cloverleaf" type deformity of the duodenal bulb remaining after healing of an ulcer. The small projections are pseudodiverticula. (D) Mucosal scar consisting of delicate converging folds (arrow) following healing of a small duodenal bulb ulcer. There is no overall deformity of the bulb in this instance.

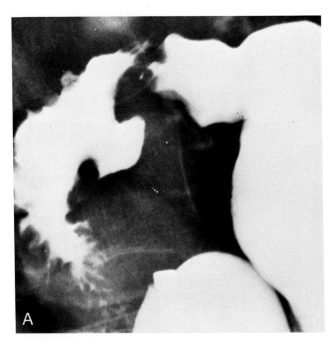

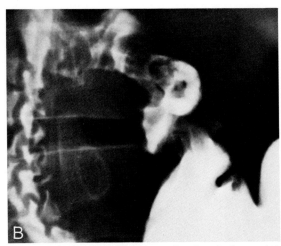

Fig. 15-9 Examples of "giant" duodenal ulcers. (A) Giant duodenal ulcer penetrating the head of the pancreas (lower arrow). A second smaller ulcer (upper arrow) is visible on the superior aspect of the duodenal bulb. (B) Giant duodenal ulcer replacing much of the contour of the bulb itself. The unchanging contour of the ulcer was apparent during fluoroscopy.

usually are not at the center of the converging folds, as would be expected with a chronic or healing ulcer.

A more subtle *duodenal ulcer scar* may occasionally be seen in a duodenal bulb that is not deformed. These scars appear as thin, delicate folds converging to a central point (Fig. 15-8D).

Giant Ulcers

When a duodenal ulcer occupies a considerable fraction of the size of the duodenal bulb, the term giant duodenal ulcer may be applied (Fig. 15-9). Giant ulcers have a serious prognostic importance in that they frequently fail to heal with medical therapy, may bleed severely, or may heal with eventual obstructive stenosis of the duodenum.

Certain giant ulcers present a diagnostic problem when large enough to in effect replace much of the wall of the bulb. These giant ulcers are occasionally overlooked because their size and shape may cause them to be mistaken for the bulb itself. Radiologically, the diagnosis is usually made by fluoroscopic observation of a large, bulb-sized collection of barium that does not undergo changes in size or contour in response to peristalsis as would the normal duodenal bulb.

Duodenal Stenosis

Because the duodenum is narrow as compared to the stomach, the healing of large duodenal ulcers and the fibrosis associated with chronic, recurrent ulcers occasionally leads to a stenosis that may partially obstruct the duodenum. Such patients may experience obstructive symptoms but the more frequent complication is gastric ulceration due to prolonged retention of gastric secretions within the stomach.

Certain factors may predispose a patient to the occurrence of multiple and/or recurrent duodenal ulcers. Patients chronically ingesting large quantities of alcohol and aspirin users are subject to an increased incidence of peptic ulcer in the duodenum, as well as in the stomach. Patients receiving corticosteroids or cancer chemotherapy also are apt to have a greater incidence of gastric and duodenal ulcers. If multiple ulcers or very large ulcers are present the possibility of Zollinger-Ellison syndrome also must be raised.

Fig. 15-10 Three examples of postbulbar ulcers. (A) Visible ulcer craters surrounded by thickened, edematous folds. (B) Postbulbar ulcer on the medial aspect of the descending duodenum with an obvious incisura visible on the opposite wall. (C) Postbulbar ulcer (arrow) visible primarily as narrowing of the duodenum due to edema surrounding the ulcer.

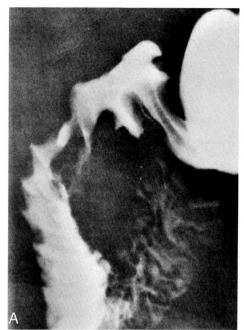

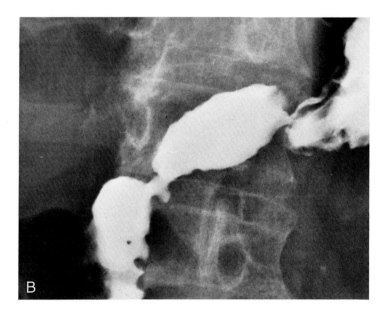

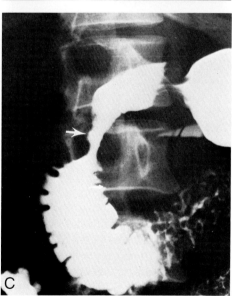

Postbulbar Ulcers

Although most duodenal ulcers are found in the vicinity of the duodenal bulb, a small fraction occur within the several centimeters of the duodenal loop distal to the bulb. Postbulbar ulcers have proven somewhat more difficult to detect radiologically than bulbar ulcers, perhaps because

of a lower degree of suspicion on the part of the radiologist and a resulting less thorough examination of the postbulbar duodenum.

Radiologically, the appearance of postbulbar ulcers differs somewhat from those occurring in the bulb. The ulcer niche may be difficult to differentiate from barium trapped between the duodenal folds normally occurring in the postbulbar area and is seldom accompanied by converging folds. The most useful signs of postbulbar ulcer (Fig. 15-10), other than identifying the crater itself, are the considerable edema usually accompanying the ulcer and the frequent presence of an incisura on the wall of the duodenum opposite the ulcer proper.

DUODENITIS

Since the advent of the fiberoptic duodenoscope, it has become apparent that duodenitis is approximately twice as frequent a cause of upper gastrointestinal symptoms than is duodenal peptic ulcer disease. The radiologic signs of duodenitis have not been completely defined, but the radiologic diagnosis of duodenitis is possible in many cases.

Nonspecific Duodenitis

Nonspecific duodenitis is a term given to the common form of duodenitis that is unassociated with infectious agents, parasites, or more generalized processes such as Crohn's disease. It appears to be more common among persons with heavy alcohol intake than in the general population. It is capable of producing ulcer-like symptoms and of causing significant gastrointestinal hemorrhage. Only a small fraction of these patients will have associated peptic ulcer disease.

The macroscopic appearance of duodenitis varies considerably from case to case, but presents certain common elements. In mild cases, there is moderate erythema of the duodenal mucosa combined with nodular thickening of the folds. In more severe cases, the duodenal mucosa becomes considerably inflamed and friable, often with multiple bleeding points and/or discrete erosions.

Radiologically, nonspecific duodenitis is usually seen as thickening and nodularity of the folds of the proximal duodenum (Fig. 15-11), in many cases combined with hyperactive peristalsis or irritability. In occasional cases, discrete duodenal erosions may be identified (Fig. 15-11D).

There are numerous entities capable of causing irregular thickening or nodule formation in the duodenum (Table 15-1). However, in most moderate or severe cases of duodenitis, the presence of duodenitis can be confidently suggested radiologically. A firm diagnosis requires endoscopy.

Crohn's Disease of the Duodenum

The presence of Crohn's disease in the duodenum without involvement elsewhere in the gastrointestinal tracts is unusual. The majority of patients with duodenal Crohn's disease will also have ileal disease and may have noticeable changes in the stomach as well.

The usual presentation of duodenal Crohn's disease is in conjunction with Crohn's disease of the distal stomach, with either a stenotic, deformed duodenum (Fig. 15-12) or with obliteration of the pyloric channel and evolution of the distal stomach and duodenum into a continuous, irregular contour. In occasional cases of duodenal Crohn's disease, isolated ulcerations in the duodenum will be seen and will require differentiation from peptic ulcer disease, which is often not possible radiologically. In these cases, endoscopic examination and biopsy generally are necessary to establish the diagnosis of Crohn's disease.

Eosinophilic and Tuberculous Duodenitis

Both tuberculous and eosinophilic gastroduodenitis may involve the proximal portion of the duodenal loop in a manner similar to Crohn's disease. Without appropriate clinical information, a radiologic diagnosis is seldom possible. Endoscopy with biopsy is usually necessary to establish these diagnoses.

Giardiasis

Infestation of the duodenum and proximal mesenteric small bowel by giardiasis is not an uncommon problem, particularly with increased travel to areas with poorly treated water supplies. The usual symptoms are crampy abdominal pain and diarrhea. Many patients will have a history of travel abroad or a recent outdoors expedition with drinking of untreated water. Infrequently, one will encounter a case of chronic giardiasis asso-

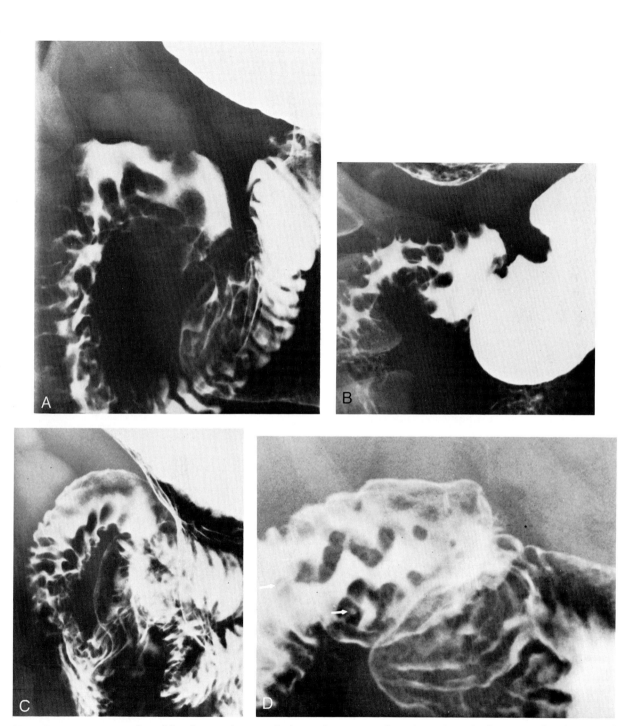

Fig. 15-11 Four examples of duodenitis. (A, B, and C) Duodenitis mainfested mainly as thickening and nodularity of duodenal folds. (D) Erosive duodenitis with visible erosions (arrows) as well as nodularity and thickening of folds.

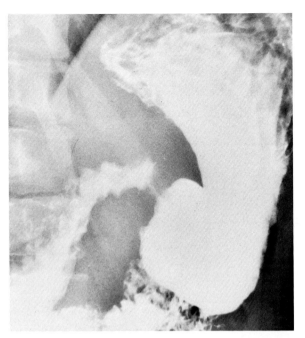

Fig. 15-12 Duodenal deformity and a stenotic pylorus due to Crohn's disease. The patient had extensive ileal involvement as well.

ciated with dysgammaglobulinemia.

Giardiasis is caused by the nonbacterial, single-celled parasite *Giardia lamblia*. Definitive diagnosis is made by identification of the active organism in duodenal or small bowel aspirates and biopsies or by identification of the active organism or its cysts in stool samples.

The radiologic appearance of giardiasis is that of thickening of folds throughout the duodenum and proximal mesenteric small bowel. The extensive involvement of the jejunum as well as the duodenum is a clue that the thickening of duodenal folds may be due to giardiasis, rather than gastric hypersecretion, chronic peptic ulcer disease, or nonspecific duodenitis. In patients with dysgammaglobulinemia, nodular lymphoid hyperplasia may be present and will superimpose a fine, nodular pattern on top of the generalized thickening of folds caused by the giardiasis.

DUODENAL HEMATOMA

Duodenal hematoma may simulate the thickened folds of an inflammatory process or it may present as a large intramural mass (Fig. 15-13), depending upon whether the blood has diffusely infiltrated the bowel wall or remained localized. Duodenal hematoma most frequently follows blunt trauma to the upper abdomen, but it may occasionally be the result of intramural bleeding in a patient receiving anticoagulants or suffering from a bleeding diathesis.

Radiologically, the more common form seen is that of diffuse thickening of folds in the duodenal loop due to infiltration of blood into the submucosal regions of the bowel wall. "Thumbprinting," a nodular impression on the barium column, is often seen in association with this presentation. A well-defined intramural mass is the less common presentation.

BENIGN NEOPLASMS AND TUMOR-LIKE CONDITIONS

True neoplasms of the duodenum are infrequently seen. Indeed, tumor-like masses and nodularities caused by hyperplasia, inflammations,

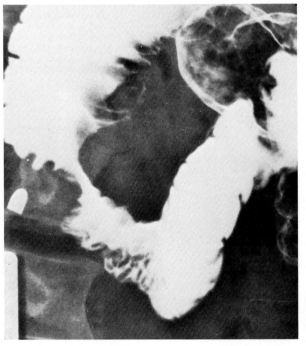

Fig. 15-13 Localized duodenal hematoma due to a gunshot wound presenting as an intramural mass with thickening of adjacent folds.

aberrant tissue and cysts are more frequent findings. Neoplasms may take origin from the surface mucosa or from a Brunner's gland.

Adenomatous Polyps

These small benign tumors occur primarily in the duodenal bulb and proximal portions of the duodenal loop, their incidence decreasing distally. In general, adenomatous polyps present as spherical lesions approximately 1 cm in size with a smooth or ovoid contour (Fig. 15-14). The vast majority sit on a broad base, with polyps on a stalk being unusual. However, gastric polyps may develop a pedicle and may prolapse into the duodenal bulb where they can be mistaken for duodenal polyps (Fig. 15-15).

Brunner's Gland Hypertrophy

Infrequently, Brunner's glands of the proximal duodenum may undergo hypertrophy, possi-

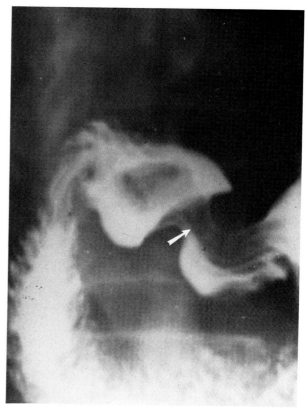

Fig. 15-15 Gastric polyp prolapsing into the duodenal bulb. The stalk of the polyp is visible as a radiolucency filling much of the pyloric canal (arrow).

bly in response to inflammation. Radiologically, one may see several polypoid filling defects in the duodenal bulb and proximal duodenal loop. Enlarged Brunner's glands are very difficult to distinguish from the nodular mucosal swellings of duodenitis.

Nonspecific Duodenitis

The nodular thickening of folds occurring in many cases of nonspecific duodenitis may produce well-defined, multiple nodular filling defects measuring up to 1 cm in size (Fig. 15-11), although usually they are smaller. As mentioned above, the appearance may closely approximate that of Brunner's gland hypertrophy, and definitive differentiation between the two conditions requires endoscopy and biopsy.

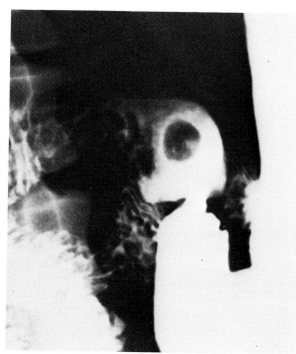

Fig. 15-14 Typical adenomatous polyps of the duodenum visible as smooth filling defects of approximately 1 cm diameter.

Table 15-2. Polypoid Lesions of the Duodenum

Nonneoplastic
  Duodenitis
  Brunner's gland hypertrophy
  Brunner's gland cyst
  Ectopic gastric mucosa
  Duplication cyst
  Aberrant pancreas
  Prominent papilla
  Aortoduodenal fistula
  Varix
  Cronkhite-Canada Syndrome
Neoplastic — Benign
  Adenomatous polyp
  Pentz-Jehgers disease
  Mesenchymal tumor
    Leiomyoma
    Lipoma
    Fibroma
    Neurilemmoma
    Neurofibroma
    Paraganglioneuroma
    Angioma
Neoplastic — Malignant
  Carcinoma
  Lymphoma
  Villous adenoma
  Carcinoid
  Leiomyasarcoma

Heterotopic Gastric Mucosa

It has recently been pointed out that heterotopic gastric mucosa may occur in the duodenal bulb and may produce numerous small filling defects closely simulating those of Brunner's gland hypertrophy and nonspecific duodenitis.

Mesenchymal Tumors

The usual assortment of tumors of mesenchymal origin occurring throughout the gastrointestinal tract is found in the duodenum as well and includes leiomyoma, lipoma, fibroma, angioma, and neurolemmoma. These benign neoplasms present as round or oval masses with a smooth surface and range up to 3 to 4 cm in size. Leiomyomas may be specifically identifiable because of their tendency to undergo central necrosis and ulceration. Lipomas are occasionally identifiable on the basis of their radiolucency and deformability.

A list of entities capable of presenting as benign-appearing small filling defects in the duodenum is presented in Table 15-2.

MALIGNANT NEOPLASMS

The duodenum is infrequently the site of malignant neoplasm. Primary duodenal malignancy and malignant invasion from adjacent sites (usually pancreatic cancer) occur with approximately equal frequency. Clear differentiation between primary and invasive malignancy of the duodenum is often impossible, even at surgery or autopsy.

Primary Carcinoma

Carcinoma of the small bowel is unusual, but it is most prevalent in the duodenum. Its appearance is similar to that of carcinoma presenting in most other locations of the gastrointestinal tract. The earliest lesions are irregular plaque-like or polypoid lesions (Fig. 15-16A). As the lesion progresses, it tends to encircle the lumen, presenting as a circumferential or "apple-core" lesion (Fig. 15-16B). Because of the small caliber of the duodenal lumen, advanced duodenal carcinomas often cause obstruction.

Invasive Pancreatic Carcinoma

Primary pancreatic and ampullary carcinomas may rapidly invade the duodenum in a manner closely simulating primary duodenal carcinoma. Indeed, if there is involvement of both the head of the pancreas and duodenum by an adenocarcinoma, it is often impossible to determine at surgery whether the tumor is of duodenal or pancreatic origin.

Radiologically, the earliest signs of invasion of the duodenum by a pancreatic carcinoma are an impression on the medial aspect of the duodenal loop accompanied by thickening and/or tethering of the duodenal folds (Figs. 15-17A and B). A double contour of the medial aspect of the duodenal loop may be caused by the indenting pancreatic mass. As the lesion progresses, however, it may encircle the duodenum (Fig. 15-17C), simulating primary duodenal carcinoma, and may eventually cause duodenal obstruction.

Lymphoma

The non-Hodgkin's variety of lymphoma may involve the duodenum primarily or secondarily.

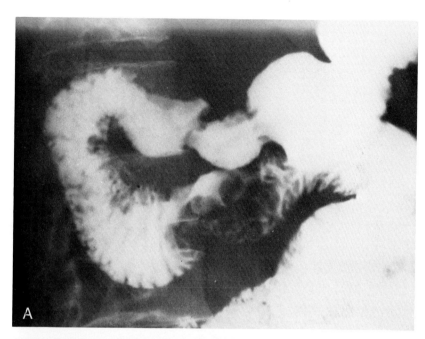

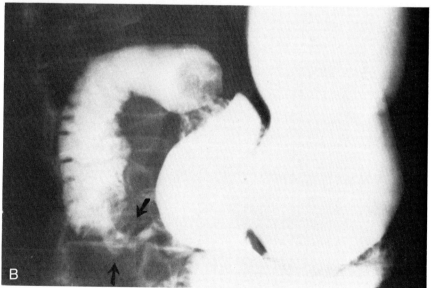

Fig. 15-16 Two carcinomas of the duodenum. (A) Polypoid lesion of the fourth portion of the duodenum. (B) Apple core lesion in the third portion of the duodenum (arrows).

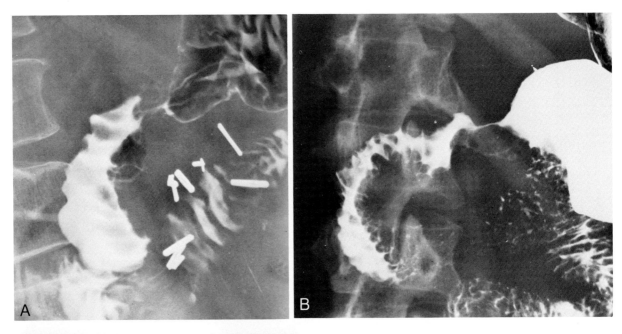

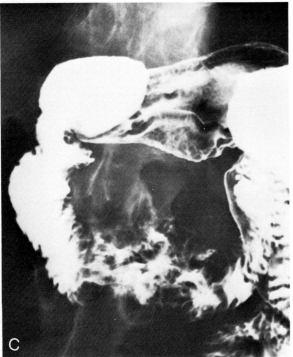

Fig. 15-17 various examples of carcinoma of the pancreas invading the duodenum. (A) Mass impinging on the medial aspect of the descending limb of the duodenum, thickening and effacing the duodenal folds. (B) Large carcinoma of the head of the pancreas causing impressions of the medial aspect of the duodenal loop and the greater curvature of the distal antrum. (C) Carcinoma of the pancreas encircling the third portion of the duodenum and destroying the normal fold pattern of that segment.

Primary involvement usually simulates carcinoma of the duodenum as described above. However, it may cause a more diffuse infiltrating process, with thickening and nodularity of folds over a consider-able length of the duodenal loop. This second form usually occurs as part of the diffuse small bowel involvement found in the Mediterranean form of gastrointestinal lymphoma.

Secondary invasion of the duodenum by malignant lymphoma occasionally occurs in advanced cases of abdominal lymphoma. In these patients, the duodenal loop is usually displaced anteriorly by lymphomatous masses in the retroperitoneal nodes. The duodenal loop is seldom invaded to the point where the normal fold pattern has been destroyed.

Leiomyosarcoma

Leiomyosarcoma is the most common of the malignant mesenchymal tumors of spindle cell origin. A presumptive diagnosis of leiomyosarcoma can be made on the basis of finding a very large smooth duodenal mass. Radiologically, these tumors appear as bulky, smoothly defined round masses, often with a central ulceration. Thus, except for their greater size, their appearance is similar to the benign leiomyoma.

EXTRINSIC MASSES

Since the duodenum is located quite centrally in the abdomen, masses developing in adjacent organs frequently impinge upon it. Many of these create a characteristic impression upon or deviation of the duodenal loop.

Pancreatic Masses

Pancreatic masses located within the head of the pancreas may visibly enlarge the entire duodenal loop if sufficiently large. However, smaller masses within the head of the pancreas may cause more localized impressions on the duodenal loop if they lie in close proximity to the duodenum. Localized dudodenal impressions create the classic Frostberg's "reverse three" sign (Fig. 15-17A). Although generally regarded as a sign of carcinoma of the head of the pancreas, the cases originally described by Frostberg included pancreatic carcinoma, ampullary carcinoma, and enlargement of the head of the pancreas by pancreatitis. Thus, any mass in the region of the head of the pancreas may create the reverse three sign, and any extrinsic impression disturbing the normal contour of the medial aspect of the duodenal loop should be considered potentially abnormal.

Liver Enlargement

Liver enlargement displaces the duodenum posteriorly, inferiorly, and to the left. Displacement of the duodenal bulb below the level of the second lumbar vertebral body or to the left of the midline, as seen on a supine film of the abdomen, is a reliable sign of the hepatomegaly. Conversely, if the duodenal bulb is well above its usual location, a small liver due to hepatic cirrhosis should be suspected.

Distension of the Gallbladder

Distension of the gallbladder occurs in patients with cystic or common duct obstruction. The enlarged gallbladder may cause an impression on the anterolateral aspect of the second portion of the duodenal loop. However, a normal gallbladder may also create a similar impression on the duodenal loop, making the diagnosis of gallbladder distension on this basis a tenuous one.

Right Renal Masses

Right renal masses may infrequently cause an impression on the posterior aspect of the second portion of the duodenal loop and may displace the duodenum anteriorly.

SUGGESTED READINGS

Structural Abnormalities

Ale G, Pompili G: The digestive tract in scleroderma: Radiologic study. II: The stomach and intestine. Radiol Med (Torino) 55:431, 1969.
Bateson EM: Duodenal and antral varices. Br J Radiol 42:744, 1969.
Brunton FJ, Bamforth J: Intraluminal diverticulum of the duodenum and choledochocele. Gut 13:207, 1972.
Dodd GD, Nafis WA: Annular pancreas in the adult. Am J Roentgenol 75:333, 1956.

Griffiths GJ, Whitehouse GH: Radiological features of vascular compression of the duodenum occurring as a complication of the treatment of scoliosis (the cast syndrome). Clin Radiol 29:77, 1978.

Hanssens JF, Moen JP: Intraluminal duodenal diverticulum. J Belge Radiol 64:425, 1981.

Itzchak Y, Glickman MG: Duodenal varices in extrahepatic portal obstruction. Radiology 124:619, 1977.

Kiernan PD, ReMine SG, Kiernan PC, ReMine WH: Annular pancreas: Mayo Clinic experience from 1957 to 1976 with review of the literature. Arch Surg 115:46, 1980.

Lee C, Mangla JC: Superior mesenteric artery compression syndrome. Am J Gastroenterol 70:141, 1978.

Marchal M, Lacombe J, Bassoulet J, Garetta L: Le diverticule endoluminal du duodenum. Ann Radiol 24:656, 1981.

Poppel MH, Marshak RH: Roentgen diagnosis of pancreatic disease. Am J Roentgenol 52:307, 1944.

Richter RM, Pochaczevsky R: Duodenal varices. Arch Surg 95:269, 1967.

Wallace RG, Howard WB: Acute superior mesenteric artery in the severely burned patient. Radiol 94:307, 1970.

Inflammatory Diseases

Balikian JP, Yenikomshian SM, Jedijian YD: Tuberculosis of the pyloro-duodenal area. Am J Roentgenol 101:414, 1967.

Eisenberg RL, Margulis AR, Moss AA: Giant duodenal ulcers. Gastrointest Radiol 2:347, 1978.

Gelfand DW, Ott DJ: Single- vs double-contrast studies: Critical analysis of reported statistics. AJR 137:523, 1981.

Gelzayd EA, Gelfand DW, Rinaldo JA: Nonspecific duodenitis: A distinct clinical entity? Gastrointest Endosc 19:131, 1973.

Kunstlinger FC, Thoeni RF, Grendell JH, et al: The radiologic appearance of erosive duodenitis: A radiographic endoscopic correlative study. J Clin Gastroenterol 2:205, 1980.

Legge DA, Carlson HC, Judd ES: Roentgenologic features of regional enteritis of the upper gastrointestinal tract. Am J Roentgenol 110:355, 1970.

Miller EM, Moss AA, Kressel HY: Duodenal involvement with Crohn's disease: A spectrum of radiographic abnormality. Am J Gastroneterol 71:107, 1979.

Mistilis SP, Wiot JF, Nedelman SH: Giant duodenal ulcer. Ann Intern Med 59:1155, 1963.

Nelson SW, Christoforidis AJ: Roentgenologic features of the Zollinger-Ellison syndrome — ulcerogenic tumor of the pancreas. Semin Roentgenol 3:254, 1968.

Rosenquist CJ: Clinical and radiographic features of giant duodenal ulcer. Clin Radiol 20:324, 1969.

Schulman A: The cobblestone appearance of the duodenal cap, duodenitis and hyperplasia of Brunner's glands. Br J Radiol 43:787, 1970.

Sim GPG: The diagnosis of craters in the duodenal cap. Br J Radiol 41:792, 1968.

Stein GN, Martin Rd, Roy RH, Finkelstein AK: Evaluation of conventional roentgenographic techniques for demonstration of duodenal ulcer craters. Am J Roentgenol 91:801, 1964.

Vaidya MG, Sodhi JS: Gastrointestinal tract tuberculosis; a study of 102 cases including 55 hemicolectomies. Clin Radiol 29:189, 1978.

Wehling H. Das Postbulbare ulcus duodeni. Radiologe 6:274, 1966.

Duodenal Hematoma

Essenhigh DM, Toland J: Duodeno-jejunal haematoma. Br J Radiol 41:349, 1968.

Slonim L: Duodenal haematoma. Aust Radiol 15:236, 1971.

Benign Neoplasm and Tumor-Like Conditions

Bellon EM, George CR, Schreiber H, Marshall JB: Pancreatic pseudocysts of the duodenum. AJR 133:827, 1979.

Boyer CW, Helfrich RB: Adenoma of the duodenal bulb: Case report. Am J Roentgenol 90:753, 1963.

Cynn WS, Rickert RR: Heterotopic gastric mucosal polyp in the duodenal bulb associated with congenital absence of the gallbladder. Am J Gastroenterol 60:171, 1973.

Dodd GD, Fishler JS, Park OK: Hyperplasia of Brunner's glands. Radiology 60:814, 1953.

Kalmar JA, Merritt CRB: Villous adenoma of the duodenum with intussusception. South Med J 73:651, 1980.

Langkemper R, Hoek, AC, Dekker W, Op den Orth JO: Elevated lesions in the duodenal bulb caused by heterotopic gastric mucosa. Radiology 137:621, 1980.

Luckmann KF, Welch RW, Schwesinger W, et al: Symptomatic duodenal duplication cyst in an adult demonstrated by endoscopic retrograde cholangiopancreatography. Am J Gastroenterol 72:153, 1979.

Malmed LA, Levin B: Villous adenoma of the duodenum. Am J Roentgenol 94:362, 1965.

McWey P, Dodds, WJ, Slota T, et al: Radiographic features of heterotopic gastric mucosa. AJR 139:380, 1982.

Meltzer AD, Ostrum BI, Isard HJ: Villous tumors of the stomach and duodenum. Radiology 87:511, 1966.

Ott DJ, Gelfand DW, Kerr RM: Aortoduodenal fistula: An unusual endoscopic and radiologic appearance simulating leiomyoma. Gastrointest Endosc 27:296, 1978.

Peison B, Benisch B: Brunner's gland adenoma of the duodenal bulb. Am J Gastroenterol 77:276, 1982.

Rutgeerts P, Hendrickx H, Geboes K, et al: Involvement of the upper digestive tract by systemic neurofibromatosis. Gastrointest Endosc 27:22, 1981.

Seymour EQ, Griffin CN, Kurtz SM: Carcinoid tumors of the duodenal cap presenting as multiple polypoid defects. Gastrointest Radiol 7:19, 1982.

Shandalakis JE, Gray SW: Smooth Muscle Tumors of the Alimentary Tract: Leiomyomas and leiomyosarcomas — a Review of 2525 Cases. Springfield, IL, Charles C Thomas, 1962.

Spellberg MA, Vucelic B: A case of Brunner's glands hyperplasia with diarrhea responsive to cimetidine. Am J Gastroenterol 73:519, 1980.

Starr FG, Dockerty MB: Leiomyomas and leiomyosarcomas of the small intestine. Cancer 8:101, 1955.

Stassa G, Klingensmith WC: Primary tumors of the duodenal bulb. Am J Roentgenol 107:105, 1969.

Waters CA: The roentgenologic diagnosis of papilloma of the duodenum. Am J Roentgenol 24:554, 1930.

Malignant Neoplasms

Alfonso A, Morehouse H, Dallemand, et al: Local duodenal metastasis from colonic carcinoma. J Clin Gastroenterol 1:149, 1979.

Blery M, Bismuth V, Bard M: Malignant tumors of the duodenum. Report of 6 cases presenting distal to the ampulla of Vater. Ann Radiol 14:543, 1971.

Cortese AF, Cornell GN: Carcinoma of the duodenum. Cancer 29:1010, 1972.

Kato O, Kuno N, Kasugai T, Matsuyama M: Pancreatic carcinoma difficult to differentiate from duodenal carcinoma. Am J Gastroenterol 71:74, 1979.

Extrinsic Masses

Berenbaum SL: Carcinoma of the pancreas: A bidirectional approach. Am J Roentgenol 96:447, 1966.

Bluth I, Vitale P: Right renal enlargement causing alterations in the descending duodenum. Radiology 76:777, 1961.

Chen H, Arger PH, Miller WT: Displacement of the duodenum by an enlarged liver. Am J Roentgenol 119:85, 1973.

Dodds WJ, Zboralske FF: Roentgenographic diagnosis of pancreatic neoplasms. Semin Roentgenol 3:242, 1968.

Frostberg N: A characteristic duodenal deformity in cases of different kinds of peri-vaterial enlargment of the pancreas. Acta Radiol 19:164, 1938.

Kattan KR, Moskowitz M: Position of the duodenal bulb and liver size. Am J Roentgenol 119:78, 1973.

Makrauer FL, Antonioli DA, Banks PA: Duodenal stenosis in chronic pancreatitis: Clinicopathological correlations. Dig Dis Sci 27:525, 1982.

Novelline RA, Ferrucci JT, Eaton SB: The results of hypotonic duodenography in the diagnosis of pancreatoduodenal cancer. J Assoc Can Radiol 26:184, 1975.

Poppel MH: The roentgen manifestations of pancreatitis. Semin Roentgenol 3:227, 1968.

Whalen JP, Evans JA, Meyers MA: Vector principle in the differential diagnosis of abdominal masses: II. Right upper quadrant. Am J Roentgenol 115:318, 1972.

Yoong P, House R: Deceptive duodenal deformity. Br J Radiol 53:1012, 1980.

16

Abnormalities of the Mesenteric Small Bowel

CONGENITAL ANOMALIES

The small intestine is subject to a variety of congenital anomalies due to the complex rotation and fixation of the intestine and its mesenteries during gestation. The most severe congenital abnormalities tend to manifest themselves during infancy. However, certain abnormalities that persist into adult life may present diagnostic difficulty radiologically or may be the belated cause of illness.

Malrotation and Related Anomalies

Malrotation and related anomalies are for practical purposes regarded as a single class of diseases from the standpoint of adult radiology. The varieties of malrotation and nonrotation are legion, but for purposes of this discussion, only the more common forms of abnormal rotation of the small intestine likely to present in the adult are described. It should be noted that in assessing a congenital malposition of the bowel radiologically, the most important elements to be discerned are the presence or absence of the ligament of Treitz, the position of the cecum, and the general location of the mesenteric small bowel.

Complete nonrotation, often termed malrotation, is the consequence of failure of the small

bowel and colon to undergo its normal counterclockwise rotation prior to fixation of the mesenteries. The result is the presence of most of the small bowel on the right side of the abdomen, with the cecum and colon being located mainly on the left (Fig. 16-1). The ligament of Treitz is often absent, and the fourth part of the abdomen accordingly may not ascend behind the stomach, with the result that the duodenal loop is incomplete. This condition may be an infrequent cause of symptoms in an adult, usually on the basis of midgut volvulus.

Paraduodenal hernias may occur in several locations adjacent to the duodenal loop, with trapping of a portion of the small intestine by the remains of the fetal dorsal mesentery. Paraduodenal hernias are the most common of internal hernias and usually present clinically as obstruction of the proximal small intestine. The usual radiologic picture is that of abnormally placed small bowel loops in the upper abdomen. These may be dilated and contain air-fluid levels on plain films if entrapped to the point of obstruction.

Encasement of the small intestine by thin sheets of mesentery or peritoneum may occur in conjunction with nonrotation and/or paraduodenal hernia or for causes that are unestablished. In its usual form, much of the proximal small bowel is encased in a thin sac of peritoneal tissue (Fig. 16-2). The diagnosis may be made by discerning that on appli-

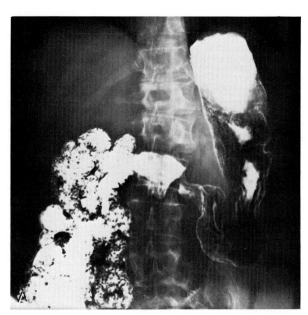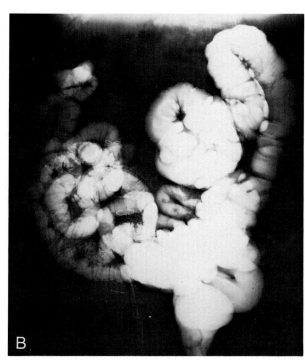

Fig. 16-1 (A) Upper gastrointestinal series showing complete nonrotation of the mesenteric small bowel, with the jejunum in the right abdomen and absence of the ligament of Treitz. (B) Barium enema in a patient with nonrotation showing the small bowel in the right abdomen and the colon on the left.

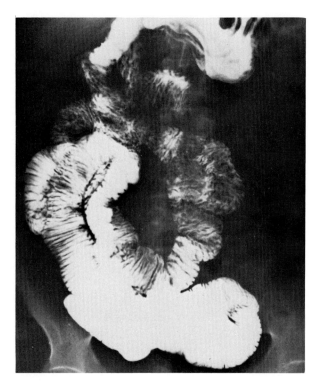

Fig. 16-2 Abnormal location of the jejunum in a patient with nonrotation and a paraduodenal hernia. Encasement of the small bowel within a sac of mesentery was found at laparotomy.

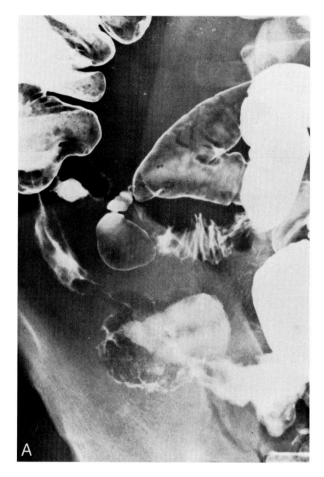

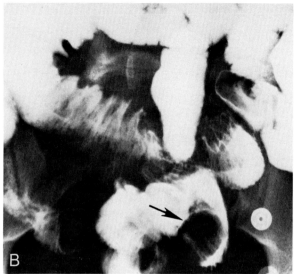

Fig. 16-3 (A) Meckel's diverticulum of the ileum shown unusually well in this example. The patient also has Crohn's disease of the distal ileum and appendix, with an associated retroperitoneal abscess. (B) Inverted Meckel's diverticulum seen as a smooth, benign-appearing mass in the ileum.

cation of compression an entire group of small bowel loops moves about the abdomen as a unit, being contained within the abnormal peritoneal sac. Also, a loop exiting the abnormal sac may be identified in the region of the duodenum. This condition is thought to be capable of causing symptoms of intermittent small bowel obstruction.

Situs inversus is an occasionally encountered anomaly that is usually asymptomatic throughout life. All of the viscera and their locations are mirror images of normal. Many of these cases are found in identical twins.

Duplication

Variable lengths of the small intestine may occasionally be paralleled by an intestinal duplication. In its most common form, the duplication does not communicate with the functioning small intestine and is manifested radiologically as an extramural mass deforming the small bowel. Very rarely, however, a duplication may communicate with the small intestine. The barium study then demonstrates an extra segment of small bowel that tends to be abnormal in appearance and may not with certainty be identifiable as small bowel or colon.

Meckel's Diverticulum

Persistence of a small segment of the vitello-intestinal duct causes formation of a Meckel's diverticulum (Fig. 16-3A), which is usually located in the ileum approximately 1.5 m proximal to the cecum. Frequently, gastric mucosa is present within a Meckel's diverticulum, and ulcerations

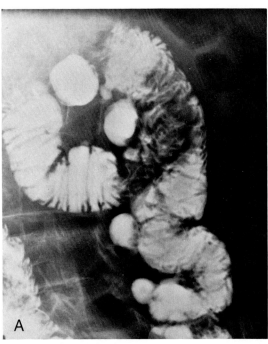 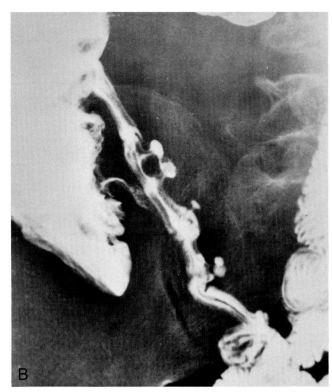

Fig. 16-4 (A) Multiple jejunal diverticula in an elderly female patient. (B) Several diverticula of the distal ileum, an unusual finding that may predispose a patient to diverticulitis of the ileum.

caused by secretions of the gastric mucosa may be a source of bleeding. Meckel's diverticulum may also invert and prolapse into the small bowel lumen, causing intussusception or partial obstruction (Fig. 16-3B).

Radiologically, Meckel's diverticulum may be demonstrated on the peroral small bowel examination, but has recently been described as being more reliably detected by means of single-contrast enteroclysis. Branching of the barium column into the neck of the diverticulum can usually be detected if the flow of barium through the ileum is carefully monitored. The barium then outlines an ovoid sac that is usually slightly larger in diameter than the adjacent small bowel.

DEVELOPMENTAL ABNORMALITIES

A variety of noninflammatory, non-neoplastic structural abnormalities may develop in the adult

that are of idiopathic origin or are the consequence of disease processes that are not primary to the small intestine itself.

Multiple Diverticula

Multiple diverticula are generally encountered in the elderly and are of unknown cause. They are seen as multiple small bowel diverticula similar in appearance to the diverticula commonly encountered in the second portion of the duodenum (Fig. 16-4A). In the small bowel, these diverticula may become large and numerous, and their clinical importance lies in the potential for stasis of small intestinal contents with bacterial overgrowth. This results in "blind loop" syndrome, which consists of crampy abdominal pain, diarrhea, and vitamin K deficiency. The bacterial overgrowth is amenable to treatment by orally administered, nonabsorbable antibiotics. The radiologic investigation of small intestinal diverticula is straightforward, since they inevitably fill with barium during the routine small bowel series.

Diverticula, single or multiple, may also occur in the terminal ileum (Fig. 16-4B). These are seldom of clinical importance except that rare cases of ileal diverticulitis have been reported, with the disease clinically simulating appendicitis.

Intussusception

Intussusception is characteristic of a pediatric population, but occasionally occurs in adults. Any entity that dilates the small bowel, such as nontropical sprue or hypothyroidism, may predispose the small bowel to transient intussusceptions. Also, a small bowel tumor that becomes largely intraluminal may become the lead mass for an intussusception.

Radiologically, intussusception appears as an excess of closely spaced circular barium shadows surrounding an ill-defined mass, the mass being the intussusceptum, or internally telescoped segment of bowel. In certain cases, linear collections of barium within the compressed lumen may be seen extending through the mass.

Adhesions

Adhesions involving the small intestine are detectable radiologically, but their diagnosis has been neglected for decades. However, the recent development of effective techniques for enteroclysis has somewhat improved this situation. Radiologically, adhesions are detectable in many patients with obstructive symptoms following abdominal surgery and may be visible as:

1. Distinct bands crossing, indenting, or "veiling" the small bowel, best shown with the bowel fully distended (Fig. 16-5A – C);
2. Immobility of small bowel loops in response to application of compression, the loops being adherent to the abdominal wall or less mobile viscera;
3. Inseparability of small bowel loops bound together by adhesions, normal loops usually being separable by compression;
4. Sharp, closely spaced reverses of course or

angulations of the small bowel (Fig. 16-5B);
5. Tenting of the wall of the small bowel due to traction by an adhesion on one wall of the bowel;
6. A narrowed segment of small bowel with intact mucosal folds; and
7. Indirect evidence of obstruction consisting of proximal dilation and a normal or decreased caliber of the small bowel distally.

Many of these signs of adhesions will be detectable on the peroral small bowel examination. However, the diagnosis of small intestinal adhesions is most readily made using enteroclysis, which distends the bowel and entails higher flow rates through the bowel. Retrograde small bowel enemas are also effective in the diagnosis of adhesions, particularly if located in the distal small bowel.

INFLAMMATORY DISEASES

Inflammatory diseases of the small bowel is an extensive category ranging from single, discrete ulcers to diffuse granulomatous processes. In most circumstances, the largest number of cases seen will be of Crohn's disease, which is also the most thoroughly described of the small bowel inflammatory diseases.

Discrete Ulcers of the Small Intestine

Discrete ulcers of the small intestine may be produced by several disease entities and may occur as single or multiple lesions.

Zollinger-Ellison syndrome may produce one or more ulcers of the jejunum, often large, and often accompanied by diffuse thickening of jejunal folds. The upper gastrointestinal findings of large or multiple gastric and duodenal ulcers, thickened gastric and duodenal folds, and massive hypersecretion will also be evident.

Potassium chloride tablets were in past years administered to patients receiving diuretics. Since it was discovered that they cause small bowel ulcers with resulting bleeding, pain, or obstructive symptoms, potassium supplements are no longer administered in tablet form.

Ischemia is a rare cause of discrete ulceration. In

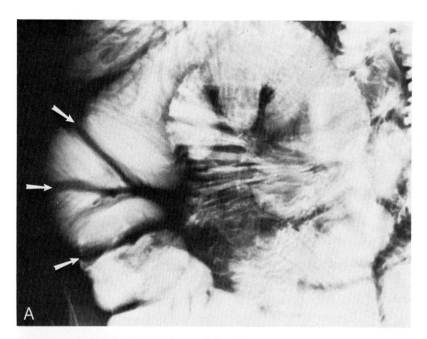

Fig. 16-5 Various manifestations of small bowel adhesions as demonstrated radiologically. (A) Several discrete bands crossing the bowel (arrows). Stretching of valvulae conniventes due to adhesions to a neighboring structure is also visible in the center of the illustration. (B) Adhesive band obstructing and angulating the distal ileum in a patient with clinical symptoms of ileostomy dysfunction. Barium suspension injected through the ileostomy is diluted by fluid retained in the dilated bowel proximal to the partially obstructing adhesion. (C) Broad adhesive band (demarcated by arrows) partially obstructing a loop of ileum.

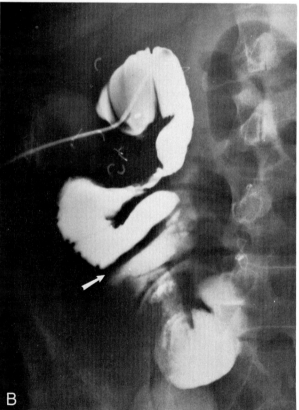

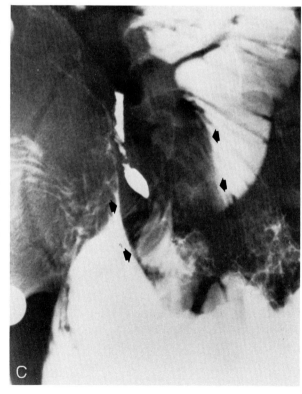

most cases, ischemia involves longer lengths of the small bowel and causes more extensive ulceration.

Crohn's Disease

Crohn's disease is the most commonly encountered serious disease of the small bowel in Western practice. It has been described as being particularly prevalent in northern Europeans and Jews of European origin, and of lower incidence in rural populations, the urban poor, and in developing nations. The etiology of Crohn's disease remains unestablished.

The macroscopic appearance of Crohn's disease is characterized by mucosal ulcerations and thickening of the wall of the bowel and adjacent areas of the mesenteries. Initial mucosal changes consist of nodular enlargement of lymphoid tissue, swelling of the valvulae conniventes, and aphthoid ulcers. Ulceration quickly becomes extensive in most cases, however, and tends to be transmural. Penetration of the wall of the bowel by ulcers is not uncommon, particularly in the small bowel and colon, and is a major cause of complications. Chronic ulceration of the ileum with subsequent fibrotic stenosis and obstruction is a second common cause of complications. Microscopically, Crohn's disease is characterized by transmural ulceration, inflammatory cell infiltrates, submucosal lymphoid aggregates, granulomas, and dilated lymph channels.

The distal ileum is involved in nearly all cases of small intestinal Crohn's disease, either alone or in combination with Crohn's disease elsewhere in the gastrointestinal tract. The second most common site of involvement is the colon, which is significantly involved in between one-fourth to one-half of cases. Complications occur in most longstanding cases of Crohn's disease and include sinus tracts and abscesses, enteroenteric and enterocolonic fistulae, ileal obstruction, and perirectal abscesses and fistulae.

Radiologically, the earliest small bowel changes of Crohn's disease are nodular enlargement of the lymphoid follicles and thickening of the valvulae conniventes, usually first seen in the terminal ileum (Figs. 16-6A and B). Several centimeters of bowel usually are involved when the process is detected. The second early change, occasionally

seen simultaneously, is the presence of aphthoid ulcers, shallow ulcerations surrounded by a raised area of edema (Fig. 16-6C).

Somewhat more advanced radiologic findings are seen at the stage in which Crohn's disease is usually first detected. Ulcers have enlarged and coalesced and involve several centimeters of ileum, often producing pseudopolyps and a "cobblestone" appearance (Figs. 16-6D and E). The ileum may be normal in caliber or slightly stenotic as a result of both the thickening of the bowel wall and the spasm accompanying the inflammatory process. The thickening of the bowel wall and adjacent mesenteric tissues may also be manifested by separation of the barium in adjacent bowel loops from the barium in the involved ileum.

In advanced cases, extensive ulceration of the distal ileum produces an almost featureless, narrowed tube. Both normal valvulae conniventes and the cobblestone pattern may be absent in most of the involved region (Figs. 16-6F and G). The narrowing of the lumen may be quite marked, usually representing spasm as well as fibrotic stenosis. The appearance of the long, slender, featureless lumen filled with barium has been termed the "string" sign. Occasionally, a film will show slight widening of the lumen as the spasm temporarily abates. The bowel wall and adjacent mesenteries are considerably thickened, and separation of normal adjacent loops from the lumen of the diseased ileum may be increased to several centimeters. In occasional severe cases, the entire small bowel may exhibit Crohn's disease (Fig. 16-6H).

The most common complication encountered radiologically is that of an ulcer perforating the wall of the diseased bowel segment leading to formation of a sinus tract or fistula, usually in the distal ileum. The typical radiographic evidence of this complication is the presence of a large inflammatory mass in the right lower quadrant of the abdomen, with adjacent bowel loops widely displaced from the area. Occasionally, sinus tracts may fill with barium and will then be detectable (Fig. 16-7A). Rarely, an adjacent abcess will be opacified with barium (Fig. 16-3A).

If a transmural ulceration of Crohn's disease penetrates an adjacent loop of small bowel or colon, an enteroenteric or enterocolonic fistula will be formed. Frequent sites of fistula formation

(Text continues on page 271)

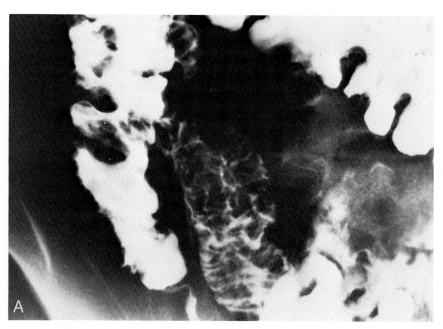

Fig. 16-6 Varied manifestations of uncomplicated Crohn's disease of the small intestine. (A and B) Early changes in the distal ileum consisting mainly of thickening of folds and nodularity. In these illustrations, ulceration has not yet become a dominant factor. (C) Early Crohn's disease of the distal ileum. A well-developed aphthoid ulcer is visible near the ileocecal valve (upper arrow) while a large, irregular ulcer is seen more proximally (lower arrows), with several adjacent tiny ulcerations. The villi are visible in the region as a velvet-like pattern.

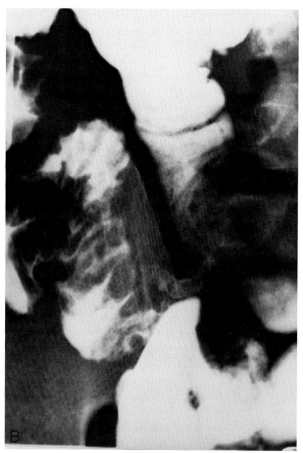

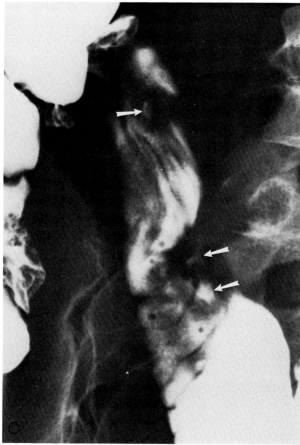

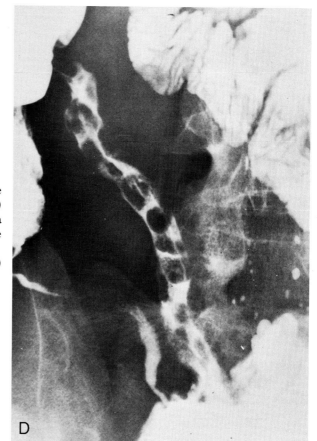

Fig. 16-6 (*continued*) (**D**) Extensive ulceration of the distal ileum resulting in formation of pseudopolyps. (**E**) Extensive ulceration forming a cobblestone pattern in a patient with Crohn's disease involving most of the mesenteric small bowel.

(*Figure continues on next page.*)

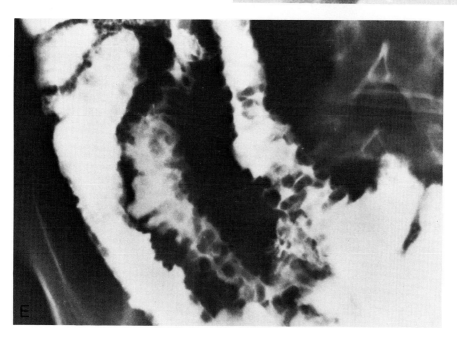

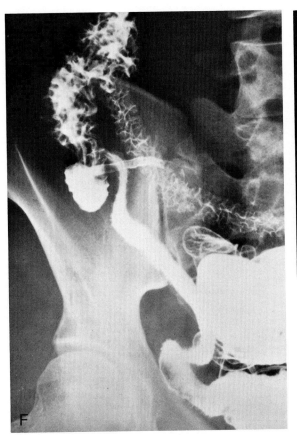

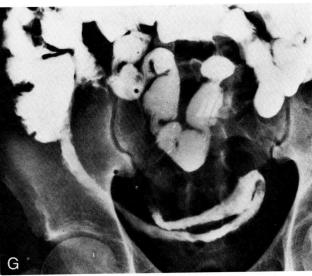

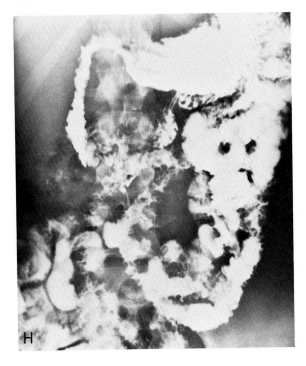

Fig. 16-6 (*continued*) (F and G) Essentially complete ulceration of the distal ileum in Crohn's disease, producing an amorphus surface pattern. The long, narrowed segment of ileum is often referred to as the "string sign." (H) Crohn's disease involving the entire small intestine.

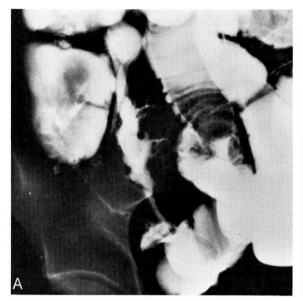
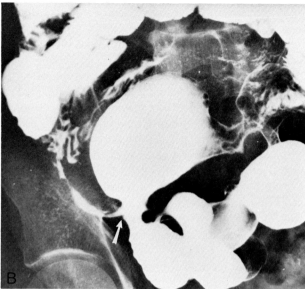
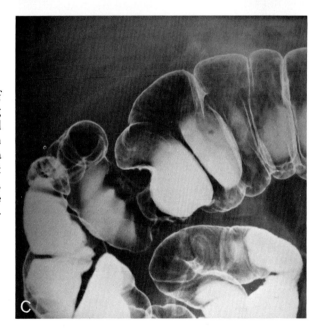

Fig. 16-7 Common complications of Crohn's disease of the small intestine. (A) Numerous sinus tracts extending from a badly diseased segment of ileum. The diseased section of bowel is separated from its neighbors by an extensive inflammatory mass. (B) Ileosigmoid fistula (arrow) in a patient with Crohn's disease. (C) Recurrent Crohn's disease following ileal resection. Thickened, nodular folds are visible in the anastomotic region. The recurrent disease involves both the ileum and the adjacent ascending colon.

are from distal ileum to sigmoid colon and from distal ileum to a more proximal loop of small bowel. Occasionally, several loops of small bowel and colon may be interconnected in an elaborate system of fistulae.

Radiologic evidence of sinus tract or fistula formation takes two forms. First, with either a sinus tract or fistula a branching of the flow of barium will be noted (Fig. 16-7B), an obvious abnormality since the gut at no point normally branches. A second sign of fistula is opacification of a distal loop of gut, such as the sigmoid colon, well before the barium column has progressed into the region by the normal route. Such early opacification is the result of filling of the more distal loop via a fistula. Closely spaced radiographs and careful spot filming may be required to demonstrate the early opacification and the barium within the fistula itself.

Obstruction is the second serious complication seen in patients with advanced Crohn's disease of the small intestine. Partial or complete obstruction may be found in patients who, after a number of years of illness, have developed a stenotic ileum.

The radiographic evaluation of small intestinal Crohn's disease is, in the author's opinion, best performed in most circumstances by the peroral small bowel examination. Although it has been claimed that the earliest changes of mucosal swelling and aphthous ulceration are more readily demonstrated with enteroclysis, it remains to be established that enteroclysis is, over a large number of cases of varying degree of severity, materially more efficacious than the peroral examination. Indeed, the slower progress of the barium column and the use of a more dense barium suspension during the peroral study may have advantages in examination of cases complicated by obstruction, sinus tracts, fistulae, or rerouting of the bowel by surgery.

Surgery of one form or another is eventually performed in many patients with longstanding regional enteritis. It may consist of resection of diseased bowel, diversion of the intestinal stream away from diseased bowel, or resection of an inflammatory mass, sinus tract, or fistula. Surgery in Crohn's disease is further characterized by frequent recurrence following resection. The radiologic findings following surgical intervention in Crohn's disease may therefore be extremely varied, and it is thus desirable to know the exact nature of any surgery prior to performing a small bowel examination.

The most common postsurgical presentation in Crohn's disease is that of the patient who has had resection of the diseased distal ileum followed by an ileoascending colostomy. The majority of these patients will be examined radiologically because of recurrence of symptoms, and any radiologic evidence of recurrent disease usually will be seen at or near the anastomosis. The radiologic changes of recurrent disease are similar to those of primary Crohn's disease, consisting of swelling of folds, thickening of the bowel wall, and ulceration (Fig. 16-7C).

An increasingly less common postoperative presentation is the patient with a side to side ileotransverse colostomy bypassing the ileal disease. This older type of surgery is seldom effective at stabilizing the patient's symptoms, and frequently there will be radiologic evidence of recurrent disease both in the terminal ileum and at the ileotransverse colostomy. In some of these patients the diseased distal ileum may eventually become obstructed, producing a blind loop syndrome with dilatation of the bypassed distal small bowel.

Tuberculosis

Tuberculosis of the small bowel may result from either hematologic spread of the organism or, more commonly, from ingestion of the organism. Infection of the bowel by the human form of tuberculosis usually occurs in patients who have open pulmonary tuberculosis and are swallowing sputum containing tubercle bacilli. In regions lacking routine pasteurization of milk, the bovine tuberculosis organism may be ingested in milk from cows with tuberculous mastitis. With infection by swallowed organisms, the usual site of small bowel involvement is the distal ileum, the organisms preferentially infecting the rich lymphoid tissue of the region. In the occasional case of hematogenous infection, initial involvement of the small bowel is more likely to be multifocal.

The radiologic appearance of the typical early tuberculous lesion is that of one or two isolated, irregular ulcers of the distal ileum, surrounded by thickened folds. Often, there is slight ileal stenosis and distortion of the valvulae conniventes due to accompanying fibrotic changes. With more extensive involvement, multiple ulcerations, fistulae, and involvement of the adjacent areas of the colon may be seen (Fig. 16-8).

Differentiation of intestinal tuberculosis from Crohn's disease is often difficult radiologically. When there has been severe inflammatory contraction of the cecum, often in a characteristically pointed fashion, a specific diagnosis of ileocecal tuberculosis may be suggested. Other characteristic findings include a thickened, gaping ileorecal valve and Stierlin's sign, a funnel-shaped junction of the terminal ileum and the ascending colon, the lumen of the cecum having been obliterated.

Histoplasmosis

Histoplasmosis in most ways imitates the patterns of tuberculosis. The organism may reach the

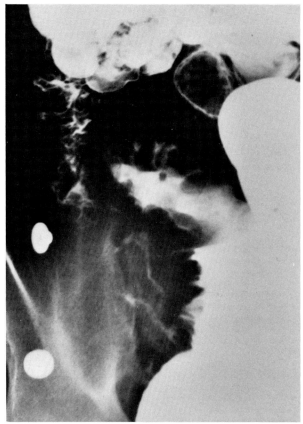

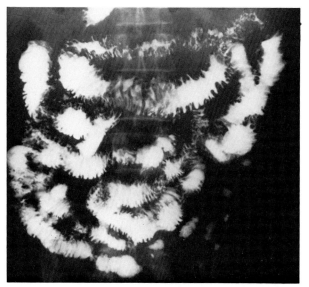

Fig. 16-9 Eosinophilic enteritis resulting in patchy thickening of small intestinal folds.

Fig. 16-8 Tuberculous of the distal ileum and cecum with transmural ulcerations and formation of several sinus tracts.

small intestine by swallowing of infected sputum or via hematogenous dissemination. The small bowel involvement may be confined to the ileum, or may be multifocal.

Radiologic findings in histoplasmosis follow two major patterns. Where hematogenous dissemination has occurred, multiple ulcerations may be detected throughout the length of the small bowel. Indeed, virtually every portion of the gastrointestinal tract may be affected by hematogenously disseminated histoplasmosis. The second pattern is that of ileocecal ulceration, deformity, and mass formation, similar to Crohn's disease or intestinal tuberculosis.

Eosinophilic Gastroenteritis

Eosinophilic gastroenteritis may be manifested in the small bowel by solitary or diffuse lesions,

most often the latter, which tend to involve segments of small intestine of variable length. Histologically, the lesions are seen as inflammatory cell infiltrates of the bowel wall dominated by eosinophils and often accompanied by a considerable fibrotic component. Ulceration occurs inconstantly.

Radiologic findings tend to mimic those of regional enteritis, with irregular thickening of folds and/or ulceration, the process involving variable lengths of bowel (Fig. 16-9). Unlike regional enteritis, however, the lesions may be found anywhere in the small bowel and there is no particular propensity for the disease to occur in the ileum.

Radiation Enteritis

Radiation enteritis may be seen following radiotherapy for almost any abdominal or pelvic malignancy, but currently the most frequent association is with radiotherapy of carcinoma of the uterine cervix. The effects of radiation on the bowel include inflammation, edema, ulceration, and fibrosis. Clinically, patients experience abdominal pain, diarrhea, gastrointestinal bleeding, and obstructive symptoms.

Radiologically, radiation fibrosis presents most frequently as a segmental thickening of the valvu-

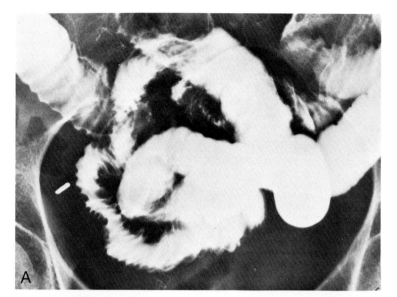

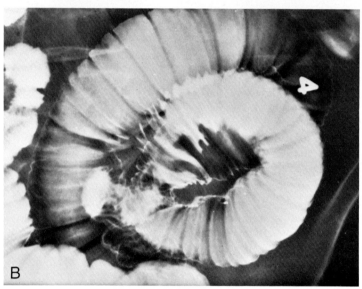

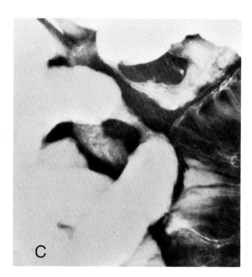

Fig. 16-10 Radiologic appearances of radiation enteritis. (A) Relatively mild radiation enteritis visible as patchy thickening of folds. (B) Moderate radiation enteritis with thickening of folds, acute agulation of the bowel due to adhesions, and partial obstruction. (C) Severe radiation enteritis with ulceration and stricture.

lae conniventes that is limited to the irradiated region (Fig. 16.10). The thickened folds are usually rather smooth, although the degree of thickening may vary considerably from fold to fold. Nodularity occurs but is infrequently the dominant finding. Although ulceration occurs during the most acute phases of radiation enteritis, it is seldom detectable radiologically. The fibrosis and adhesions accompanying radiation enteritis produces characteristic findings that include immobility of the bowel, stenoses, acute angulations, and thickening of the bowel wall.

DIFFUSE NONINFLAMMATORY, NON-NEOPLASTIC DISEASES

Diffuse noninflammatory, non-neoplastic diseases may be described as affecting substantial lengths of bowel and as having a noninflammatory, non-neoplastic origin. Most are characterized by infiltration or deposition of fluid, amorphous substances, or cellular materials in the wall of the bowel. Many are among that group of diseases traditionally described as "malabsorbtion" syndromes.

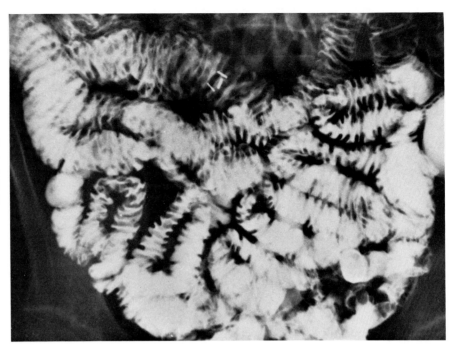

Fig. 16-11 Edema of the small intestine due to hypoalbumenia. The valvulae conniventes are thickened rather uniformly throughout the small intestine.

Small Bowel Edema

Small bowel edema may occur if the serum albumin falls below approximately 2.5 mg percent. With sufficient hypoalbuminemia, fluid migrates from the capillaries into the extracellular space, resulting in tissue edema. Most often, this is the consequence of hepatic cirrhosis, chronic renal failure, or malnutrition. A virtually identical end result occurs when capillary hydrostatic pressure exceeds the normal osmotic pressure of the blood, as in patients with corporal edema accompanying right heart failure. In all of the above circumstances, the small bowel participates in a process that also includes edema of the somatic tissues as well as ascites and other serous effusions.

Radiologic signs of small bowel edema mainly reflect the presence of excess fluid in the submucosal and mucosal tissue layers. This causes an extensive and rather uniform thickening of the valvulae conniventes (Fig. 16-11). The thickening of folds is usually seen over the entire length of the mesenteric small intestine. In severe cases there may be excessive fluid within the lumen of the bowel, and the barium then becomes dilute and may flocculate if an unstable preparation has been used for the examination.

In many cases, ascites will also be present and will be manifested as an inconstant separation of small bowel loops as well as a centering of loops in the anterior midabdomen. The ascites may also impart an overall grey, groundglass appearance to the abdomen and may cause the normally visible inferior margins of the liver and spleen to be absent.

Intestinal Lymphangiectasia

Intestinal lymphangiectasia, also known as Gordon's protein-losing enteropathy, is a rare disease with most of the same radiographic appearances of small bowel edema due to other causes. The basic abnormality is loss of serum proteins from dilated lacteals within the small bowel mucosa. This leads to hypoproteinemia and subsequent edema of the small bowel and other tissues. As with small bowel edema of other origins, there is swelling of the mucosal folds throughout the entire small intestine, but with a more marked severity and uniformity (Fig. 16-12).

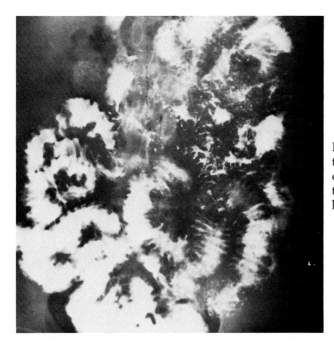

Fig. 16-12 Thickening of folds and a "wet" bowel due to Gordon's protein-losing enteropathy. In the presence of considerable fluid within the lumen of the small intestine, the unstable barium in this examination has flocculated.

Small Bowel Ischemia

Small bowel ischemia may result in intramural edema and hemorrhage. The overall result is that of thickening of the valvulae conniventes in a rather uniform fashion over a variable length of small intestine. The distribution of findings is not as generalized as the entities described above. The folds become club-shaped, rounded, or blunted, depending on the extent of thickening of individual valvulae conniventes (Figs. 16-13A and B). The space between the valvulae conniventes is often narrowed, creating a "stacked coin" appearance (Fig. 16-13A). Where larger submucosal collections of blood have occurred, folds may be obliterated and discrete accumulations of blood may assume the tumor-like appearance that has been termed "thumbprinting" (Fig. 16-13B).

If ischemia is severe, the ischemic mucosa may ulcerate extensively, forming a featureless tube in the region of the ulceration (Fig. 16-13C). If the patient survives, these areas may then become stenotic. In most cases, however, the intramural blood is rather rapidly absorbed, and the appearance of the intestinal mucosa returns to normal. Intestinal ischemia is most often seen in elderly patients with advanced atherosclerosis.

Intramural Hemorrhage

Intramural hemorrhage unaccompanied by ischemia presents virtually the same radiologic appearances as small bowel ischemia and is seen mainly in patients receiving anticoagulants, in patients with Henoch-Schoenlein purpura, in patients who have suffered blunt abdominal trauma, in hemophiliacs, and in patients with pancreatitis. However, these cases rarely progress to the stages of extensive ulceration and stenosis. With amelioration of the underlying abnormality, radiologic findings regress.

Amyloid Disease

Amyloid disease may affect the small bowel in its primary or secondary form. The abnormally staining collections of amyloid are usually deposited in the region of mucosal and submucosal vessels. With extensive involvement, however, many of the normal histologic features of the mucosa are replaced by amyloid material. Clinically, intestinal amyloidosis is characterized by intestinal blood loss, abdominal pain, and signs of obstruction. The

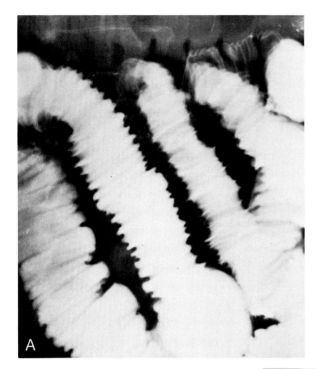

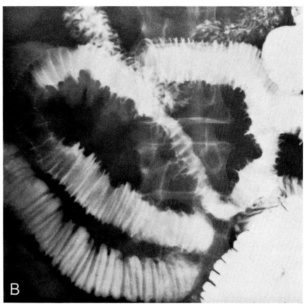

Fig. 16-13 Varied manifestations of small intestinal ischemia. (A) Segmental thickening of the valvulae conniventes, which are spaced unusually close together. (B) Severe thickening of valvulae conniventes as well as "thumbprinting" caused by submucosal accumulations of blood in a patient with small bowel ischemia. Thickening of the bowel wall causes apparent separation of small intestinal loops. (C) Segmental loss of folds and ulceration in a patient with small intestinal ischemia.

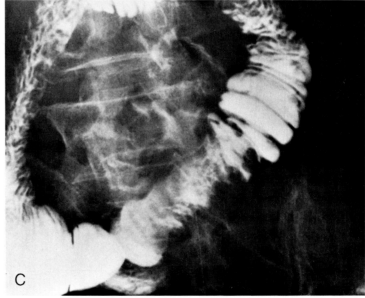

diagnosis is usually established on the basis of small bowel biopsy, with histologic demonstration of amyloid deposits.

Radiologically, there is patchy, irregular thickening of valvulae conniventes in the affected areas. Ulceration and nodule formation are not characteristic radiologic findings. Occasionally, deposits of amyloid are sufficiently heavy throughout the small bowel that peristalsis is virtually absent, and the bowel becomes greatly dilated.

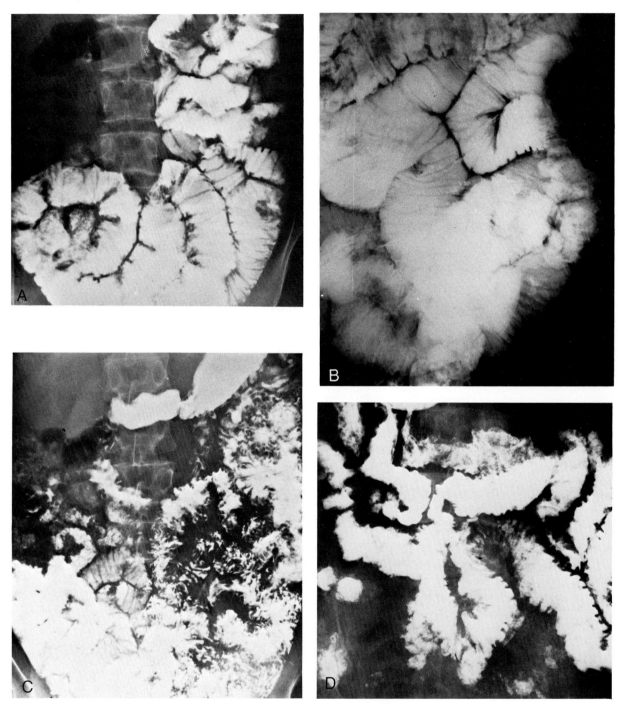

Fig. 16-14 Several examples of nontropical sprue. (A and B) Examples of dilatation of the small bowel with normal-appearing valvulae conniventes. (C) Moderate flocculation of barium in the face of malabsorption due to use of an unstable suspension. (D) An example of the ''moulage sign'' in which featureless streams of barium are seen. This sign is considered to be relatively specific for sprue.

Gluten-Induced Enteropathy

Gluten-induced enteropathy, or nontropical sprue, is caused by sensitivity of the small bowel to the glutens in certain grains. Histologically, inflammatory cell infiltrates permeate the mucosa and submucosa, and there is virtually complete loss of the villi. However, most of these changes are on the microscopic or semimicroscopic level, with little macroscopic alteration of the appearances of the mucosal folds.

Clinically, patients with nontropical sprue suffer malnutrition due to inability of the small intestinal mucosa to absorb a wide variety of nutrients. Fat malabsorption in particular is marked. Careful exclusion of gluten-bearing foodstuffs from the diet usually results in partial or complete remission.

Radiologically, nontropical sprue is primarily characterized by dilatation of the small intestine throughout its entire length (Fig. 16-14A and B). The normally feathery pattern of the jejunum may be absent due to its distention by unabsorbed food materials and copious mucus. The valvulae conniventes remain normal in appearance, they may be minimally thickened in a smooth and uniform manner, or they may be absent over much of the length of the small intestine. Even with the most stable barium preparations, there is likely to be flocculation and sedimentation due to retained foodstuffs and secretions (Fig. 16-14C). In severe cases, tenacious mucus may coat the bowel wall so thickly that the barium cannot outline the valvulae conniventes. This produces amorphous collections of barium in the center of the bowel lumen known as the "moulage" sign, a finding relatively specific for nontropical sprue (Fig. 16-14D).

The major complication of nontropical sprue of interest radiologically is the delayed development of mesenteric or intestinal lymphosarcoma after 10 to 20 years of treatment and remission. Lymphosarcoma should be suspected in any patient with longstanding sprue whose disease unexpectedly becomes refractory to treatment. Since these lymphosarcomas may develop in the mesentery, rather than in the bowel itself, radiologic evidence may consist of an abdominal or retroperitoneal mass displacing bowel. Those malignancies developing in the bowel wall proper can be expected to exhibit the full spectrum of the changes seen in small intestinal lymphosarcoma.

Scleroderma

Scleroderma affects the small intestine in a substantial fraction of those patients who eventually manifest gastrointestinal consequences of the disease. The underlying process is a variable and patchy destruction of the muscularis propria of the small intestine that produces the structural and functional changes detected radiologically.

The radiologic changes in scleroderma of the small intestine are of two general varieties. First, there may be a dilatation of the bowel that tends to involve the proximal small intestine most severely (Fig. 16-15). Rather striking dilatation of the duodenum and jejunum are often seen, usually without similar changes in the ileum. In the dilated regions, the valvulae conniventes are straightened and are either normal in thickness or very slightly thickened. They are also situated more closely together than usual, with a striking parallelism that may be described as resembling railroad ties. In patients with a severely dilated bowel, intermittent intussusceptions may be detected during the examination.

Second, many of these patients develop a variety of wide-mouthed diverticulum that is specific for scleroderma. These diverticula are generally 2 to 4 cm in diameter, with a hemispherical configuration. They open directly into the bowel lumen and are without the neck-like opening associated with most gastrointestinal diverticula (Fig. 16-15B).

The loss of smooth muscle and resulting functional abnormality also contribute to decreased peristalsis and a lengthened transit time. Peristalsis may be virtually absent in those segments of the bowel that are widely dilated, and transit times may be several times longer than those in normal patients. In its most severe manifestations, scleroderma of the small bowel may result in intestinal pseudo-obstruction.

Whipple's Disease

Whipple's disease is an increasingly rare entity characterized by infiltration of the small intestinal mucosa by macrophages containing a glycoprotein that reacts positively to periodic acid-Schiff (PAS) stain. It is thought to be caused by a bacteria-like organism and responds to antibiotic therapy. The

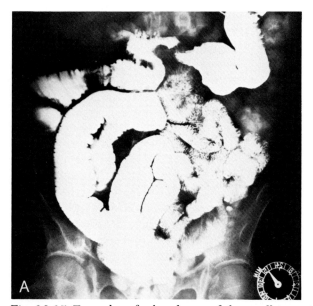
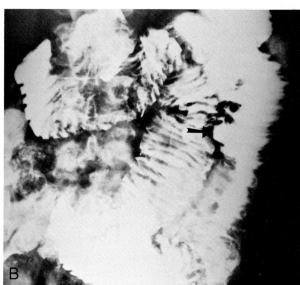

Fig. 16-15 Examples of scleroderma of the small intestine. (A) Dilatation of the proximal small intestine with a normal-appearing ileum in a patient who also has nonrotation of the bowel. (B) Dilatation of the duodenum and jejunum with closely spaced valvulae conniventes. A wide-mouthed diverticulum (arrow) is also visible.

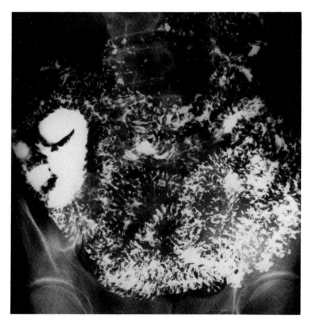

Fig. 16-16 An example of Whipple's disease, a rare entity since the advent of antibiotics. This example of several decades ago shows the uniformly distributed irregular thickening of the valvulae conniventes. Malabsorption has caused flocculation of an unstable barium suspension.

clinical presentation is that of diarrhea, steatorrhea, pain, weight loss, abdominal distension, lymphadenopathy, and epidermal pigmentation.

Radiologically, the small intestine may be dilated, and the valvulae conniventes in Whipple's disease are irregular and mildly nodular in contour (Fig. 16-16). The small bowel is usually uniformly involved from end to end. Evidence of marked malabsorption will usually be seen in the form of flocculation of the barium, with an occasional moulage sign. Because of its increasing rarity, Whipple's disease is a radiologic curiosity, rather than a significant diagnostic possibility.

Nodular Lymphoid Hyperplasia

Nodular lymphoid hyperplasia is mainly seen in patients with congenital or acquired hypogammaglobulinemia, usually of the variety demonstrating IgA deficiency. In these patients, the normally microscopic submucosal lymphoid follicles throughout the small bowel hypertrophy, enlarging to 1 or 2 mm in diameter. Radiologically, they are visible as innumerable tiny masses on the mucosal surface, involving the entire small intestine from pyloric channel to ileocecal valve (Fig. 16-17). The appearance of these nodules has been described as "sand-like." Since most of these patients also have chronic giardiasis, the tiny nodules may be superimposed on folds that are already thickened by inflammation.

PARASITIC DISEASES

As a class, parasitic diseases may be the most frequently occurring disorders of the small intestine when considered on a world-wide basis. Most of the parasites that colonize the small bowel are worms of one variety or another. In developed nations within the temperate climatic zone, parasitic infestation of the small bowel in an adult may be an infrequent event. At the other extreme, a significant fraction of the population of an undeveloped tropical or subtropical region may harbor one or more varieties of intestinal parasites at any given moment.

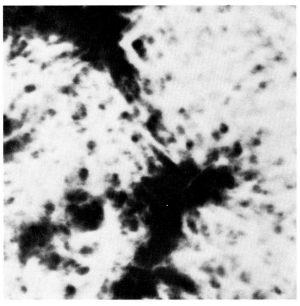

Fig. 16-17 Nodular lymphoid hyperplasia of the small intestine visible as innumerable 1 to 2 mm nodules superimposed on the valvulae conniventes.

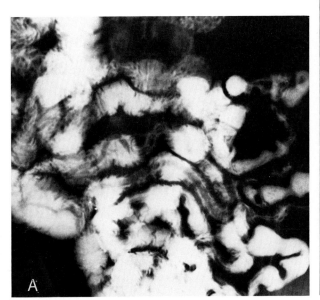
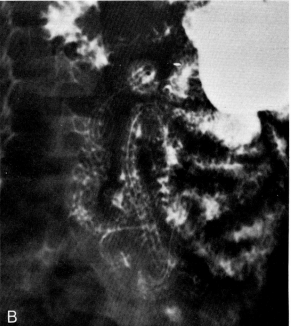

Fig. 16-18 Two examples of ascariasis. **(A)** The worm appears as a slender, pencil-sized filling defect within the barium column. **(B)** Barium visible within the gastrointestinal tracts of several ascarids.

Ascariasis

Ascariasis, or infestation of the small bowel with *Ascaris lumbricoides*, is endemic in many areas of the world, but it is only infrequently seen in adults in developed nations. The typical radiologic appearance of ascarids outlined by the barium in the small intestine is that of one or more worm-like objects of the approximate length and diameter of a slender pencil outlined by the barium (Fig. 16-18A). Barium may be ingested by the ascarids and be visible within their gastrointestinal tract (Fig. 16-18B). The mucosal pattern of the small bowel itself is usually normal.

In severe cases, the worms may be sufficiently numerous as to cause partial intestinal obstruction. In this circumstance, matted balls of tangled worms may be visible during the small bowel study or on plain films of the abdomen. Ascarids may also migrate into the biliary tract where their presence causes biliary tract obstruction, cholangitis, and cholecystitis.

Strongyloidiasis

Strongyloidiasis is widespread in tropical and subtropical regions and may be associated with severe malnutrition. Radiologic abnormalities are extremely varied and are the result of both hypoalbuminemia and inflammatory changes caused by the helminth and its ova. The hypoalbuminemia may be seen radiologically as thickening of valvulae conniventes throughout the small bowel. However, individual cases of strongyloidiasis with severe parasitic invasion of the bowel wall may exhibit nodularity, loss of normal folds, ulceration, or localized dilatation in the areas of the small bowel more severely affected.

Teniasis

Infestation of the small intestine by the pork tapeworm, *Tenia solium,* or the beef tapeworm, *Tenia saginata,* may produce cramping abdominal pain or anemia that leads to radiologic investigation of the small bowel. The tapeworms may occasionally be visible during a small bowel series as long, very slender radiolucencies extending through several loops of the small intestine. The mucosa remains normal in appearance.

With the pork tapeworm, *T solium*, a generalized larval infestation of the body may also develop, a process known as cysticercosis. The larvae encyst and eventually calcify. Small ovoid calcifications may then be visible in tissues throughout the body, including the brain.

Giardiasis

Giardiasis is an infestation of the duodenum and proximal mesenteric small bowel by the microscopic parasite *Giardia lamblia*, usually acquired from unsanitary water supplies. After ingestion, the parasites attach themselves to the mucosa of the proximal small intestine, provoking an inflammatory response.

The radiologic appearance of giardiasis is that of rather uniform thickening of mucosal folds throughout most of the small bowel (Fig. 16-19). The changes are always most intense in the duodenum and jejunum. In an uncomplicated case, the swelling of folds is rather smooth. However, this appearance is greatly altered in patients with nodular lymphoid hyperplasia and gammaglobulin deficiency, who are chronically infested with *G lamblia* due to their immunodeficiency. In these patients, the valvulae conniventes are both swollen by the giardiasis and made irregular by the superimposed fine nodularity of the lymphoid hyperplasia.

Trichinosis

Trichinosis is an infestation of skeletal muscle by the encysted larval form of *Trichinella spiralis,* which is acquired by eating inadequately cooked pork. The ingested larvae burrow into the mucosa of the proximal small bowel where they mature and the females begin producing larvae. The larvae penetrate the small intestinal mucosa and enter the circulation, encysting in skeletal muscles and causing weakness, stiffness, and muscle pains. However, while the larvae are penetrating the intestinal mucosa, an inflammatory response is also produced in the small intestine. Radiologic changes may be noted in the small intestine during the several week period of larva production, and consist of patchy thickening of the valvulae conniventes.

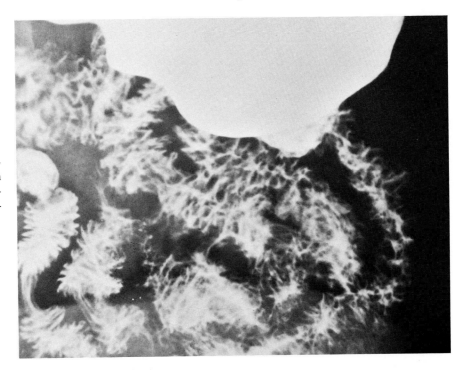

Fig. 16-19 Thickening of jejunal folds in a patient with giardiasis acquired by drinking water from streams during a camping trip.

Schistosomiasis

Schistosomiasis as it affects the gastrointestinal tract is mainly a disease of the colon and rectum. However, small bowel involvement has been reported in *Schistosoma mansoni* infestations. The overall appearance has been likened to that of regional enteritis, with a similar tendency to involve the distal ileum. Small intestinal schistosomiasis has also been described as causing obstruction and malabsorption.

DIFFERENTIAL DIAGNOSIS OF GENERALIZED SMALL BOWEL ABNORMALITIES

It is obvious from the foregoing discussion that a variety of diseases are capable of causing widespread radiologic abnormality of the small intestine and thus often require differentiation from each other. Many of these diseases have traditionally been included among the group of entities known as "malabsorption" syndromes when discussed in the radiologic literature. However, most do not in fact cause malabsorption, a diagnosis best established by laboratory tests.

Generalized small bowel disease is best investigated by means of the peroral small bowel examination. The barium employed should be an extremely stable, viscous, small particle preparation that is resistant to flocculation by abnormal intestinal contents. Since many patients with generalized intestinal diseases will have malabsorption, a fact usually already established clinically, it adds little to confirm the existence of malabsorption on the basis of demonstrating the flocculation of a poorly suspended barium suspension. It is more important that the barium remain in suspension and thus remain capable of demonstrating the structural abnormalities that may allow a more specific diagnosis. Since several of the more common generalized small bowel abnormalities causing malabsorption are characterized by dilatation, the author does not use enteroclysis in this particular application, as the examination itself artificially dilates the small bowel.

Table 16-1 presents a list of the rather numerous generalized diseases of the small bowel causing radiologic abnormalities that may require differentiation from one another. My approach to the differential diagnosis of these diffuse small bowel abnormalities is somewhat more simple than many previously advocated. In this approach, the gener-

Table 16-1. Diffuse Diseases of the Small Intestine

Inflammatory
  Crohn's disease
  Tuberculosis
  Histoplasmosis
  Eosinophilic gastroenteritis
  Radiation injury
  Peritonitis
  Pancreatitis
  Zollinger-Ellison syndrome
Noninflammatory
  Edema due to hypoproteinemia, heart failure
  Intestinal lymphangiectasia (Gordon's enteropathy)
  Ischemia
  Hemorrhage
  Nontropic sprue (gluten–induced enteropathy)
  Scleroderma
  Whipple's disease
  Nodular lymphoid hyperplasia
  Cronkhite-Canada syndrome
Parasitic
  Strongyloidiosis
  Giardiasis
  Schistosomiasis
  Trichinosis
Neoplastic
  Diffuse lymphosarcoma
  Metastatic carcinoma
  Carcinoid tumor

alized small bowel diseases are divided into three groups, each having a dominant overall appearance. Within these groups, further differentiation is attempted on the basis of the radiologic characteristics of the individual disease entities as well as the clinical history.

Diseases Mainly Characterized by Dilatation

In diseases mainly characterized by dilatation, the small bowel is uniformly or segmentally dilated to a considerable degree. However, major abnormalities of the valvulae conniventes are usually absent radiologically.

Nontropical sprue, or gluten-induced enteropathy, produces a rather uniform dilatation of virtually all of the small bowel from the ligament of Treitz to the distal ileum (Figs. 16-14A and B). The valvulae conniventes are either normal or minimally and smoothly thickened and are uniform in appearance. There is usually flocculation of the barium even when a stable preparation has been used (Fig. 16-14C). When seen, the moulage sign is strongly suggestive of the diagnosis of sprue (Fig. 16-14D).

Pancreatic malabsorption due to chronic pancreatitis occasionally produces a small bowel series having many of the appearances of sprue, but of lesser degree. The small bowel becomes mildly dilated in a rather uniform manner. The valvulae conniventes remain normal in appearance. Occasionally there is flocculation of the barium suspension due to unabsorbed intestinal contents. However, the dilatation and signs of malabsorption are less striking than in sprue, and the moulage sign is not seen.

Scleroderma involving the small intestine is also characterized by dilatation, often locally more marked than in sprue. The dilatation in scleroderma tends to be less uniformly distributed and is generally localized to the proximal small bowel. The widely dilated duodenum and/or jejunum, with closely spaced, parallel valvulae conniventes, is a rather specific appearance suggesting this disease (Fig. 16-15). Scleroderma is also identifiable in certain cases by the presence of wide-mouthed diverticula. A further characteristic is greatly decreased peristalsis with a very long transit time.

Drug effects may simulate the appearance of nontropical sprue or pancreatic malabsorption, since the anticholinergic and narcotic classes of pharmaceuticals may cause dilatation of the bowel with decreased peristalsis. In these cases, evidences of intestinal malabsorption, such as flocculation or the moulage sign, are absent and it is usually possible to establish that the patient has been receiving a pharmaceutical capable of causing decreased peristalsis.

Hypothyroidism in its more severe forms may also cause a generalized dilatation of the small intestine. The valvulae conniventes remain normal. The dilatation of the bowel can be quite marked and transit of barium is slowed.

Ileus and distal obstruction also cause dilatation of the small bowel. Patients examined within the first few weeks following a laparotomy often exhibit a residual ileus with noticeable dilatation of the small bowel. More challenging is the diagnosis of partial small bowel obstruction, since the offending adhesions or neoplasm may be difficult to demonstrate radiologically. In cases of suspected partial obstruction, enteroclysis may be helpful in identifying the site and cause of the obstruction (Fig. 16-20).

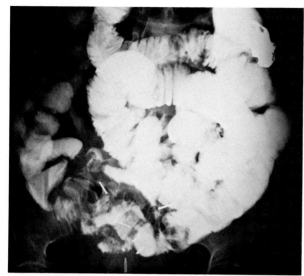

Fig. 16-20 Dilatation of the proximal small bowel due to partial obstruction. The findings in the distal small intestine were due to a combination of recurrent pelvic neoplasm, adhesions, and radiation enteritis.

Diseases Exhibiting Smooth, Uniform Thickening of Valvulae Conniventes

A large group of diseases is characterized by a relatively smooth thickening of the valvulae conniventes over much or all of the small intestine. In many of these the small bowel will be "wet," but the severe malabsorption found in an entity such as nontropical sprue will be absent, and flocculation of the barium will not usually be a dominant factor if a stable barium suspension has been used. Many of these diseases resemble each other radiologically, and considerable reliance must often be placed on available clinical information so as to narrow the range of diagnostic possibilities.

Intestinal edema thickens the valvulae conniventes in a relatively uniform manner throughout the mesenteric small intestine (Fig. 16-11). Minor variation of thickness from fold to fold does not exclude this entity, however. In profile, the folds may assume a somewhat club-shaped contour, and may appear more closely spaced than usual. The bowel is often slightly "wet," with visible dilution of the barium, but marked flocculation of a stable barium separation is seldom seen. Clinical association with hepatic cirrhosis, chronic renal disease, or right heart failure is helpful in making the diagnosis.

Intestinal lymphangiectasis, or Gordon's enteropathy, mimics most of the findings of severe intestinal edema. Folds are thickened strikingly and in a very uniform manner (Fig. 16-12). The bowel is "wet," and dilution of the barium may be marked. Knowledge of the patient's fecal protein loss is helpful in establishing radiologic confirmation of the disease.

Ischemia and hemorrhage of the bowel thicken the valvulae conniventes in a relatively smooth fashion, but the involvement is segmental rather than generalized as in intestinal edema (Fig. 16-13). There is usually some variation in the degree of fold thickness in the involved region, but nodularity is not often a significant factor. When present, thumbprinting and the stacked coin appearance may be helpful at arriving at a specific diagnosis. A history of episodic abdominal pain with bleeding or of anticoagulant therapy is helpful.

Radiation enteritis also produces a relatively smooth thickening of the small intestinal folds, although the thickness of individual folds tends to vary considerably within the affected region (Fig. 16-14). Fibrotic stenoses, acute angulations, and thumbprinting may also be present. Because of the history of radiation treatment, diagnosis is seldom a problem. The major task that may face the radiologist is one of excluding intraperitoneal recurrence of neoplasm.

Zollinger-Ellison syndrome may often be accompanied by thickening of folds in the duodenum and jejunum, apparently a response to the massive gastric hypersecretion. Ulcers may be found in the distal duodenum and proximal jejunum, where their presence is distinctly unusual. Because of the remarkable findings usually present in the stomach and duodenum, the nature of the changes in the mesenteric small bowel is usually recognized.

Interloop abscess or peritonitis may extensively thicken the folds in the small bowel; the thickness is due to secondary inflammation and edema of the bowel wall.

Pancreatitis produces thickening of the folds in the proximal jejunum by a very similar process.

Giardiasis thickens the mucosal folds of the duodenum and proximal mesenteric small bowel. The thickening may be variable from one fold to another, but the thickened folds lack any appreciable nodular component in the uncomplicated case (Fig. 16-19). However, when giardiasis is found in association with *intestinal lymphoid hyperplasia,* a mixed pattern of fine nodularity and thickened folds is produced.

Trichinosis may present radiologically as thickened folds in the small intestine if the examination is performed at the stage in which the parasites are migrating through the intestinal mucosa. The resulting inflammation produces a patchy but relatively diffuse thickening of the mucosal folds.

Diseases Characterized by Irregular or Nodular Enlargement of Mucosal Folds

A third group of entities is characterized by thickening of the valvulae conniventes that is far more irregular or nodular than in those diseases just described. Although many of these resemble each other radiologically, a specific diagnosis is aided by their association with the presence of the same disease process in other organ systems or by a distinct natural history. Differentiation may also be possible on the basis of their distribution within the small intestine and specific radiologic signs.

Diffuse lymphosarcoma of the small intestine is the premier example of a disease that thickens folds in a nodular and irregular manner throughout the small intestine (see Fig. 16-25C). Nonuniform growth of the malignancy infiltrating the wall of the small bowel is the cause of the irregularity and nodularity. Although a severe and extensive case of Crohn's disease (Fig. 16-6H) may mimic this disease, no other entity regularly produces such a major distortion of the fold pattern. Recognition of the malignant nature of the process is aided by the detection of discrete tumor masses when present.

Extensive Crohn's disease may closely simulate the diffuse form of lymphosarcoma, since in very severe cases, Crohn's disease may involve virtually the entire small bowel. The combination of thickening of the bowel wall, irregular thickening of the valvulae conniventes, and nodularity (Fig. 16-6H) may be strikingly similar to lymphosarcoma. Usually, however, many years of an increasing severity of Crohn's disease has been present, allowing differentiation from lymphosarcoma on the basis of the natural history of the disease.

Eosinophilic gastroenteritis may cause an irregular and nodular thickening of valvulae conniventes in a patchy distribution over variable lengths of small bowel (Fig. 16-9). Its appearance can be described as similar to that of a mild case of Crohn's disease, but occurring in the wrong locations. The diagnosis may be confirmed by a small bowel biopsy showing eosinophilic infiltration or by the presence of eosinophilia in the peripheral circulation.

Whipple's disease presents with a more uniformly distributed nodularity and irregularity of the valvulae conniventes than the foregoing entities (Fig. 16-16). The folds are only moderately thickened in most cases, and there is neither ulceration nor mass formation.

Nodular lymphoid hyperplasia produces a very fine nodularity of the valvulae conniventes that is rather specific for this entity because of the extremely small size of the nodules (Fig. 16-17). The nodularity of lymphoid hyperplasia in the small bowel seldom exceeds 1 to 2 mm in diameter.

BENIGN NEOPLASMS

The small bowel is subject to the same variety of benign neoplasms as found in the esophagus, stomach, and duodenum, although adenomatous polyps of the mesenteric small intestine are rare. Benign tumors of the small intestine are typically smooth, round or oval masses, appearing radiologically to be of mucosal or intramural origin (Fig. 16-21). For the complete list of benign tumors and tumor-like conditions likely to be encountered in the small bowel, reference should be made to Table 16-2. The most frequent are leiomyoma and lipoma. Of these, the lipoma can usually be diagnosed specifically because it is soft and deformable and sometimes detectably radiolucent. When multiple polypoid lesions are demonstrated, particularly if they are on a stalk, they will most likely represent Peutz-Jehgers disease (Fig. 16-22), and similar lesions are likely to be found elsewhere in the gastrointestinal tract.

Endometriosis

Endometriosis may simulate the presence of a benign neoplasm and is a consideration whenever a

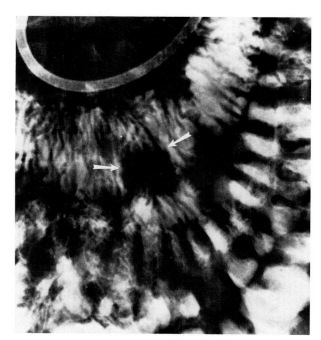

Fig. 16-21 Small leiomyoma (arrows) found in the proximal jejunum by enteroclysis.

Table 16-2. Benign-Appearing Small Bowel Mass Lesions

Non-neoplastic
  Duplication
  Intraluminal diverticulum
  Inverted Meckel's diverticulum
  Submucosal hemorrhage
Benign neoplasm
  Leiomyoma
  Lipoma
  Fibroma
  Angioma
  Neurilemmoma
  Carcinoid
  Pentz-Jegher's syndrome
  Endometriosis
Malignant
  Carcinoid
  Hematogenous metastasis
  Direct metastasis

benign-appearing, mass-like lesion is encountered in the distal small bowel. As a result of repeated bleeding into the pelvic cavity, patients with endometriosis often have extensive pelvic adhesions, which may render the pelvic loops of small bowel immobile.

MALIGNANT NEOPLASMS

Malignancies of the small intestine are less common than elsewhere in the gastrointestinal tract. Unfortunately, the resulting low order of suspicion for small bowel malignancies often causes them to be overlooked on radiologic examinations.

Carcinoid Tumors

Also known as argentifinomas, these neoplasms arise from silver-staining cells found at the base of the crypts of Lieberkuhn and are said to be the most common of small bowel neoplasms. Unlike other small bowel neoplasms, carcinoid tumors

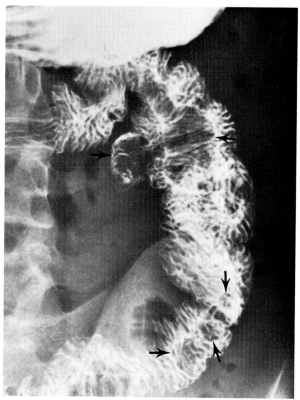

Fig. 16-22 Several polypoid neoplasms of the proximal small intestine due to Peutz-Jehgers disease (arrows). The large polyp in the upper portion of the illustration is on a visible stalk.

occur most frequently in the distal small bowel. The majority of carcinoid tumors encountered are asymptomatic and are found incidentally at surgery or autopsy. However, approximately one-third of carcinoid tumors produce symptoms referable to the mechanical effects of the neoplasm or its liberation of serotonin. In *carcinoid syndrome,* resulting from serotonin release by the tumor, the patient may experience a variable combination of flushing, wheezing, diarrhea, and right heart failure. Generally, carcinoid syndrome does not occur unless the tumor has metastasized to the liver.

Carcinoid tumors are difficult to classify as benign or malignant on the basis of either their macroscopic appearances or histologic findings. The natural history of the tumor itself best determines the final evaluation, and thus all carcinoid tumors are considered to have malignant potential. However, the majority of small intestinal carcinoid tumors have the macroscopic appearances of benign tumors, being smoothly contoured polypoid lesions of modest size, while only a minority have the gross pathologic characteristics of frank malignancies.

Radiologically, the appearance of a carcinoid tumor may vary from that of a benign, polypoid lesion to a large, irregular, and frankly malignant-appearing mass (Fig. 16-23). Whether the radiologic characteristics are benign or malignant, suspicion of carcinoid tumor of the small intestine should be raised whenever a mass lesion is encountered in the distal ileum. A further characteristic of malignant carcinoid tumors is their ability to excite a dense, scirrhotic reaction in their immediate environs. This produces peculiar angulations and separations of ileal loops as well as thickening of mucosal folds. When multiple carcinoid tumors are present, this wild appearance may be produced over much of the length of the small intestine.

Adenocarcinoma

Adenocarcinoma occurs infrequently in the mesenteric small bowel, particularly as compared to its incidence in the esophagus, stomach, and colon. It is most frequently found in the jejunum. Radiologically, small intestinal carcinomas have all

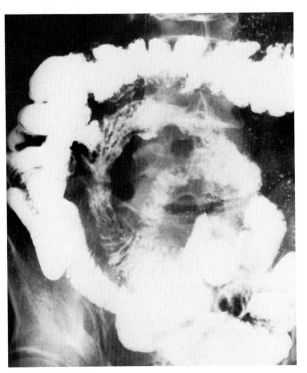

Fig. 16-23 Large malignant-appearing carcinoid tumor of the distal ileum. Carcinoid tumors may vary in appearance from small benign-appearing lesions to frank malignancies.

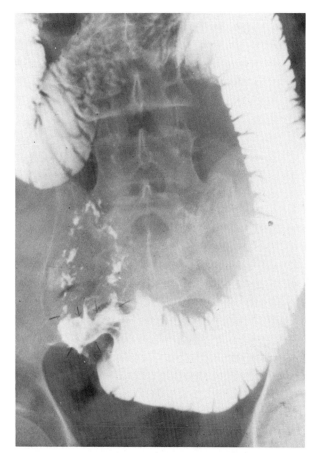

Fig. 16-24 Circumferential adenocarcinoma of the jejunum causing virtually complete obstruction.

of the expected characteristics of a gastrointestinal malignancy. Early lesions are polypoid or plaque-like masses. However, they quickly encircle the small bowel lumen, producing an irregular, partially obstructing lesion (Fig. 16-24). When partial obstruction is present, carcinomas are usually easy to locate and detect radiologically. However, small nonobstructing intestinal carcinomas may be very difficult to diagnose on a typically cursory peroral small bowel examination. Enteroclysis, since it allows fluoroscopically monitored filming of the entire small bowel, is the preferred method for detection of these small, localized lesions. The usual clinical presentation of small bowel carcinoma is that of bleeding or obstruction.

Lymphoma

Lymphoma of the small bowel occurs in two forms, discrete and diffuse. The most common type in Western practice is that of the discrete lesion having many of the gross-pathologic and radiologic appearances of a carcinoma. However, lymphomas of the small bowel tend to be much bulkier lesions than carcinomas, and they may have a very large necrotic center, forming an irregular cavity in the midst of the lesion. (Figs. 16-25A and B). The large mass of the tumor is often apparent and displaces adjacent bowel loops. Unlike small intestinal carcinoma, lymphomas rarely cause obstruction.

The diffuse form of small bowel lymphosarcoma occurs mainly in patients of Near Eastern extraction, and has been referred to as the "Mediterranean" form of the disease. It usually presents with involvement of the entire small intestine. Valvulae conniventes over most or all of the mesenteric small bowel and duodenum are thickened and/or nodular, and the wall of the bowel is thickened (Fig. 16-25C). In slightly more advanced cases, distinct masses may be identified. With severe, full thickness involvement of the bowel wall, segments

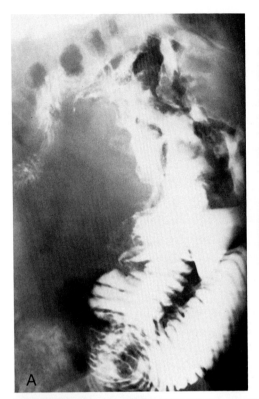

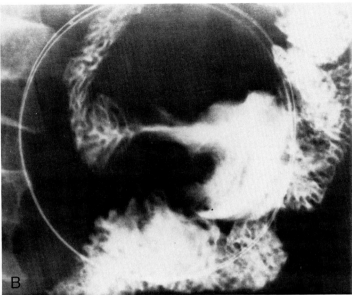

Fig. 16-25 Various examples of lymphosarcoma of the small intestine. (A) Bulky necrotic lymphosarcoma of the jejunum with a large, irregular cavity filling with barium. (B) Discrete lymphosarcomatous tumor of the jejunum with an "apple core" appearance similar to a carcinoma. (C) Diffuse lymphosarcoma of the small intestine of the "Mediterranean" variety. The thickening of folds and separation of bowel loops is due to infiltration of tumor in the bowel wall. (D) Aneurysmal dilatation of the small intestine at the duodenal-jejunal junction (arrow) due to segmental involvement of the intestine by lymphosarcoma. Several other similar dilated areas were visible elsewhere in the small bowel.

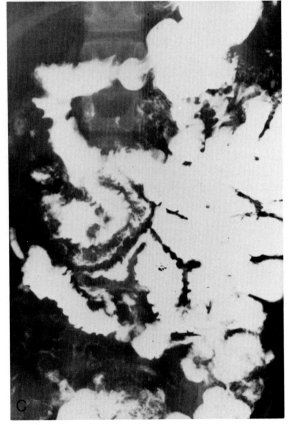

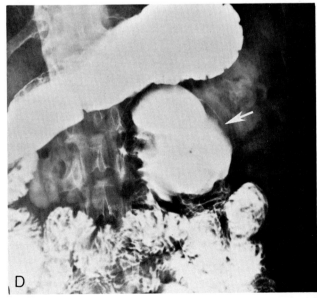

of bowel may become dilated and featureless, a phenomenon termed *aneurysmal dilatation* (Fig. 16-25D). In severe cases, considerable evidence of malabsorption may be present. The diffuse form of lymphosarcoma has been described in association with immunoglobulin disorders.

Diffuse lymphoma also occurs in patients who have had longstanding nontropical sprue, or gluten-sensitive enteropathy. After many years, there may be clinical deterioration in spite of maintenance of a gluten-free diet. The radiologic appearance of the small bowel may then change from that typical of sprue to an appearance more characteristic of small intestinal lymphosarcoma.

Metastatic Carcinoma

Metastatic carcinoma affects the small bowel with approximately the same incidence as primary malignancies. Malignant neoplasms may metastasize to the small intestine via either hematogenous dissemination or direct extension.

With blood-born metastases, the earliest manifestation is usually that of multiple submucosal or intramural nodules (Figs. 16-26A and B). However, these may then destroy the overlying mucosa, becoming more ragged in appearance, or they may encircle the bowel lumen in a manner characteristic of primary small bowel carcinoma or lymphoma. The most frequent blood-born metastatic lesions are carcinoma of the breast and malignant melanoma. Occasionally, particularly with malignant melanoma, the central portion of metastatic nodules may become necrotic, producing a target or bullseye appearance.

Direct invasion of the small bowel by malignancies originating in adjacent organs is more frequent than hematogenous metastases. The origins of the invading malignancies most often include the colon, ovary, uterine cervix, stomach, and pancreas. Small bowel invasion is often the preterminal event in patients dying of abdominal carcinomatosis.

Radiologically, the appearance of direct invasion is usually the result of a combination of effects (Figs. 16-26C–E). The mass effect of the abdominal tumor displaces the small bowel, which may be adherent and draped partially around it. Where the tumor has invaded most of the thickness of the bowel wall, it may assume the appearance of an intramural lesion. A scirrhous reaction may duplicate the appearances of non-neoplastic adhesions, producing stenoses, acute angulations, tenting, and partial or complete obstruction. It is thus occasionally necessary, in a postoperative patient, to determine whether abnormalities of this variety are the result of postoperative adhesions, radiation enteritis, or recurrent intraabdominal malignancy. In the latter case, intramural or extramural tumor masses are sought as signs of the recurrent neoplasm.

EXTRINSIC MASSES

Because the small bowel is mobile and extends throughout the abdomen, any mass impinging on the abdominal cavity is likely to cause its displacement. Certain characteristic presentations of small bowel displacement by extrinsic masses should be noted.

Mesenteric Cysts

Mesenteric cysts may present a unique appearance when they occur in the midportion of the mesenteric small bowel. They tend to spread the small bowel loops around their periphery in a manner outlining the cyst. The lack of any associated abnormality of the valvulae conniventes is a clue to the benign nature of the mass.

Pelvic Masses

Pelvic masses, particularly of the female reproductive organs, generally displace the ileum upward and out of the pelvis as they enlarge.

Pancreatic Masses

Pancreatic masses, specifically those in the body and tail of the pancreas, may inferiorly displace the small bowel at the ligament of Treitz.

(Text continues on page 294)

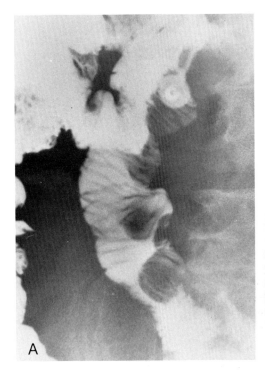

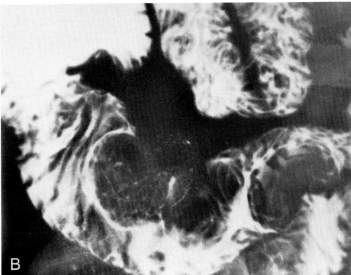

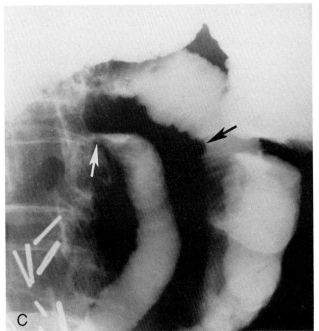

Fig. 16-26 The variable appearances of metastatic neoplasm involving the small intestine. (A) Multiple submucosal nodules due to hematogenous spread of malignancy. (B) Submucosal and intramural nodules due to metastatic melanoma. (C) Intramural nodule (black arrow), separation of loops, and virtually complete obstruction (white arrow) with proximal dilatation in a patient with abdominal carcinomatosis.

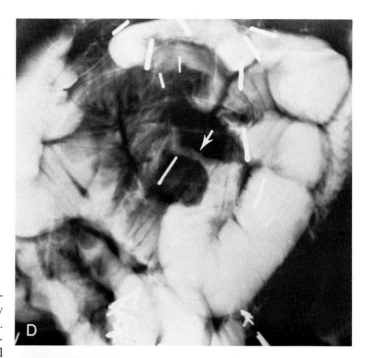

Fig. 16-26 (*continued*) (D) Circumferential narrowing due to invasion by adjacent, recurrent neoplasm (arrow). (E) Submucosal intramural and extramural masses deforming the bowel and separating adjacent loops. The findings were due to carcinoma of the breast, extensively metastatic to the serosa, bowel wall, and mesentery.

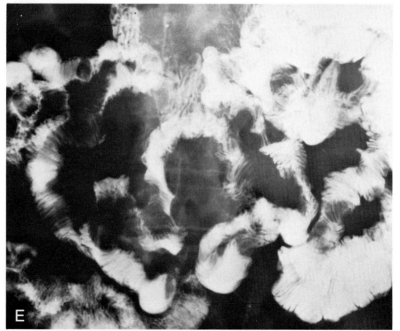

Massive Hepatomegaly or Splenomegaly

Massive hepatomegaly or splenomegaly is capable of displacing the small bowel inferiorly. With sufficient enlargement of the liver or spleen, the inferior borders of the enlarged organ may be outlined by adjacent small bowel loops rather than the colonic flexures.

SUGGESTED READINGS

Congenital Anomalies and Developmental Abnormalities

Bartram CI: The radiological demonstration of adhesions following surgery for inflammatory bowel disease. Br J Radiol 53:650, 1980.

Baskin RH, Mayo CW: Jejunal diverticulosis. A clinical study of 87 cases. Surg Clin North Am 32:1185, 1952.

Basu R, Forshall I, Rickham PP: Duplications of the alimentary tract. Br J Surg 47:477, 1961.

Berdon WE, Baker DH, Bull S, Santulli TV: Midgut malrotation and volvulus. Radiology 96:375, 1970.

Carlson HC: Small intestinal intussusception: An easily misunderstood sign. Am J Roentgenol 110:338, 1970.

Christensen N: Jejunal diverticulosis. Am J Surg 118:612, 1969.

Cohen MD, Lintott DJ: Transient small bowel intussusception in adult coeliac disease. Clin Radiol 29:529, 1978.

Dalinka MK, Wunder JF: Meckel's diverticulum and its complications, with emphasis on roentgenologic demonstration. Radiology 106:295, 1973.

Dott NM: Anomalies of intestinal rotation: Their embryology and surgical aspects. Br J Surg 11:251, 1923.

Estrada RL: Anomalies of Intestinal Rotation and Fixation (Including Mesentericoparietal Hernias). Springfield, IL, Charles C Thomas, 1958.

Favera BE, Franciosi RA, Akers DR: Enteric duplications. Thirty seven cases: Vascular theory of pathogenesis. Am J Dis Child 122:501, 1971.

Freeny PC, Walker JH: Inverted diverticula of the gastrointestinal tract. Gastrointest Radiol 4:57, 1979.

Frieden JH, Kaplan L: Duplication of the terminal ileum with intussusception in an adult. Am J Gastroenterol 73:523, 1980.

Houston CS, Wittenborg MH: Roentgen evaluation of anomalies of rotation and fixation of the bowel in children. Radiology 84:1, 1965.

Maglinte DDT, Elmore MF, Isenberg M, Dolan PA: Meckel's diverticulum: Radiologic demonstration by enteroclysis. AJR 134:925, 1980.

Miller KB, Naimark A, O'Connor JF, Bouras L: Unusual roentgenologic manifestations of Meckel's diverticulum. Gastrointest Radiol 6:209–215, 1981.

Sellink JL: Radiological Atlas of Common Diseases of the Small Bowel. Leiden, Stenfert Kroese, 1976, pp 355–362.

Turley K: Right paraduodenal hernia: A source of chronic pain in the adult. Arch Surg 114:1072, 1979.

Wiot JF, Spitz HB: Small bowel intussusception demonstrated by oral barium. Radiology 97:361, 1970.

Inflammatory Diseases

Boley SJ, Allen AC, Schultz, L, Schwartz S: Potassium induced lesions of the small bowel. II. Pathology and pathogenesis. JAMA 193:1001, 1965.

Brombart M, Massion J: Radiologic differences between ileocecal tuberculosis and Crohn's disease. Am J Dig Dis 6:589, 1961.

Bruneton JN, Faure X, Bourry J, et al: A radiologic study of chronic radiation-induced injuries of the small intestine and colon. Fortschr Röntgenstr 136:129, 1982.

Burhenne HJ, Carbonne JV: Eosinophilic (allergic) gastroenteritis. Am J Roentgenol 96:332, 1966.

Carlson HC: Localized nonspecific ulceration of the small intestine. Radiol Clin North Am 7:97, 1969.

Carrera GF, Young S, Lewicki AM: Intestinal tuberculosis. Gastrointest Radiol 1:147, 1976.

DeDombal FT, Burton I, Goligher JC: Recurrence of Crohn's disease after primary excisional surgery. Gut 12:519, 1971.

Ekberg O, Lindstrom C: Superficial lesions in Crohn's disease of the small bowel. Gastrointest Radiol 4:389, 1979.

Gershon-Cohen J, Kremens V: X-ray studies of the ileocecal valve in ileocecal tuberculosis. Radiology 62:251, 1954.

Haberkern CM, Christie DL, Haas JE: Eosinophilic gastroenteritis presenting as ileocolitis. Gastroenterology 74:896, 1978.

Hildell J, Lindstrom C, Wenckert A: Radiographic appearance in Crohn's disease. I. Accuracy of radiographic methods. Acta Radiol Diag 20:609, 1979.

Hildell J, Lindstrom C, Wenckert A: Radiographic appearances in Crohn's disease. IV. The new distal ileum after surgery. Acta Radiol Diag 21:221, 1980.

Kelvin FM, Gedgaudas RK: Radiologic diagnosis of Crohn's disease (with emphasis on its early manifestations). CRC Crit Rev Diagn Imaging, 16:43, 1981.

Marshak RH: Granulomatous disease of the intestinal tract. Radiology 114:3, 1975.

Marshak RH, Lindner AE: Radiology of the small intestine. Philadelphia, WB Saunders, 1976, pp 179–245.

Mason GR, Dietrich P, Friedland GW, Hanks GE: The radiological findings in radiation-induced enteritis and colitis: A review of 30 cases. Clin Radiol 21:232, 1970.

Muhletaler CA, DeSoto L, Gerlock AJ, Pendergrass HP: Radiographic manifestations of gastrointestinal tuberculosis. Revista Interamericana Radiol 4:123, 1979.

Nolan DJ: Radiology of Crohn's disease of the small intestine: A review. J Royal Soc Med 74:294, 1981.

Nolan DJ, Gourtsoyiannis NC: Crohn's disease of the small intestine: A review of the radiological appearances in 100 consecutive patients examined by a barium infusion technique. Clin Radiol 31:597, 1980.

Nolan DJ, Piris J: Crohn's disease of the small intestine. A comparative study of the radiological and pathological appearances. Clin Radiol 31:591, 1980.

Schulman A, Morton PCG, Dietrich BE: Eosinophilic gastroenteritis. Clin Radiol 31:101, 1980.

Sellink JL: Radiological Atlas of Common Diseases of the Small Bowel. Leiden, Stenfert Kroese, 1976, pp 171–202.

Vaidya MG, Sodhi JS: Gastrointestinal tuberculosis: A study of 102 cases including 55 hemicolectomies. Clin Radiol 29:189, 1978.

Werbeloff Z, Novis BH, Banks S: The radiology of tuberculosis of the gastrointestinal tract. Br J Radiol 46:329, 1973.

Diffuse Noninflammatory, Non-Neoplastic Diseases

Bluestone R, MacMahon M, Dawson JM: Systemic sclerosis and small bowel involvement. Gut 10:185, 1969.

Clemett AR, Marshak RH: Whipple's disease: Roentgen features and differential diagnosis. Radiol Clin North Am 7:105, 1969.

Crooks DJM, Brown WR: The distribution of intestinal nodular lymphoid hyperplasia in immunoglobulin deficiency. Clin Radiol 31:701, 1980.

Dodds WJ, Spitzer RM, Friedland GW: Gastrointestinal roentgenographic manifestations of hemophilia. Am J Roentgenol 110:413, 1970.

Farthing MJG, McLean AM, Bartram CI, et al: Radiologic features of the jejunum in hypoalbuminemia. AJR 136:883,1981.

Hale CH, Schatzki R: The roentgenological appearance of the gastrointestinal tract in scleroderma. Am J Roentgenol 51:407, 1944.

Handel J, Schwartz S: Gastrointestinal manifestations of the Schonlein-Henoch syndrome. Am J Roentgenol 78:643, 1957.

Hodgson JR, Hoffman HN, Huizenga KA: Roentgeno-logic features of lymphoid hyperplasia of the small intestine associated with dysgammaglobulinemia. Radiology 88:883, 1967.

Kemp-Harper RA, Jackson DC: Progressive systemic sclerosis. Br J Radiol 38:835, 1965.

Khilnani MT, Marshak RH, Eliasoph J, Wolf BS: Intramural intestinal hemorrhage. Am J Roentgenol 92:1061, 1964.

Kumar P, Bartram CI: Relevance of the barium follow-through examination in the diagnosis of adult coeliac disease. Gastrointest Radiol 4:285, 1979.

Kuoff M, Lindner AE, Marshak RH: Intussusception in sprue. Am J Roentgenol 103:515, 1968.

Marshak RH, Khilnani M, Eliasoph J, Wolf BS: Intestinal edema. Am J Roentgenol 101:379, 1967.

Marshak RH, Lindner AE: Malabsorption syndrome. Semin Roentgenol 1:128, 1966.

Marshak RH, Wolf BS, Cohen N, Janowitz HD: Protein-losing disorders of the gastrointestinal tract. Radiology 77:893, 1961.

Masterson JB, Sweeney EC: Role of the small bowel follow through examination in the diagnosis of coeliac disease. Br J Radiol 49:660, 1976.

Philips RL, Carlson HC: The roentgenographic and clinical findings in Whipple's disease: A review of 8 patients. Am J Roentgenol 123:268, 1975.

Pock-Steen OC: Roentgenologic changes in protein-losing enteropathy. Acta Radiol 4:681, 1966.

Reinhart JF, Barry SF: Scleroderma of the small bowel. Am J Roentgenol 88:687, 1962.

Schultz G, Zeller C, Pauline D, et al: Radiologic features of small bowel involvement in Henoch-Schönlein syndrome of the adult. J Radiol 63:315, 1982.

Schwartz S, Boley S, Schultz L, Allen A: A survey of vascular diseases of the small intestine. Semin Roentgenol 1:178, 1966.

Shimkin PM, Waldmann TA, Krugman RL: Intestinal lymphangectasia. Am J Roentgenol 110:827, 1970.

Werbeloff L, Bank S, Marks IN: Radiological findings in protein-losing gastroenteropathy. Br J Radiol 42:605, 1969.

Wolf BS, Marshak RH: Segmental infarction of the small bowel. Radiology 66:701, 1956.

Parasitic Diseases

Louisy CL, Barton CJ: The radiological diagnosis of strongyloides stercoralis enteritis. Radiology 98:535, 1971.

Marshak RH, Ruoff M, Lindner AE: Roentgen manifestations of giardiasis. Am J Roentgenol 104:557, 1968.

Monroe LS, Norton RA: Roentgenographic signs produced by *Toenia saginata*. Am J Dig Dis 7:519, 1962.

Newman CM, Aron BS: Roentgen diagnosis of tapeworm

infestation. J Mt Sinai Hosp NY 28:91, 1961.

Strijk SP, Rosenbuch G: Radiologic findings in parasitic infection of the small bowel. J Belge Radiol 3:233, 1981.

Yoshida T, et al: Strongyloides stercoralis hyperinfection: Sequential changes of gastrointestinal radiology after treatment with thiabendazole. Gastrointest Radiol 6:223, 1981.

Differential Diagnosis of Generalized Small Bowel Abnormalities

Osborn AG, Friedland GW: A radiological approach to the diagnosis of small bowel disease. Clin Radiol 24:281,1973.

Swischuk LE: Mucosal patterns in diffuse disease of the small bowel. Med Rad Photo 47:34, 1971.

Benign Neoplasms

Bruneton JN, Drouillard J, Roux P, et al: Lieomyoma and leiomyosarcoma of the digestive tract — a report of 45 cases and review of the literature. Eur J Radiol 1:291, 1981.

Dodds WJ: Clinical and roentgen features of the intestinal polyposis syndromes. Gastrointest Radiol 1:127, 1976.

Ekberg O, Ekholm S: Radiography in primary tumors of the small bowel. Acta Radiol Diag 21:79, 1980.

Macafee CHG, Greer HL: Intestinal endometriosis. J Obstet Gynaec 67:539, 1960.

Skandalakis JE, Grey S, Shepherd D, Bourne F: Smooth Muscle Tumors of the Alimentary Tract. Springfield, IL, Charles C Thomas, 1962.

Malignant Neoplasms

Balthazar EJ: Carcinoid tumors of the alimentary tract. Gastrointest Radiol 3:47, 1978.

Bancks NH, Goldstein HM, Dodd GD: The roentgenologic spectrum of small intestinal carcinoid tumors. Am J Roentgenol 123:274, 1975.

Boijsen E, Kaude J, Tylen U: Radiologic diagnosis of ileal carcinoid tumors. Acta Radiol Diag 15:65, 1974.

Chang SF, Burrell MI, Brand MH, Garsten JJ: The protean gastrointestinal manifestations of metastatic breast carcinoma. Radiology 126:611, 1978.

Ekberg O, Ekholm S: Radiology in primary small bowel adenocarcinoma. Gastrointest Radiol 5:49, 1980.

Goldstein HM, Beydoun MT, Dodd GD: Radiologic spectrum of melanoma metastatic to the gastrointestinal tract. AmJ Roentgenol 129:605, 1977.

Good CA: Tumors of the small intestine. Am J Roentgenol 89:685, 1963.

Hudson HL, Margulis AR: Roentgen findings of carcinoid tumors of the gastrointestinal tract: Report of 12 recent cases. Am J Roentgenol 91:833, 1964.

Joffe N: Symptomatic gastrointestinal metastases secondary to bronchogenic carcinoma. Clin Radiol 29:217, 1978.

Libshitz HI, Lindell MM, Dodds GD: Metastases to the hollow viscera. Radiol Clin North Am 20:487, 1982.

Marshak RH, Wolf BS, Eliasoph J: The roentgen findings in lymphosarcoma of the small intestine. Am J Roentgenol 86:682, 1961.

Norfray J, Calenoff L, Zanon B Jr: Aneurysmal lymphoma of the small intestine. Am J Roentgenol 119:335, 1973.

Raiford T: Tumors of the small intestine. Arch Surg 25:122, 1932.

Ramos L, et al: Radiological characteristics of primary intestine lymphoma of the "Mediterranean" type: Observations on 12 cases. Radiology 126:379, 1978.

Samuel E: Radiology of serosal malignancy. Clin Radiol 20:113, 1969.

Smith SJ, Carlson HC, Gisvold JJ: Secondary neoplasms of the small bowel. Radiology 125:29, 1977.

Vuori JVA, Vuori MK: Radiological findings in primary malignant tumors of the small intestine. Ann Clin Res 3:16, 1971.

Wagner KM, Thompson J, Herlinger H, Caroline D: Thirteen primary adenocarcinomas of the ileum and appendix: A case report. Cancer 49:797, 1982.

Zornoza J, Dodd GD: Lymphoma of the gastrointestinal tract. Semin Roentgenol 15:272, 1980.

Zornoza J, Goldstein HM: Cavitating metastases of the small intestine. Am J Roentgenol 129:613, 1977.

17

Abnormalities of the Colon

STRUCTURAL ABNORMALITIES

Anomalies of Rotation and Fixation

Most colonic anomalies are produced by abnormal rotation and fixation of the colon during fetal development. The major consequences likely to be encountered radiologically in adults are as follows:

Nonrotation of the colon results in all or most of the colon lying in the left side of the abdomen while the right side of the abdominal cavity is occupied by small intestine (Fig. 17-1A). The ligament of Treitz is usually absent. Patients with this anomaly are subject to an increased incidence of volvulus of the small intestine and/or colon, which may occur during adult life.

Hyporotation of the colon results in the cecum being located in the right upper quadrant of the abdomen (Fig. 17-1B). The major importance of this finding is that such patients may present with upper abdominal symptoms during an attack of appendicitis.

Hyper-rotation of the colon results in an elongated ascending colon, with the cecum being on a mesentery and freely movable. In these patients, the cecum usually lies crosswise in the midabdomen or extends down into the pelvis. Cecal volvulus is an occasional complication.

Duplication

Duplication is a rare anomaly in which a variable length of colon may be duplicated and lies adjacent to it. The duplicated segment is usually not in continuity with the main lumen of the colon. The most frequent radiologic finding is indentation or displacement of the colon by a round or sausage shaped adjacent mass. In the rare instance where the lumen of the duplicated segment fills with barium, the interior of the duplication usually has an appearance unlike the normal colon. The extra loop of bowel opacified may thus present a confusing picture in which its identity may be difficult to establish radiologically.

Adult Hirschsprung's Disease

In a small minority of cases, Hirschsprung's disease may escape detection during childhood. In time, such patients develop an enormous colon that fills most of the abdomen. On barium examination, the aganglionic distal colon and rectum is narrow, suddenly greatly widening near the transition zone between aganglionic and normal colon (Fig. 17-2). These patients should be examined with single-contrast technique and should not be

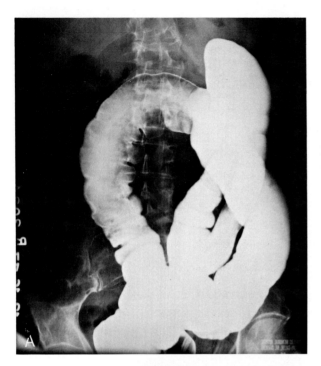

Fig. 17-1 (**A**) Nonrotation of the colon, with almost all of the colon lying on the left side of the abdomen. The small bowel is seen as air shadows in the right side of the abdominal cavity. (**B**) Hyporotation of the colon presenting with the cecum in the right upper quadrant of the abdomen.

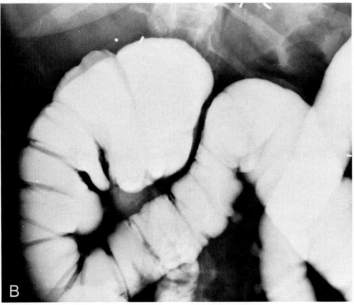

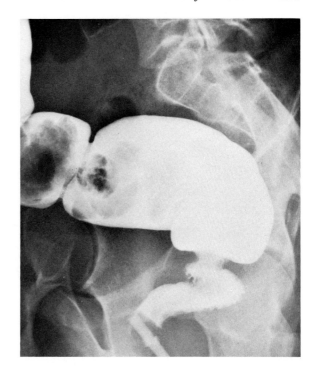

Fig. 17-2 Adult Hirschsprung's disease. The aganglionic distal rectum is contracted, while the normal colon is dilated.

given laxatives or otherwise prepared prior to the barium enema, since the transition between collapsed distal colon and fecal-filled proximal colon will be lost. When the distal colon has been filled and the transition zone demonstrated, the barium should be stopped to avoid formation of a barium-stool concretion within the dilated fecal-filled colon proximal to the diseased segment.

Cecal Volvulus

In patients with a mobile cecum, the result of hyper-rotation of the colon during gestation, the proximal ascending colon may twist at the junction between the fixed and mesenteric portions of the ascending colon. The diagnosis of volvulus may be made on plain films of the abdomen, which show a large, oval air-filled viscus stretching transversely across the abdomen. The small bowel is dilated and air-fluid levels are seen. If barium examination is performed, the point of rotation in the ascending colon can usually be identified. Due to the danger of cecal rupture, however, barium enema should be avoided in these patients unless the diagnosis cannot otherwise be established.

A variant of cecal volvulus is herniation of a mobile cecum through the foramen of Winslow into the lesser sac (Fig. 17-3). The herniated cecum produces an abnormal collection of gas in the left upper quadrant of the abdomen behind the stomach. The diagnosis may be confirmed by either barium enema or small bowel examination. If obstruction is not present, barium will fill the abnormally located cecum.

Sigmoid Volvulus

In elderly individuals, the sigmoid colon may become dilated and tortuous. This is associated with a propensity for volvulus of the sigmoid colon, the twist usually occurring near the root of its mesentery. When volvulus occurs, the sigmoid colon becomes greatly distended with air, producing the appearance of two dilated loops lying side by side in the abdomen, extending from the left lower to the right upper quadrant. The overall plain film appearance of the dilated sigmoid colon has been described as resembling a "coffee bean."

A barium enema may be performed on these patients for both diagnostic and therapeutic pur-

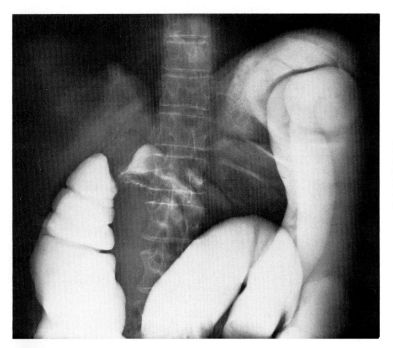

Fig. 17-3 Herniation of a mobile cecum through the foramen of Winslow. The herniated cecum lies in the lesser sac behind the stomach and splenic flexure of the colon.

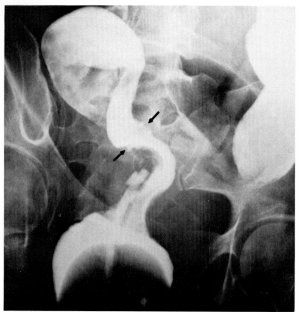

Fig. 17-4 Volvulus of the sigmoid colon at the moment of untwisting during barium enema. The point of twist can be seen as spiral folds at the rectosigmoid junction (arrows).

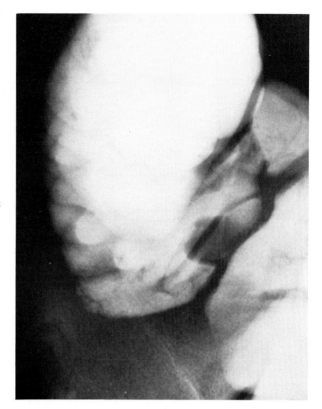

Fig. 17-5 Inverted appendiceal stump. Except for its location, it is indistinguishable from a sessile polyp.

poses. Diagnostically, the barium examination shows a peaked or twisted appearing partial or complete obstruction to the retrograde flow of barium in the distal sigmoid region. This is the actual point of obstruction caused by the sigmoid twist (Fig. 17-4). Therapeutically, the hydraulic pressure of the barium suspension often causes the volvulus to partially or completely untwist. When this occurs, the barium suddenly floods past the obstruction into the dilated sigmoid colon.

Ileosigmoid Knot

Rarely, a loop of small bowel, usually ileum, becomes twisted around the root of the sigmoid mesentery with a firmness sufficient to cause both sigmoid and ileal obstruction. On barium enema, the appearance is one of sigmoid obstruction similar to that of sigmoid volvulus. However, the hydraulic pressure of the enema will be insufficient to uncoil the affected loops of bowel or open the

obstruction. An additional finding will be dilatation of small bowel loops due to the coexisting ileal obstruction.

Inverted Appendiceal Stump

During appendectomy, most surgeons invert the stump of the resected appendix. The inverted tissue may duplicate the appearance of a 1- to 2-cm polypoid lesion on the inferior or medial aspect of the cecum (Fig. 17-5). The major importance of this finding is potential confusion with a polypoid neoplasm occurring in the same region.

Retrocecal Appendix

In many patients, the appendix lies in a retrocecal position, with certain radiologic consequences. First, the retrocecal appendix may indent the tip of the cecum as it courses around and behind that

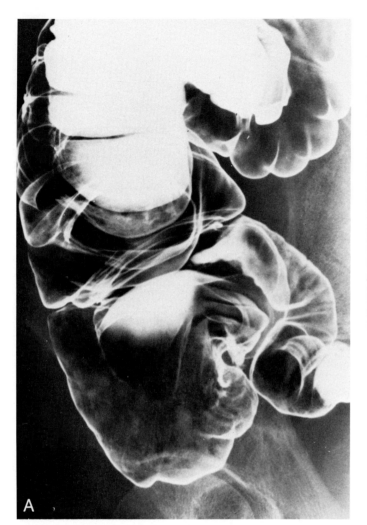

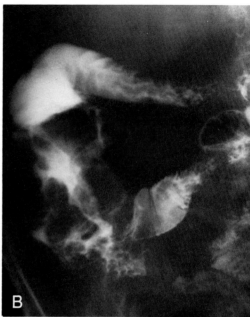

Fig. 17-6 (A) Retrocecal appendix causing a notch on the inferior-medial aspect of the cecum, as well as a linear indentation on its posterior wall. (B) Carcinoma-like appearance of the cecum and ascending colon due to a large pericolonic abscess caused by a ruptured retrocecal appendix.

structure, a finding of no particular significance per se (Fig. 17-6A). Second, in patients in whom the appendix has ruptured and produced a large peri-appendiceal abscess, the inflammatory reaction surrounding the cecum and ascending colon may very occasionally mimic the appearance of a large, circumferential carcinoma or lymphoma (Fig. 17-6B).

Intussusception

Intussusception, mainly a pediatric phenomenon, occurs in adults almost exclusively in association with a lead mass, usually a neoplasm. The most common presentation in adults is a colocolic intussusception in which a carcinoma acts as the lead mass. However, intussusceptions in adults may occur in association with almost any variety of polypoid neoplasm.

The radiologic features of colonic intussusception parallel those in the small bowel, with certain variations. The most common presentation is that of an obstructing or partially obstructing intraluminal mass composed of the lead mass plus the intussusception (Fig. 17-7A). The slender, streak-like lumen through the intussusception may or may not be demonstrable (Fig. 17-7B). Also, because of the crowding of circular folds in the colon, a coiled-spring effect may be present (Fig. 17-7C).

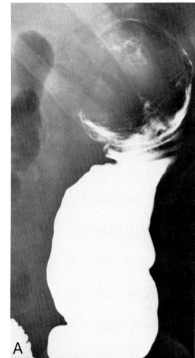

Fig. 17-7 (A) Obstructing intussusception with carcinoma of the colon as the lead mass. (B) Intussusception associated with carcinoma of the colon. Thin longitudinal lines of barium traverse the telescoped segment of colon. (C) Coiled-spring appearance caused by telescopic shortening of the colon during intussusception.

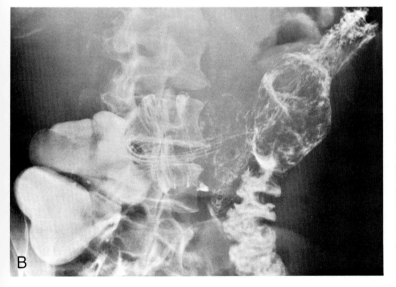

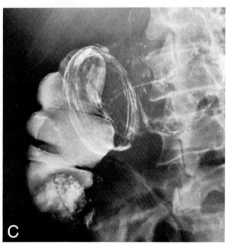

Diseases Causing Colonic Distention

Noninflammatory distention of the colon may be encountered under a variety of circumstances, mostly in association with disease processes that are not primary to the colon. In most instances, the diagnosis of the associated disease process has been made, or the necessary information is available from the patient. With one or two exceptions, there is little about the radiologic appearance of the distended colon to allow a specific diagnosis. Except as noted, all of these present radiologically as colonic distention without ulceration, often with loss of the haustral markings. A listing of those

**Table 17-1. Disorders Causing Bland
Colonic Distention**

Cathartic abuse
Megacolon of the insane
Neuromuscular disease
Spinal cord lesion
Drug-induced megacolon
Hirschsprung's disease
Scleroderma
Porphyria
Hypothyroidism
Adrenal insufficiency
Electrolyte imbalance
Amyloidosis
Idiopathic intestinal pseudo-obstruction
Mucoviscidosis
Sprue
Polyarteritis nodosa
Chaga's disease

diseases associated with bland colonic distention is presented in Table 17-1. The more important are discussed below.

Cathartic colon is the consequence of longstanding abuse of laxatives. There is usually both moderate colonic distention and loss of haustral markings. If loss of haustral markings is the predominant finding, the radiologic appearance may resemble chronic inactive ulcerative colitis.

Psychogenic colonic distention (megacolon of the insane) is found among inmates of mental institutions and produces an increase in colonic diameter, usually with retention of haustral markings. Its development is attributed to infrequent defecation. Similar colonic distention may be found among nursing home residents, in patients with spinal cord lesions, and in patients with neuromuscular disorders such as multiple sclerosis, amyotrophic lateral sclerosis, Parkinson's disease, and senility.

Scleroderma may cause colonic distention and more specifically produces characteristic wide-mouthed diverticula, most frequently in the transverse colon. These unique diverticula are formed by the merging of two or more haustral compartments as the result of loss of the intervening folds (Fig. 17-8). The development of colonic distention and the wide-mouthed diverticula is attributed to degeneration of smooth muscle in the colon wall.

Chaga's disease may present with megacolon and is the result of destruction of the colonic myenteric plexuses by the causative organism *Trypanosoma cruzi*. Colonic distention is manifest only in the chronic form of the disease, which is endemic to parts of South America.

Sprue and *mucoviscidosis* may present with bland colonic distention on barium enema. Both are associated with malabsorption and a bulkier than normal colonic contents.

Porphyria is a familial disorder of porphyrin metabolism characterized by obstipation and intermittent bouts of abdominal pain. Plain films taken during these abdominal crises may show dilated large and small bowel and air-fluid levels visible on upright or decubitus films. The chronic obstipation is associated with an enlarged colon as seen on barium enema.

Intestinal pseudo-obstruction is a rare condition of uncertain etiology characterized by chronic ileus with intermittent obstructive crises and a widely dilated small and large intestine. The diagnosis may be suspected on plain films showing signs of ileus with an unusual degree of dilatation of the large and small bowel. The greatly dilated colon is also demonstrable by barium enema.

INFLAMMATORY DISEASES

The colon is subject to a wide variety of inflammatory diseases. The most common of these in

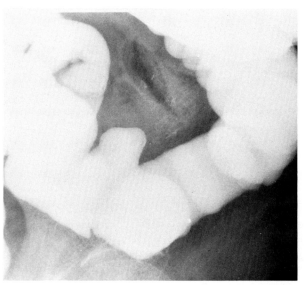

Fig. 17-8 Wide-mouthed diverticulum of the sigmoid colon in a patient with scleroderma.

Western radiologic practice, ulcerative colitis and Crohn's disease, remain of uncertain etiology. Diverticulosis and diverticulitis, examples of a developmental structural abnormality leading to localized inflammation, are also common in developed countries and may be caused by a low residue, highly refined diet. Tuberculosis, amebiasis, bacillary dysentery, and parasitic infestations are the dominant inflammatory diseases in less developed regions of the world.

Ulcerative Colitis

Ulcerative colitis remains of unknown cause and is a disease primarily of the mucosa and submucosa. Initially, the mucosa assumes a hyperemic and granular macroscopic appearance while histologically, small crypt abscesses may be visible. These then enlarge and produce small, numerous, discrete ulcers. However, the ulcers rapidly tend to become confluent, leaving raised, inflamed islands of mucosa that have been labeled *pseudopolyps*. In severe cases, the mucosa may be entirely destroyed. The haustral pattern of the colon disappears early in the course of the disease. Following prolonged activity, considerable fibrosis with shortening and stenosis may result.

Ulcerative colitis almost invariably commences in the distal colon and rectum, and with further involvement the zone of transition from diseased to normal mucosa progresses proximally toward the cecum until the entire colon is involved. With severe, total involvement of the colon, the terminal ileum may become diseased as well, exhibiting inflammatory thickening of the folds, dilatation, and occasional ulceration, changes that have been labeled *backwash ileitis.* With severe colonic and ileal involvement, the ileocecal valve may become dilated and may cease to exist as a well-defined, functioning structure.

With remission, the mucosa may re-ephithelialize the previously ulcerated areas, but the regenerated mucosa is often atrophic in appearance. Furthermore, remaining islands of the original mucosa persist as raised, polypoid features often labeled *mucosal tags.* With remission, the haustral pattern may be re-established to a variable degree.

Clinically, the onset of ulcerative colitis is characterized by bloody diarrhea and abdominal pain as well as systemic signs of illness such as fever,

pallor, anemia, and weight loss. When the disease is both extensive and very active, the patient may be extremely ill. Ulcerative colitis usually responds to treatment with parenteral corticosteroids, steroid enemas, nonabsorbable sulfa drugs, dietary changes, and supportive therapy. In the first few years, the course of the disease is marked by alternating remission and recrudescence. However, after several years, the disease may become almost permanently quiescent or "burnt out." In these latter patients, complication of the disease by carcinoma becomes the greatest consideration.

Ulcerative colitis is unique among colonic inflammatory diseases in that it carries a markedly increased risk of colonic carcinoma. The risk increases with the duration of the disease. After 10 years duration of ulcerative colitis, the risk of carcinoma becomes a major consideration in patient management, and patients may be advised to have their colon surgically removed.

Earliest radiologic evidence of ulcerative colitis consists of a fine granularity of the rectal and distal colonic mucosa and is most easily detected with the double-contrast barium enema (Fig. 17-9A). Usually, the rectum is decreased in caliber, even at this early stage. Also, loss of the haustral markings and the rectal folds will be detectable in the diseased segment. Usually, a distinct area of transition can be detected between the abnormal, granular mucosa of the diseased regions and the more proximally located normal, smooth colonic mucosa.

When the disease progresses beyond the stage of mucosal granularity, the small ulcers developing from crypt abscesses are readily detectable both with full column and double-contrast barium enemas (Figs. 17-9B and C). Since the ulcers tend to be innumerable, they are visible on films of the barium-distended colon as tiny outpouchings of barium seen in profile, no more than 1 or 2 mm in size. On postevacuation films, the ulcers are seen as small collections of barium between the collapsed folds. On double-contrast films, the ulcers are visible mainly en face.

As the ulcers enlarge and coalesce, pseudopolyps become visible radiologically. These appear as numerous polypoid filling defects of 5 to 10 mm in overall size, surrounded by ulcerations dividing the pseudopolyps from each other (Fig. 17-9D). With more extensive ulceration, the colon may become devoid of mucosa, its appearance reduced to that of a featureless tube. In almost all cases of

(*Text continues on page 308*)

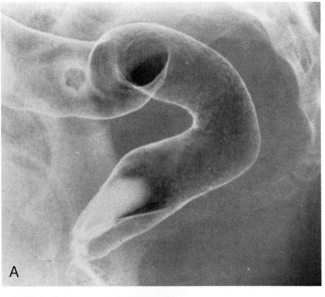

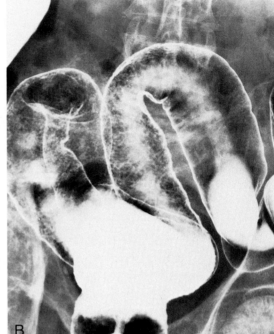

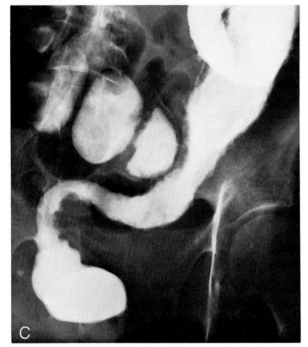

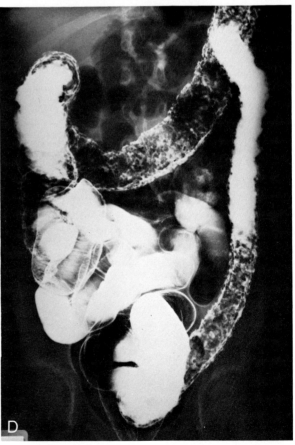

Fig. 17-9 (A) Early ulcerative colitis with granular appearance of the rectal mucosa. Transition to normal mucosa is noted in the sigmoid region, near the small fecal clump. Note the narrowed caliber of the rectum, the absence of rectal valves, and the separation of the rectum from the sacrum. (B) More extensive involvement of the rectum and sigmoid colon in ulcerative colitis. A coarsely granular surface is apparent, and small ulcerations are visible both en face and in profile. (C) Extensive involvement of the rectum, sigmoid colon, and descending colon in ulcerative colitis, as seen on a single-contrast examination. (D) Severe pancolitis in a patient with active ulcerative colitis. Ulcerations and pseudopolyps are visible throughout the colon. Note that the distal ileum is free of disease.

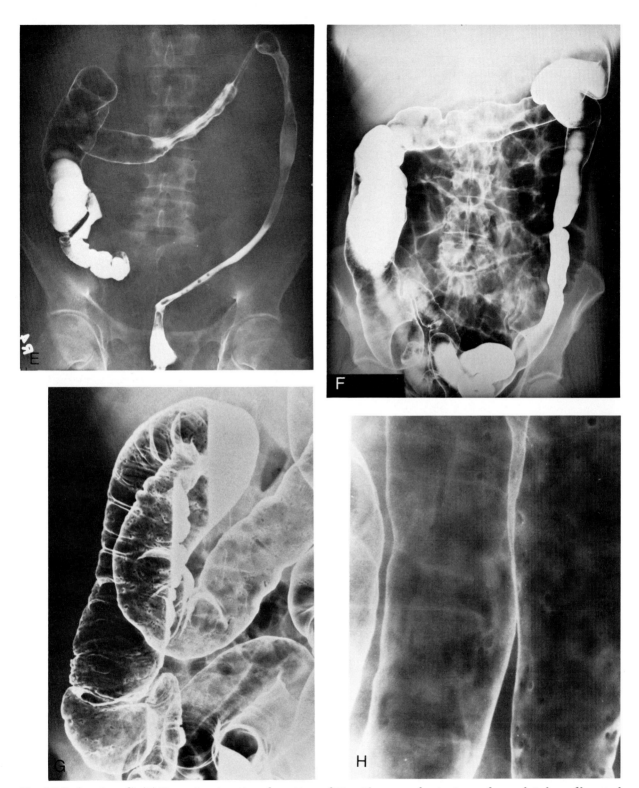

Fig. 17-9 *(continued)* (E) Extensive, inactive ulcerative colitis with severe shortening and complete loss of haustral markings, the so-called lead pipe colon. (F) Inactive chronic ulcerative colitis with smooth mucosa and slight return of haustral markings. Note the dilated terminal ileum and patulous ileocecal valve, characteristic of reflux or ''backwash'' ileitis. (G) Small, round and filiform mucosal tags in inactive ulcerative colitis. The intervening mucosal surface is smooth. (H) Mucosal tags in inactive ulcerative colitis, with an otherwise smooth mucosal surface.

ulcerative colitis involving the entire colon, significant narrowing of the rectum will be seen, with resulting increased distance between the rectum and the anterior surface of the sacrum (Fig. 17-9A). In addition, haustral markings are inevitably absent, and the colon in its entirety becomes considerably shortened. The lack of haustration and the shortening and narrowing all contribute to the pipe-like or "lead pipe" appearance of the colon in advanced ulcerative colitis (Fig. 17-9E).

With healing, radiologic evidence of ulceration disappears. The mucosal surface may become quite smooth or may retain a mildly granular appearance. Haustral markings often return (Fig. 17-9F), although usually to a limited extent. Polypoid mucosal tags may occasionally be visible, at times in considerable numbers (Fig. 17-9G and H). With recurrent bouts of activity and subsequent healing, stricture may develop.

Colonic Metaplasia.   It has recently been appreciated that the mucosa in longstanding chronic ulcerative colitis may undergo a premalignant metaplasia that is detectable endoscopically, though requiring histologic verification. These metaplastic regions may occasionally be detectable radiologically as patches of irregular nodularity.

Carcinoma complicating ulcerative colitis has a high mortality rate since the tumor has a propensity to metastasize early. Furthermore, the tumor often has appearances uncharacteristic of carcinomas occurring under more normal circumstances. Carcinoma developing in chronic ulcerative colitis often has the tapering, ill-defined margins more frequently associated with stricture. The frequent resemblance of these carcinomas to strictures is unfortunate, since true stricture may also complicate chronic ulcerative colitis. Thus, carcinoma may be indistinguishable from stricture in ulcerative colitis patients, and any constricting lesion must therefore be investigated by colonoscopy with biopsy.

Toxic dilatation of the colon (toxic megacolon) is a life threatening complication of ulcerative colitis. The colon becomes widely dilated, with extensively ulcerated, paper-thin walls. The patients are very ill and have signs of extreme systemic toxicity. Perforation often ensues, with disastrous and occasionally fatal results. The radiologic diagnosis of toxic dilatation of the colon is most appropriately

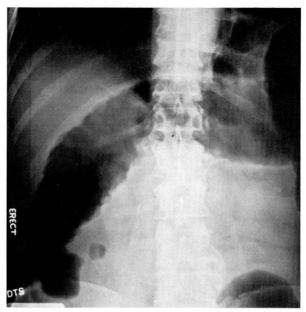

Fig. 17-10 Dilated shaggy-appearing transverse colon in a patient with toxic megacolon due to ulcerative colitis.

made on plain films of the abdomen, which usually show a dilated colon with an irregular, nodular inner surface (Fig. 17-10). Under no circumstance should a barium investigation of the colon be attempted in these patients. Although toxic megacolon is encountered most frequently in association with ulcerative colitis, other disease processes are capable of presenting with toxic megacolon and these are listed in Table 17-2.

Radiologic Investigation.   The radiologic investigation of ulcerative colitis can be performed using either the full column or double-contrast technique. The double-contrast study has advantages in the very earliest stages of the disease, being best able to show the minimal granularity of the distal colonic and rectal mucosa that is often

Table 17-2. Causes of
Toxic Megacolon

Ulcerative colitis
Crohn's disease
Amebic dysentery
Bacillary dysentery
Typhoid fever
Cholera
Pseudomembranous enterocolitis

the first radiologic sign of ulcerative colitis. However, many radiologists maintain that these earliest stages are also demonstrable on full column examinations as loss of haustral markings and subtle marginal irregularity or on postevacuation films as a finely nodular thickening of folds.

Certain precautions should be exercised in examining patients with ulcerative colitis. First, rectal balloons should never be employed, since ulcerative colitis weakens the rectal wall and use of a balloon-type enema tip is an invitation to rectal perforation. Even without a balloon, insertion of the enema tip should be very carefully performed to avoid piercing the anterior wall of the rectum. Second, a barium enema should be avoided in active acute ulcerative colitis. Performance of a barium enema on an acutely ill patient may convert ordinary ulcerative colitis into toxic dilatation of the colon. Double-contrast studies may be particularly implicated in this process due to the greater distention usually achieved. Whatever technique is used, overdistension of the colon with barium and/or air should be assiduously avoided.

Preparation of an ulcerative colitis patient for barium enema should be as gentle as possible. A satisfactory routine includes surgical liquid diet for 36 to 48 hours, 10 oz of magnesium citrate the evening of the examination, and final cleansing of the colon with a single normal saline enema the morning of the study. Vigorous purgation and repeated cleansing enemas are contraindicated.

Certain steps can be taken to make these patients more comfortable during the examination. First, as mentioned above, insertion of the tip should be gentle and balloon catheters avoided. Second, 0.5 mg of intravenously administered glucagon will ameliorate the painful spasms often accompanying the barium enema, allowing a more satisfactory examination. Finally, a full column barium enema should be prepared using normal saline rather than water, an isotonic barium suspension being less irritating than water to the unusually sensitive colonic mucosa.

Ulcerative Proctitis

Ulcerative proctitis is similar to ulcerative colitis, but tends to remain localized to the rectum

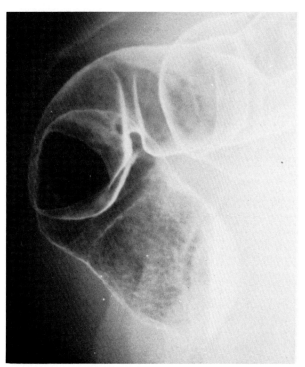

Fig. 17-11 Ulcerative proctitis. Granularity of the mucosal surface identical to ulcerative colitis is confined to the rectal region.

and sigmoid colon throughout the life of the patient. The radiologic findings in ulcerative proctitis are identical to those of the mild and intermediate forms of ulcerative colitis, but are restricted to the rectum and sigmoid colon (Fig. 17-11). Ulcerative proctitis usually does not produce the severe systemic illness or complications of ulcerative colitis. Also, no increased incidence of carcinoma of the distal colon or rectum has been reported. The radiologic evaluation of ulcerative proctitis is best performed using double-contrast technique and, as with ulcerative colitis, balloon-equipped enema tips should be avoided.

Crohn's Disease of the Colon (Granulomatous Colitis)

Colonic involvement is found in approximately one-fourth to one-half of patients with Crohn's disease of the terminal ileum. Usually, the pathologic changes are limited to the right side of the

(*Text continues on page 312*)

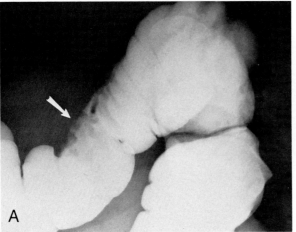

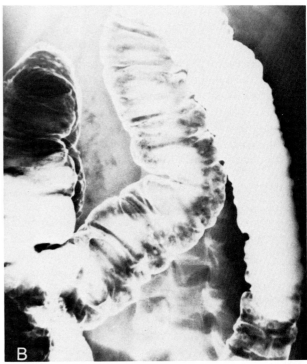

Fig. 17-12 (A) Segmental Crohn's disease in the transverse colon. Aphthous ulcers (arrow) are visible along with local loss of normal haustral configuration. The aphthous ulcers are seen en face as small ulcerations surrounded by radiolucent margins, and in profile as small projections of barium. (B) Innumerable aphthous ulcers, surrounded by halos of edema, in a patient with extensive Crohn's disease of the colon.

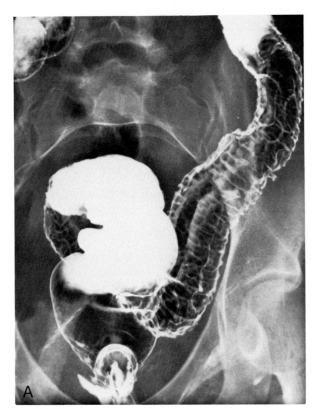

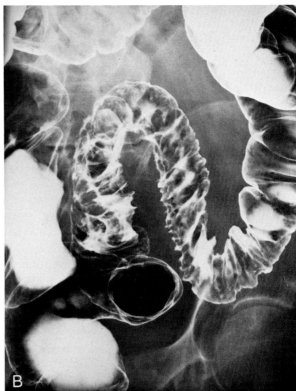

Fig. 17-13 (A and B) Cobblestone patterns of Crohn's disease of the colon as seen on double-contrast studies of the sigmoid region. Note that in both of these cases, the rectum is spared severe involvement.

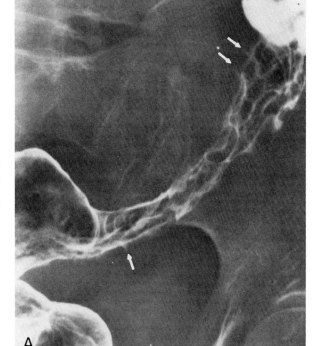

Fig. 17-14 (A) Crohn's disease of the descending colon with ''rose thorn'' ulcerations. (B) Crohn's disease of the cecum with deep ulcerations.
(*Figure continues on next page.*)

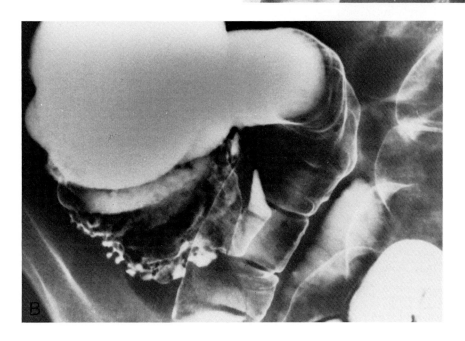

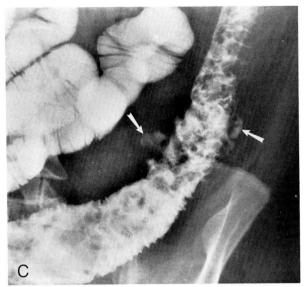

Fig. 17-14 *(continued)* (C) Severe Crohn's disease of the descending colon. Transmural ulceration has resulted in perforation (arrows).

colon in regions adjacent to the ileocecal valve, but extensive involvement of the colon is not uncommon. Extensive Crohn's disease of the colon without ileal involvement is unusual, however.

In contrast to the continuous involvement of ulcerative colitis, colonic Crohn's disease tends to exhibit patchy or segmental involvement, with unaffected "skip areas" being present between the lesions. Involvement is likely to be predominantly right-sided, and in the majority of cases severe radiologic changes are not present in the rectum. This is in contradistinction to ulcerative colitis in which the rectum is usually severely involved.

The pathologic changes of Crohn's disease of the colon are similar to those found in Crohn's disease of the ileum. Inflammatory infiltrates, lymphoid aggregates, granulomas, aphthoid ulcers, and eventually deep transmural ulcers characterize the histologic findings.

The ulcers in granulomatous colitis are of a different variety than in ulcerative colitis. Earliest ulcerations are usually aphthoid in character. However, in more advanced cases, a peculiar combination of linear and transverse ulceration produces the "cobblestone" appearance characteristic of Crohn's disease in both the small bowel and colon. The cobblestones are the islands of normal

mucosa separated by the longitudinal and transverse ulcers and are to a certain extent analagous to the pseudopolyps of ulcerative colitis. Ulceration in Crohn's disease of the colon is further characterized by its transmural nature, with a propensity to penetrate the wall and create paracolonic sinus tracts paralleling and intercommunicating with the colonic lumen.

Unlike ulcerative colitis, loss of haustral markings in Crohn's disease of the colon is confined to the ulcerated regions. Unless colonic involvement is total, intervening regions of unaffected colon with normal haustral markings will be visible. Furthermore, except in cases with marked rectal involvement, the caliber of the rectum in patients with colonic Crohn's disease will be normal.

The earliest radiologic changes in Crohn's disease of the colon consists of minute nodules, caused by enlarged lymphoid aggregates beneath the mucosal surface. These rapidly ulcerate, producing the characteristic aphthoid ulcers, which are minute collections of barium surrounded by a radiolucent halo of edema (Fig. 17-12). The extent of involvement may be quite minimal, and the disease process may be radiologically evident only on the basis of scattered aphthoid ulcers and small nodules.

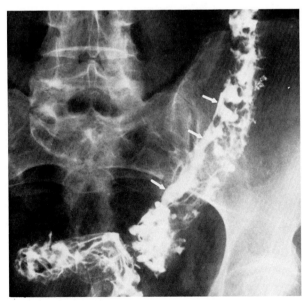

Fig. 17-15 Pericolonic sinus tract (arrows) in a patient with severe Crohn's disease.

With a more advanced disease, ulcerations tend to become confluent, causing the cobblestone appearance already described (Fig. 17-13). Haustral markings in the involved areas usually disappear. Deep ulcerations, far deeper than in ulcerative colitis, may be visible (Fig. 17-14). If ulcers have penetrated the wall of the colon, barium may fill sinus tracts, which tend to parallel the lumen of the colon (Fig. 17-15). Even in cases with advanced changes in the colon, there are often intervening areas of the colon showing a normal appearance, known as "skip" areas (Fig. 17-16).

A further radiologic characteristic of Crohn's disease of the colon is the production of pseudodiverticula. These are sac-like areas of relatively normal colon wall, partially or completely surrounded by diseased regions. Fibrosis in the diseased tissue surrounding an area of normal colonic wall causes a contraction that results in a sac-like projection of the normal area (Fig. 17-16). The process is similar to development of duodenal pseudodiverticula in patients with peptic ulcer disease.

In addition to establishing the colonic findings in Crohn's disease, it is important to investigate the terminal ileum, since most patients with Crohn's disease with colonic involvement will also have disease in the terminal ileum. Demonstration of

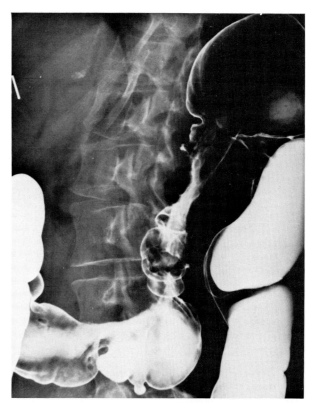

Fig. 17-16 Segmental Crohn's disease of the transverse colon. Skip areas are visible within the involved segment. Extensive scarring has produced pseudodiverticula.

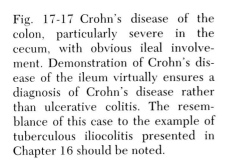

Fig. 17-17 Crohn's disease of the colon, particularly severe in the cecum, with obvious ileal involvement. Demonstration of Crohn's disease of the ileum virtually ensures a diagnosis of Crohn's disease rather than ulcerative colitis. The resemblance of this case to the example of tuberculous iliocolitis presented in Chapter 16 should be noted.

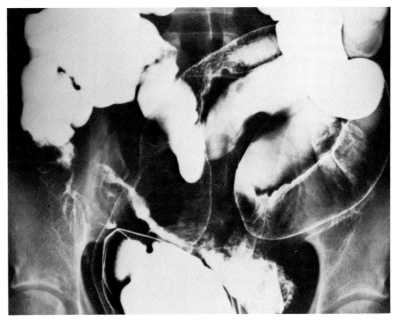

typical changes of Crohn's disease in the ileum is one of the more certain means of establishing that the pathologic process in the colon is in fact Crohn's disease rather than ulcerative colitis (Fig. 17-17).

The radiologic investigation of early Crohn's disease of the colon is best performed using double-contrast technique. The double-contrast examination most readily demonstrates the small nodules and aphthoid ulcers characteristic of early involvement. However, once the ulcers are numerous or deep, these patients should probably be investigated using single-contrast technique. Not only is the single-contrast examination faster and therefore easier for the patient, but reflux of the terminal ileum and filling of any sinus tracts or fistulae that may be present is accomplished with greater certainty. As with ulcerative colitis, balloon catheters should be avoided, and glucagon should be employed to relax the colon for greater patient comfort. The barium suspension employed should be prepared using normal saline for the same reason.

Unlike ulcerative colitis, Crohn's disease of the colon is not accompanied by a significantly increased incidence of colonic carcinoma or toxic dilatation. However, both have occasionally been reported in association with colonic Crohn's disease.

Differentiation between Ulcerative Colitis and Crohn's Disease

When inflammatory bowel disease is first encountered and a definitive diagnosis has not been established endoscopically or histologically, the radiologist may be confronted with the necessity of differentiating between ulcerative colitis and Crohn's disease of the colon. The signs of both diseases, and their characteristic differences, have been reasonably well established and may be summarized as follows:

1. *Distribution.* In ulcerative colitis, the disease is predominantly left-sided at first and then progresses proximally without skip areas to involve the entire colon. In Crohn's disease, skip areas of preserved normal mucosa are characteristic, and the disease is often predominantly right-sided.

2. *Rectal involvement.* In ulcerative colitis, the rectum is involved early in the disease, with a granular mucosal pattern, narrowing, and loss of the normal rectal valves. The only common exception to this is in patients who have been receiving steroid enemas, which may produce a local remission confined to the rectum. In Crohn's disease, the rectum is usually spared severe involvement, although it is not uncommon to see isolated ulcers.

3. *Character of ulcerations.* In ulcerative colitis, the ulcers tend to be of limited and uniform depth, since they do not penetrate the muscularis propria. In Crohn's disease, ulcers are of variable depth, some quite deep and fully penetrating the wall of the colon. The deep ulcers of Crohn's disease are often termed "rose-thorn ulcers," as compared to the shallow, slightly undermining "collar-button" ulcers of ulcerative colitis.

4. *Ileal involvement.* The terminal ileum is usually not diseased during the initial stages of ulcerative colitis, although with severe disease of the entire colon ileal involvement may be present and will be characterized by swelling of ileal folds, ileal dilatation, and patulousness of the ileocecal valve. In colonic Crohn's disease, many patients will have the typical cobblestone or stenotic changes of Crohn's disease in the terminal ileum.

5. *Wall thickness.* The thickness of the colonic wall is often discernible as a stripe of water density tissue lying between the barium-filled lumen and fat-containing pericolonic structures. It is normal or only slightly increased in thickness in ulcerative colitis, since the disease spares the muscularis propria. In regions of the colon affected by Crohn's disease, the colonic wall will usually be greatly thickened.

6. *Sinuses or fistulae.* The presence of a sinus tract or fistula is strong evidence of Crohn's disease.

Although the above discusses the differential diagnosis of the two most common forms of colitis, the wide variety of entities causing colitis or a colitis-like radiologic appearance must also be kept in mind. These may mimic many of the findings in ulcerative colitis or Crohn's disease and are listed in Table 17-3.

**Table 17-3. Differential Diagnosis
of Colitis and Similar Lesions**

Noninfectious diseases
    Ulcerative colitis
    Crohn's disease
    Ischemic colitis
    Radiation colitis
    Pseudomembranous colitis
Infectious or communicable diseases
    Amebic dysentery
    Bacillary dysentery
      Shigellasis
      Salmonellosis
      Typhoid fever
      Campylobacter enterocolitis
    Tuberculosis
    Actinomycosis
    Lymphogranuloma venerum
    Strongyloidiasis
    Schistosomiasis
Neoplastic diseases
    Scirrhous carcinoma
    Lymphoma

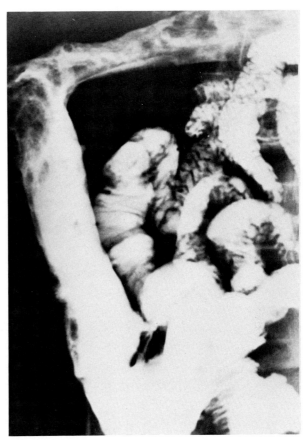

Fig. 17-18 Amebic colitis of longstanding duration with ulcerative colitis-like changes in the right colon.

Amebiasis

Clinically symptomatic infection of the colon by *Entamoeba histolytica* is not uncommon in regions where sewage disposal and water treatment are absent or imperfect. The basic lesion in amebiasis is an undermining mucosal ulcer, the margins of which may contain the organism. The extent of the disease within the colon is variable, including universally scattered small ulcers, locally severe involvement, and extensive colonic ulceration. With chronicity, stricture or an inflammatory mass may form, the latter being known as an ameboma.

Radiologically, amebiasis may resemble ulcerative colitis, Crohn's disease of the colon, or carcinoma, depending on the extent and distribution of colonic involvement (Fig. 17-18). In certain cases, the ulcers may resemble those of ulcerative colitis in that they may be widely distributed and of uniform depth. When the disease is segmental, it may closely resemble Crohn's disease. Where chronic amebiasis has produced a stricture, the narrowing is often sharply demarcated and irregular, resembling carcinoma. An ameboma, a mass of fibrous and inflammatory tissue, may similarly resemble a carcinoma.

In developed countries, a major hazard of amebiasis is that it may be unsuspected, unless a history of travel to an endemic area is obtained. Since amebiasis may resemble ulcerative colitis or Crohn's disease, an unrecognized case may be treated with corticosteroids, with dire consequences. Diagnosis of this type of case may be complicated by the frequent difficulty in recovering the amebic organism from the patient's feces during an active phase of the disease.

Tuberculosis

Tuberculosis of the colon is usually the result of ingestion of the tubercle bacillus either from cavitating pulmonary tuberculosis or in unpasteurized milk from a cow with tuberculous mastitis. It may less frequently result from hematogenous spread of the organism. The disease is characterized by

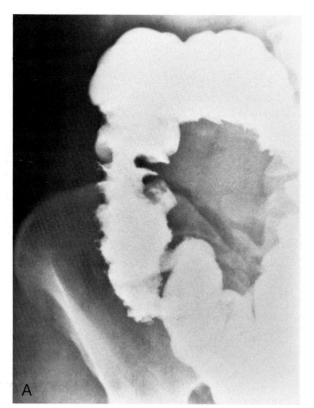 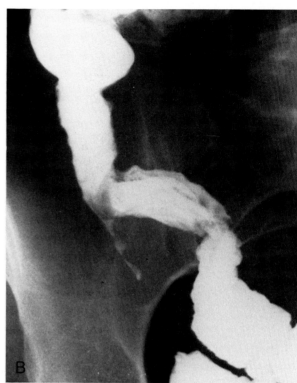

Fig. 17-19 (A) Tuberculosis of the proximal colon in an active stage showing many deep ulcerations. The appearance is indistinguishable from that of Crohn's disease. (B) Chronic ileocecal tuberculosis with almost total obliteration of the cecum. The pointed cecal remnant and gapping ileocecal valve are classic findings of tuberculosis. The transformation of the ileum and ascending colon into a continuous lumen is known as Stierlin's sign.

irregular ulceration of the colonic wall, of variable depth and distribution (Fig. 17-19A). In most cases, distribution of the disease is segmental, and thus tuberculosis may be impossible to differentiate from Crohn's disease of the colon. Indeed, until regional enteritis was identified as a distinct pathological and clinical entity, clinicians and pathologists did not distinguish between the two diseases.

A characteristic radiologic appearance is seen in certain cases in which the involvement is confined to the distal ileum and cecum. In these cases, the cecum assumes a contracted, pointed appearance considered typical of tuberculosis and the diagnosis can be strongly suggested (Fig. 17-19B). However, in regions where tuberculosis of the colon is endemic, the great variability in the radiologic appearance of the disease is appreciated.

Schistosomiasis

Schistosomiasis, also known as *bilharzia*, is a major cause of gastrointestinal and urinary tract pathology, with almost worldwide distribution. The causative organism is a circulatory fluke occurring in three major varieties. *Schistosoma mansoni* (Near East, Africa, West Indies, South America) and *S japonicum* (China, Japan, the Phillippines) affect mainly the colon. *Schistosoma haematobium* (Portugal, Africa, the Near East, India) affects the urinary bladder.

Schistosomiasis is acquired by wading in fresh water infested with larvae, which penetrate the skin and migrate via the lungs to the abdominal venous system. The mature flukes then release eggs that lodge in and clog the venules. By means of lytic enzymes, the eggs migrate through the

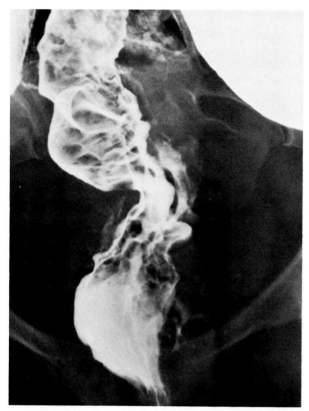

Fig. 17-20 Lymphogranuloma venerum. The rectum is narrowed, and in this case perforation has occurred.

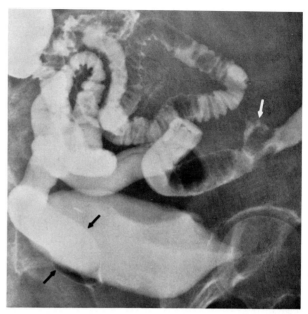

Fig. 17-21 Radiation proctosigmoiditis with marked narrowing of the rectum and sigmoid colon (black arrows). Radiation necrosis and perforation has occurred in the distal descending colon (white arrow), an unusual complication.

tissues, causing a combination of pseudoabscesses, granulomas, and dense fibrosis.

On barium enema, the most common finding is induration of the distal colon wall, best appreciated on postevacuation films. However, more severe cases may exhibit destruction of the haustral pattern, mucosal irregularity, and polypoid masses, often involving extensive segments of the colon and rectum.

Bacillary Dysentery

Shigella, typhoid, and parathyroid organisms are the usual causes of bacillary dysenteries severe enough to cause significant colonic ulceration. Findings range from relatively few, shallow punctate ulcers to extensive ulceration of the entire colon. In general, the appearance bears similarities

to universal ulcerative colitis, but without the shortening and narrowing of the colon typically encountered in ulcerative colitis. *Campylobacter* enterocolitis, caused by *Campylobacter fetus jejuni*, shows a similar ulcerative colitis-like appearance. In these entities, the colon usually returns to normal after appropriate antibiotic therapy.

Lymphogranuloma Venerum

A generalized infection of the pelvic tissues, lymphogranuloma venerum secondarily involves the rectum and sigmoid colon. The typical case shows narrowing of the rectum radiologically, with shortening and loss of haustral markings in the sigmoid colon in more extensive cases. Transmural ulcers may also be seen (Fig. 17-20), and very rarely a network of sinus tracts may be formed. The severe narrowing of the rectum seen in most cases is quite characteristic of the disease radiologically, and is often more marked than that usually seen in ulcerative colitis. Only radiation proctocolitis commonly produces a similarly marked degree of rectal stenosis.

Radiation Proctocolitis

Aggressive radiation therapy of organs adjacent to the colon, usually in the case of carcinoma of the cervix or prostate, may produce both an acute and chronic inflammatory response in the rectum and distal colon. Radiation acutely produces severe mucosal erythema with small ulcerations that are rarely detectable radiologically. Rarely, radiation necrosis and transmural ulceration may occur (Fig. 17-21). The usual radiologic finding in chronic radiation proctocolitis is progressive narrowing of the affected regions. Stenosis of the sigmoid and rectum due to radiation proctocolitis may occasionally be severe enough to cause partial or complete obstruction.

Solitary Ulcer and Stercoral Ulcer

Solitary and stercoral ulcers are rare, isolated ulcers of the colon of uncertain etiology. The major importance of the solitary ulcer is that, along with its surrounding edema, it may resemble an adenocarcinoma. The usual solitary ulcer is a deep lesion measuring 1 or 2 cm in extent that may sit on an indurated mass of considerable size. Stercoral ulcers are shallow ulcers that result from stasis of colonic contents behind a chronically obstructing lesion.

Ischemic Colitis

Ischemia of the colon is a disease of the elderly, usually the result of atherosclerotic vascular obstruction. Significant occlusion of vessels in the distribution of both the superior and inferior mesenteric arteries is generally necessary to produce ischemic colitis, since the colon is richly provided with collateral circulation. When it develops, ischemic colitis tends to occur in the descending or transverse colon, near the junction between the superior and inferior mesenteric arterial systems. In most cases, occlusions of vessels in both systems

can be demonstrated arteriographically. However, the location of the colonic ischemia often does not correlate closely with the location of the vascular occlusions.

Radiologic findings in ischemic colitis mimic those of ischemia in the small bowel, with swelling of folds and thumbprinting (Fig. 17-22) often best visible on postevacuation films. Where ulceration occurs, the radiologic appearance may be similar to that of segmental Crohn's disease of the colon (Fig. 17-23A). However, events usually progress to either complete resolution or to more extensive ulceration and colonic stenosis (Fig. 17-23B). The natural history of the disease process may be as important as the radiologic, endoscopic, or histologic findings, since occasionally these may be almost indistinguishable from granulomatous colitis.

Diverticular Disease

The term *diverticular disease* can be taken to mean either diverticulosis or its occasional sequel, diverticulitis. While there may be controversy on the subject, many gastroenterologists and radiologists are now convinced that there is an inconstant progression from spastic colon to diverticulosis to diverticulitis.

Spastic Colon and Prediverticular Disease. Spastic colon implies a symptom complex consisting of crampy abdominal pain with diarrhea, constipation, or both. Prediverticular disease refers to an observed hypertrophy of the circular muscle bundles of the sigmoid colon that produces a distinct sawtoothed contour that is also often seen in association with fully developed diverticulosis. Clinically, a significant fraction of patients referred for evaluation of spastic colon symptoms are found to have either diverticulosis or prediverticular changes in the sigmoid colon. However, it should be cautioned that the association between spastic colon and prediverticular changes is an inconsistent one. Also, the use of the term *prediverticular change* cannot be rigorously justified, since it is likely that many individuals with this radiologic picture never develop diverticulosis.

Diverticulosis. The presence of significant numbers of diverticula of the colon can be expected in approximately 20 percent of patients over the age of 50. Figures compiled from a variety

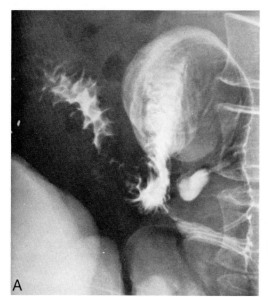

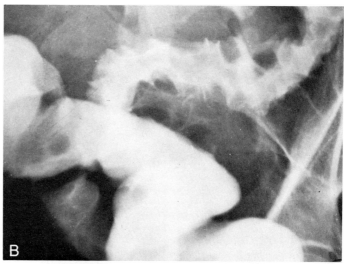

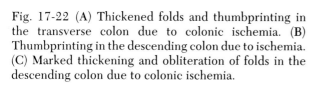

Fig. 17-22 (A) Thickened folds and thumbprinting in the transverse colon due to colonic ischemia. (B) Thumbprinting in the descending colon due to ischemia. (C) Marked thickening and obliteration of folds in the descending colon due to colonic ischemia.

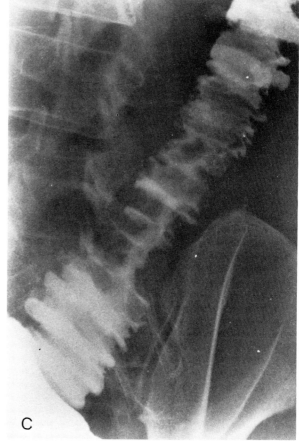

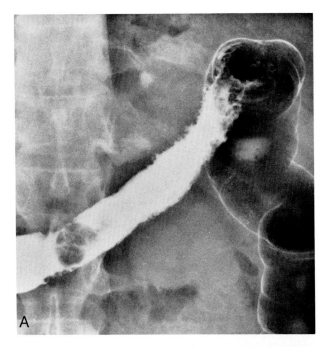

Fig. 17-23 **(A)** Segmental ulceration of the transverse colon due to ischemia. The appearance is easily confused with that of Crohn's disease. A large polyp is present in the diseased area. **(B)** Stricture of the splenic flexure due to an episode of ischemia.

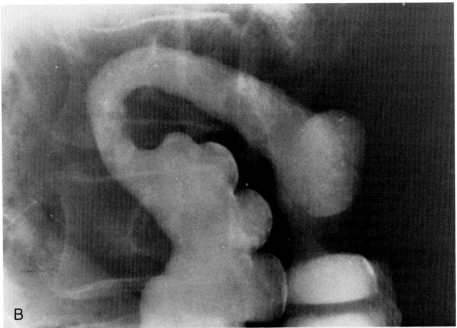

of sources suggest that it is a disease of Western urban society, and that it is rare or unknown in rural and less developed populations. There is a strong suggestion that refined diets low in fiber or roughage may be a causative factor. Spasm and increased intraluminal pressure, related to circular muscle hypertrophy and hyperactivity, can be demonstrated manometrically and pathologically in patients with diverticulosis.

Diverticula may occur anywhere in the colon proximal to the peritoneal reflection demarcating sigmoid colon from rectum. However, the location

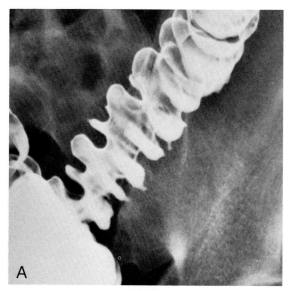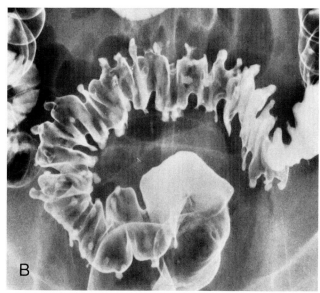

Fig. 17-24 (A) Very early diverticulosis. Note the thickened transverse muscle bundles. (B) Florid sigmoid diverticulosis of typical appearance.

of diverticula predominantly in the sigmoid colon is seen in the majority of patients. Clinically, left sided diverticula are most often the cause of diverticulitis while severe bleeding is often associated with right sided diverticula.

The earliest radiologic changes of diverticulosis are small diverticula, consisting of outpouchings of the mucosa and muscularis mucosa (Fig. 17-24A), which are known to occur where small arteries penetrate the muscle layers of the colonic wall. Initially, diverticulum formation may be intermittent and may be seen only in response to increased intraluminal pressure during colonic contraction. Indeed, radiologists may witness the appearance of small diverticula during colonic contraction, followed by their disappearance during relaxation or distension. However, most diverticula observed radiologically are already fixed in position.

In more established cases, there are thickened, deeply indented and closely spaced transverse bands with diverticula extending from between the indenting muscle bands. Eventually, the diverticula become larger and more numerous, reaching an average size of 0.5 to 1.0 cm (Fig. 17-24B). In an occasional case, the entire length of the colon may be populated by diverticula.

The closely spaced, deeply indented markings seen in association with diverticulosis are due to hypertrophic circular muscle bands, as well as persistent contraction of both the circular and longitudinal muscles. This creates a shortened colonic segment with a narrowed lumen having large, deeply indented, closely spaced folds with relatively little intervening space, the so-called sawtooth appearance.

Diverticulitis. The presence of colonic diverticula may become complicated by development of diverticulitis. The inflammatory process begins in the mucosa of the diverticulum and produces a small perforation, with subseqent peridiverticular inflammatory response and abscess formation. In most cases, the process is confined to a very small area immediately adjacent to the perforated diverticulum and healing ensues. However, the perforation may penetrate beyond the confines of the colon into the pericolonic fat or into the peritoneal cavity. The clinical picture of diverticulitis is largely determined by the extent and location of the perforation. The consequences of significant perforation include intramural inflammatory mass or abscess, pericolonic abscess, limited peritonitis, and generalized peritonitis.

When a patient has had repeated attacks of diverticulitis, fibrous tissue may be generated within and around the wall of the colon. Eventually, a fixed, fibrotic constriction of the colonic lumen

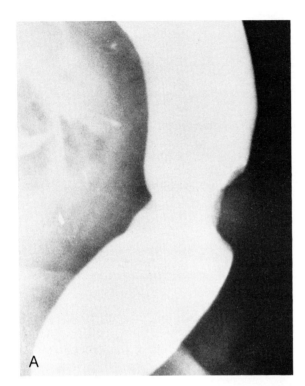

Fig. 17-25 (A) Intramural inflammatory mass caused by diverticulitis, unusual in that the disease process apparently occurred in the patient's single colonic diverticulum. (B) Diverticulitis with inflammatory infiltration of the colonic wall (arrows).

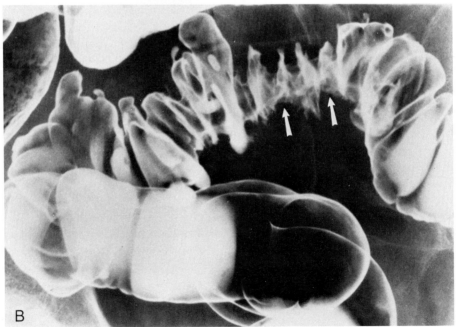

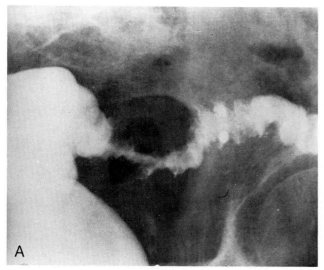
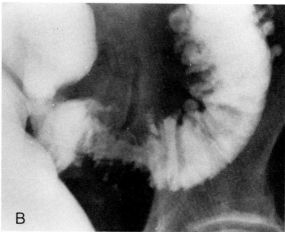

Fig. 17-26 (A) Pericolonic abscess with displacement and narrowing of the diseased segment. (B) Pericolonic abscess with narrowing of the sigmoid colon and distortion of diverticula in the region.

will result. At this stage, the patient's clinical picture may become dominated by symptoms of obstruction.

Most cases of minor perforation of diverticula cannot be detected radiologically. Thus, many patients with diverticulosis and the lower abdominal pain and fever characteristic of diverticulitis will not have radiologically detectable disease. However, where more significant diverticular perforation has taken place, the disease process is usually detectable radiologically. Fleischner very methodically described the radiologic signs of diverticulitis, which may be summarized as follows:

1. *Intramural inflammatory mass or abscess* is detectable radiologically as an intramural mass, producing a smooth, well-demarcated swelling within the colonic wall (Figs. 17-25A and B).

2. *Pericolonic abscess* produces a poorly demarcated impression on the colon, usually in the sigmoid region (Figs. 17-26A and B). Often, diverticula in the area will appear to be stretched toward the center of the mass.

3. *Barium outside the colon* within a sinus tract or abscess cavity is solid evidence of diverticulitis (Figs. 17-27A and B). Occasionally a pericolonic sinus may parallel the wall of the bowel, interconnecting several diverticula.

4. *Fixed narrowing of the colon* in an area of diverticula may be a sign of fibrosis within and around the colonic wall due to repeated attacks of diverticulitis (Fig. 17-28).

Diverticulitis must often be differentiated from colonic carcinoma, since both may be seen as an irregular, constricting lesion on barium enema. However, the diagnosis of diverticulitis can be suspected radiologically if one can detect intact mucosal folds within the involved area, since the colonic mucosa remains intact in diverticulitis but is destroyed by a circumferential carcinoma.

Differentiation of diverticulitis from certain cases of granulomatous colitis occurring in the elderly may also be necessary. In both entities, longitudinal sinus tracts connecting several diverticula may be seen. In diverticulitis, the disease process is localized in the immediate environs of the sinus tract, and the mucosa in the region is essentially intact. In granulomatous colitis, however, extensive mucosal ulceration is usually visible, both in the region of the sinus tract and elsewhere in the colon. Although granulomatous colitis may occasionally develop in areas of diverticulosis, most elderly patients presenting with this peculiar form of sinus tract will in fact have diverticulitis rather than Crohn's disease.

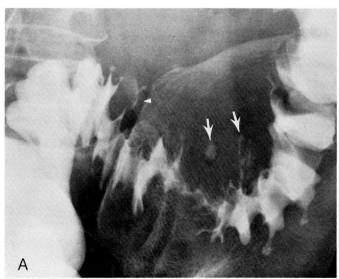
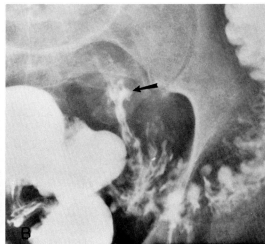

Fig. 17-27 (A) Pericolonic abscess with barium visible outside the lumen of the colon within the abscess (arrows). (B) Perforation of the sigmoid colon in diverticulitis, with an extensive tract (arrows). (Fig. B from Gelfand DW: Complications of gastrointestinal radiologic procedures: I. Complications of routine fluoroscopic studies. Gastrointest Radiol 5:293, 1980.)

The radiologic investigation of patients with significant diverticular disease, particularly suspected diverticulitis should, in my opinion, be pursued via the single-contrast barium enema for

Fig. 17-28 Fixed inflammatory stricture of the colon due to diverticulitis.

two major reasons. First, if perforation has occurred, it will be most readily demonstrated by the presence of barium, rather than air, in the paracolonic sinus tract or abscess. Experience with colonic perforation during the double-contrast enema has shown that air preferentially exits through a perforation and is difficult to detect fluoroscopically or radiographically. Second, performance of double-contrast barium enemas in patients with numerous diverticula should in general be avoided, since even in experienced hands detection of polypoid lesions among the diverticula is unreliable.

BENIGN NEOPLASMS

Adenomatous Polyps

Present in approximately 10 to 15 percent of carefully performed double-contrast barium enemas and in a similar percentage of autopsy specimens, adenomatous polyps are the most frequent significant colonic lesions likely to be detected radiologically. They are believed to be the precursors of colon carcinomas, with many small polyps containing nests of malignant cells on histologic inspection. Indeed, there are recorded radiologic observations of typically benign-appearing small

Table 17-4. Solitary Polypoid Lesion in the Colon

Adenomatous polyp
Hyperplastic polyp
Lipoma
Spindle cell tumor
Carcinoma
Villous adenoma
Carcinoid tumor
Hamartoma
Endometrioma
Metastatic lesion
Duplication cyst
Ameboma

polyps evolving over a period of years into frank colonic carcinomas. Their detection and prophylactic removal are therefore of considerable importance. Although adenomatous polyps are the most common small colonic lesions seen on barium enema, a variety of neoplastic and non-neoplastic entities may also present as solitary polypoid lesions, and these are listed in Table 17-4.

Considerable attention has been paid to the radiologic differentiation between benign and malignant polyps. This was a crucial matter in the days preceding the availability of colonoscopic polypectomy, since laparotomy was required to extirpate a suspected small polypoid carcinoma. The differentiation between benign and malignant polyps remains of some importance, however, and the determination depends on evaluation of the following characteristics:

1. *Size* (Fig. 17-29). Polyps under 1 cm have a relatively small statistical chance (1 to 2 percent) of being carcinomatous, while those over 1 cm carry an increasingly significant incidence of malignancy. The great majority of polyps under 0.5 cm size will be hyperplastic lesions totally devoid of malignant potential.

2. *Shape and surface characteristics* (Fig. 17-30). Benign polyps tend to be exquisitely round or oval, with an extremely smooth surface. Any polyps not meeting these criteria should be suspected of being malignant.

3. *Presence of a stalk* (Fig. 17-31). A well-defined stalk, particularly a long, slender one, is an excellent sign of a benign lesion. Polyps that are plaque-like or on a broad base are more likely to be malignant. Change in the length or breadth of a polyp's stalk raises the question of malignant infiltration of the stalk.

4. *Change in size.* Polyps doubling their size in less than 3 years have a significant probability of malignancy.

Certain radiographic signs associated with polyps should be mentioned. The "target sign" con-

Fig. 17-29 Small hypertrophic polyp of the descending colon.

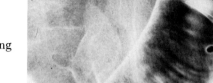

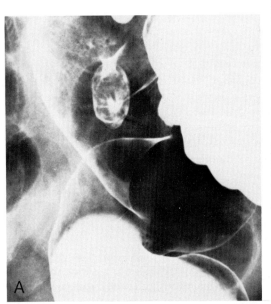
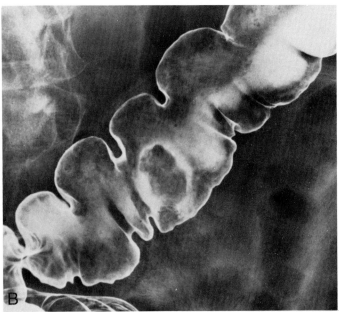

Fig. 17-30 (A) Benign adenomatous polyp of the sigmoid colon. The exquisitely smooth oval shape and narrow stalk strongly suggests the benign nature of the lesion. (B) Irregular polyp on a broad stalk, which proved to be adenocarcinoma.

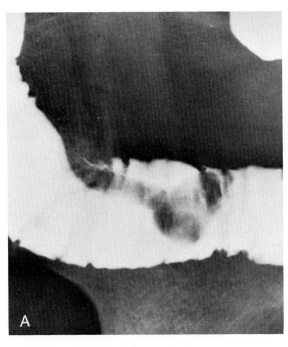
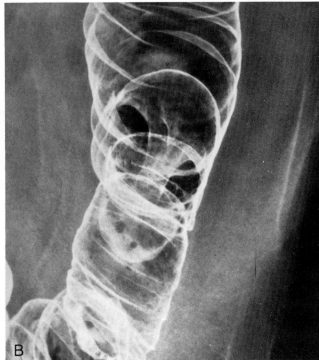

Fig. 17-31 (A) Polyp on a long stalk in the sigmoid-descending colon junction. A long slender stalk is seldom seen in malignant lesions. If malignancy is found in the head of the polyp, the long, thin stalk indicates lack of invasion of the stalk. (B) Benign adenomatous polyp on a slender stalk, as shown on a double-contrast examination.

sists of concentric circles caused by superimposition of the shadows of the head and stalk of a polyp when seen en face with the beam traversing the long axis of the pedicle (Fig. 17-32A). A "ring shadow" is produced by a barium-covered polyp located on a nondependent wall of the colon as seen during a double-contrast enema (Fig. 17-32B). The "bowler hat sign" is produced when a hemispherical sessile polyp is seen obliquely during double-contrast barium enema; the barium covers the polyp and encircles its base, producing an appearance similar to that of a bowler hat (Fig. 17-32C).

Differentiation of polyps from diverticula on double-contrast examinations may pose a problem when there is extensive diverticulosis, but several helpful indicators may be used. First, diverticula will usually fill with barium on one or more films while a polyp will usually be seen to displace barium. Second, the outer margins of the circular shadow of a diverticulum are usually very cleanly etched, since the barium is confined by a smooth mucosal surface, while the meniscus of barium surrounding a sessile polyp may be less well-defined peripherally (Fig. 17-32C). Third, diverticula are flexible and change size during the course of an examination, particularly with the application of compression, while polyps are solid and unchanging. Fourth, the air contained within a diverticulum may create an added radiolucency where it overlaps the lumen of the colon, while a polyp displaces the air within the colonic lumen, creating a shadow of lesser radiolucency (Fig. 17-32C).

Detection of small polyps is best pursued using the double-contrast barium enema. This is an area of gastrointestinal radiology where double-contrast technique has been shown, by a considerable accumulation of data, to be superior to full column examinations. Both the preparation for the examination and its performance have been described elsewhere. It is sufficient to say that the examination and patient preparation must both be meticulous if the great majority of polyps are to be detected.

Hyperplastic Polyps

Hyperplastic polyps are small non-neoplastic polypoid excrescences of the colonic mucosa that are generally less than 0.5 cm in diameter (Fig. 17-29). They cause no symptoms, and their major implication for the radiologist is that they cannot be differentiated from adenomatous polyps of the same size. Because most polyps under 0.5 cm are hyperplastic, because the incidence of malignancy in tiny adenomatous polyps is infinitesimal, and because small bits of retained detritus are common on double-contrast enemas, many gastrointestinal radiologists avoid making a diagnosis of adenomatous polyps for objects smaller than 5 mm unless the colon is absolutely clean.

Polyposis Syndromes

Several varieties of multiple polyposis syndromes have been described, both hereditary and nonhereditary. Certain of these syndromes are rarities, but at least one of them, familial polyposis, occurs quite regularly and carries significant implications for the affected individuals and their offspring. A summary of entities capable of presenting as colonic polyposis is presented in Table 17-5.

Familial polyposis is a hereditary disease manifesting itself as innumerable adenomatous polyps of the colon, generally appearing during the patient's second decade. Malignant transformation occurs in virtually 100 percent of untreated patients, and these carcinomas commonly become manifest at approximately 30 to 40 years of age. The disease has an autosomal dominant inheritance with very high penetrance, and the great majority of patients will thus have a family history of colonic polyps or of the death of several ancestors from colonic carcinoma. The accepted treatment is total proctocolectomy or colectomy with an ileorectal anastomosis. In the latter case, the retained rectal segment must be periodically inspected and any developing polyps removed.

Radiologically, the early stage of the disease shows innumerable, small sessile polyps, best demonstrated on double-contrast examinations. As the disease progresses, the individual polyps enlarge and may develop stalks. In older patients, carcinoma is likely to be encountered (Fig. 17-33) and several carcinomas may actually develop simultaneously. Many older patients first present radiologically as a frank colonic carcinoma accompanied

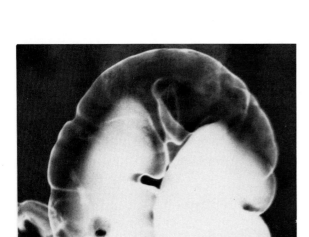

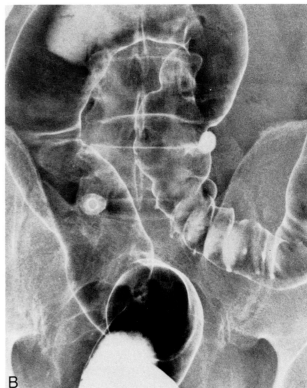

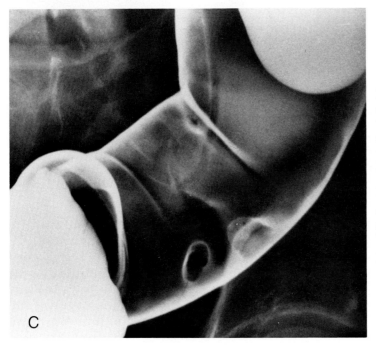

Fig. 17-32 (A) "Target sign" formed by a sigmoid polyp. The head of the polyp causes the larger circle, while the stalk forms the smaller, more dense inner circle. The eccentricity of the target's bull's-eye is typical. (B) Ring shadow and target sign formed by a polyp and its stalk hanging from the anterior wall of the sigmoid colon during a double-contrast examination. (C) Two polyps of the sigmoid colon, one sessile and the other on a broad stalk. The sessile polyp, situated more proximally, is forming a "bowler hat" sign.

Table 17-5. Multiple Polypoid Lesions in the Colon

Neoplastic diseases
　Multiple adenomatous polyps
　Familial polyposis
　Gardner's syndrome
　Turcot's syndrome
　Peutz-Jehgers disease
　Lipomatous polyposis
　Neurofibromatosis
　Lymphoma
　Metastases
Non-neoplastic diseases
　Pseudopolyps—ulcerative colitis, Crohn's disease
　Lymphoid hyperplasia
　Multiple metaplastic polyposis
　Cronkhite-Canada syndrome
　Colitis cystica profunda
　Pneumatosis cystoides intestinalis

by innumerable smaller polyps.

Recently, it has been demonstrated that occasional patients with familial polyposis will have similar changes elsewhere in the gastrointestinal tract, particularly in the stomach. In cases presented to date, the appearance of the gastric polyps has not differed greatly from the appearance of the colonic polyps, although the gastric polyps are often hyperplastic.

Gardner's syndrome is another hereditary syndrome presenting with multiple adenomatous polyps of the colon. However, these patients also exhibit bone and soft tissue changes consisting of sebaceous cysts, benign mesenchymal tumors, and multiple osteomas. The disease is transmitted as an autosomal dominant, and carries the same high risk of carcinoma of the colon as familial polyposis.

Turcot syndrome is a third variant of familial polyposis associated with central nervous system tumors, usually glioblastomas. Most of these patients die of their central nervous system malignancy. Due to the extreme rarity of the disease, the exact method of hereditary transmission has not been determined. Radiologically, the polyps of this syndrome are indistinguishable from those of familial polyposis.

Peutz-Jeghers syndrome consists of multiple hamartomatous polyps occurring in the stomach, small bowel, and colon. The lesions may be scattered or numerous. They are accompanied by pigmented areas on the lips and buccal mucosa. Occasionally, polyps are also found in the urinary and respiratory tracts.

The most common site of polyps in Peutz-

Jeghers disease is in the small bowel, with a lesser incidence in the stomach, colon, and rectum. The polyps range in size from a few millimeters to several centimeters in diameter, and they often are on long pedicles. There is no particular malignant potential associated with the polyps of Peutz-Jeghers syndrome.

Cronkhite-Canada syndrome is a rare syndrome consisting of generalized gastrointestinal polyposis in association with ectodermal abnormalities. The syndrome is nonhereditary and develops in the middle or advanced years. The polyps tend to be extremely numerous and occur throughout the gastrointestinal tract, including the esophagus. Histologically, they are similar to juvenile polyps. Ectodermal abnormalities include alopecia, atrophy of the nails, and hyperpigmentation. The disease is accompanied by diarrhea, vomiting, abdominal pain, hypoproteinemia, and electrolyte disturbances.

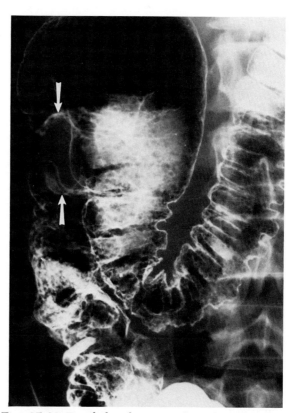

Fig. 17-33 Familial polyposis coli with innumerable small sessile polyps. A large carcinoma (arrows) is partially visible in the ascending colon.

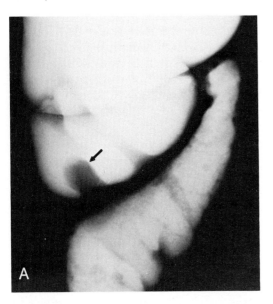

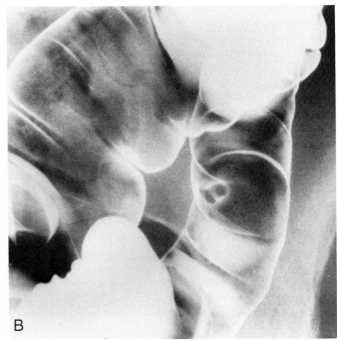

Fig. 17-34 (A) Small lipoma of the cecum (black arrow) with a smooth contour and broad base. The lesion was deformable by compression at fluoroscopy. (B) A lipoma of the descending colon originally diagnosed radiologically as an adenomatous polyp. Small lipomas cannot be differentiated from adenomatous polyps radiologically.

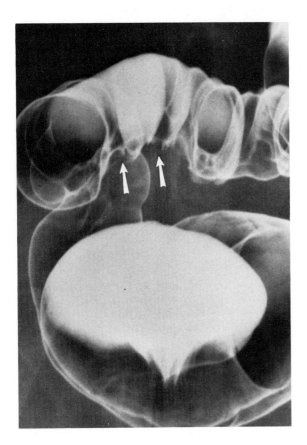

Fig. 17-35 Endometriosis of the sigmoid colon (arrows). The endometrial tissue has infiltrated the wall of the colon. Endometriosis may also present as a discrete intramural lesion.

Mesenchymal Tumors

The usual assortment of intramural mesenchymal tumors occurs in the colon as elsewhere in the gastrointestinal tract. However, for several reasons, special mention should be made of lipoma of the colon. First, lipomas appear to be more frequently diagnosed in the colon than elsewhere in the gastrointestinal tract. Second, there is predilection for colonic lipomas to form polypoid lesions, often on a broad stalk (Fig. 17-34). Small lipomas are quite common and are usually radiologically indistinguishable from adenomatous polyps, the diagnosis being established only at colonoscopy. Finally, the larger lipomas, as elsewhere in the gastrointestinal tract, are deformable in response to peristalsis or the radiologist's application of compression.

Endometriosis

Not uncommonly, pelvic endometriosis will result in endometrial implants of significant size on the wall of the distal colon. As these enlarge and are incorporated into the wall of the colon, they may present radiologically as benign-appearing intramural or extrinsic tumors (Fig. 17-35). Clinically, they are associated with abdominal pain and gastrointestinal bleeding during menstrual periods.

MALIGNANT NEOPLASMS

The considerable incidence of malignant neoplasms in the colon has already been implied in the discussion of adenomatous polyps. Indeed, carcinoma of the colon is the most common malignancy of the gastrointestinal tract in most Western nations. While many carcinomas of the colon are thought to arise within polyps that are relatively static in appearance for many years, others manifest themselves as frank carcinoma from the onset.

The incidence of carcinoma is quite low until the fifth decade of life. From then onward, the risk of developing carcinoma rises rapidly until it levels off at approximately the age of 70. It has always been maintained that carcinomas were far more frequent in the sigmoid colon and rectum than in the more proximal segments of the colon. However, a less concentrated distribution has been described in series collected in more recent years, perhaps due to the greater ease of accurately examining the entire colon both colonoscopically and radiologically.

The radiologic evaluation of the colon for carcinoma is best performed using double-contrast technique. Single-contrast technique is also quite effective in demonstrating the larger polypoid and circumferential lesions. However, if carcinoma of the colon is to be most effectively detected in its earliest and potentially most curable stages, the ability of the double-contrast barium enema to outline small polypoid and plaque-like colonic lesions should be employed.

The radiologic appearance of colon carcinoma in its earliest stages is that of a small plaque-like or polypoid lesion (Fig. 17-36). There is a tendency for early carcinoma to be flat and irregular in contour, occasionally with a depressed center. In a slightly more advanced stage, adenocarcinoma is seen as a larger polypoid lesion on a broad base, usually with an irregular surface.

Eventually, most carcinomas of the colon will encircle the lumen of the colon, producing the typical "apple core" lesion (Fig. 17-37). The lumen through the lesion is usually narrowed and irregular, reflecting the irregular surface of a fungating malignancy. Sharp demarcation from the surrounding wall of the colon is usually present, with an overhanging edge or "shelf" visible.

Many circumferential carcinomas will be obstructing the colon when first discovered, and it may be difficult to coax the barium through the lesion (Fig. 17-38). Nevertheless, it is important to attempt the radiologic delineation of the contours of the lesion so as to establish its identity. However, it is also important to avoid putting large quantities of barium proximal to an obstructing lesion, since the barium may inspissate in that location, complicating the patient's care.

When carcinomas are large and have eroded through the wall of the colon, they may become necrotic, introducing the possibility of colonic perforation during barium enema. This is an unusual complication of colon carcinoma, and it may give rise to an alarming radiologic examination. In this circumstance, the pressure of the barium enema may cause the necrotic lesion to burst, with free

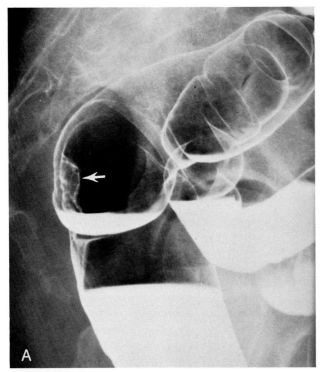

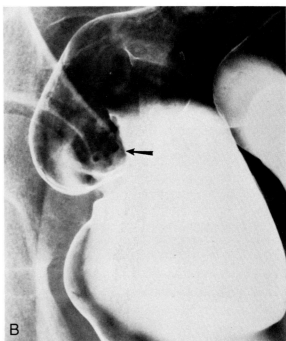

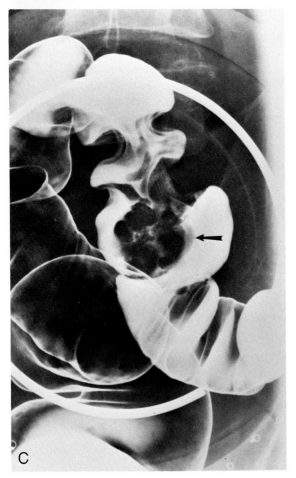

Fig. 17-36 (A and B) A plaque-like adenocarcinoma of the posterior wall of the rectum as seen on lateral and oblique films (arrows). (C) Adenocarcinoma of the sigmoid colon presenting as a large, irregular polypoid lesion (arrows).

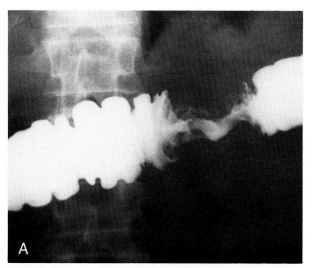 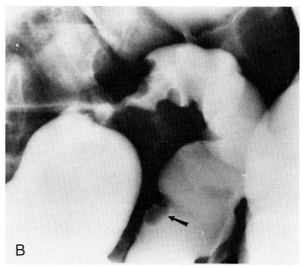

Fig. 17-37 (A and B) Typical apple-core lesion of the sigmoid colon. A sentinel polyp (arrow) is visible proximal to the carcinoma (arrow).

flow of barium suspension into the peritoneal cavity. Other than avoiding the use of excessive pressure during all barium enemas, and avoiding the use of barium in patients already suspected of having peritonitis, there is, unfortunately, little that a radiologist can do to anticipate and prevent this event when it occurs.

Carcinoma of the colon, particularly large polypoid lesions, may also form the lead mass of an intussusception. Indeed, intussusception of the colon is extremely rare in adults except in the presence of a tumor acting as a lead mass. Radiologically, it may be difficult to differentiate the neoplasm forming the lead mass from the intussusceptum itself. Nevertheless, any colonic intussusception encountered in a adult should be suspected of harboring a neoplasm, and most often it will be adenocarcinoma.

Fig. 17-38 A large, partially obstructing carcinoma of the distal colon. A certain degree of judgment must be exercised in deciding whether to attempt examination of the remainder of the colon proximal to an obstructing lesion. A large, extensive lesion of this appearance should also be suspected of being a lymphoma.

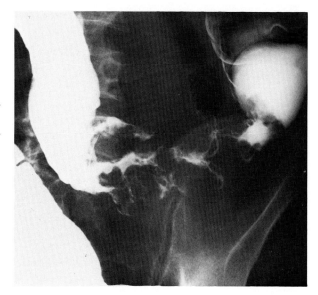

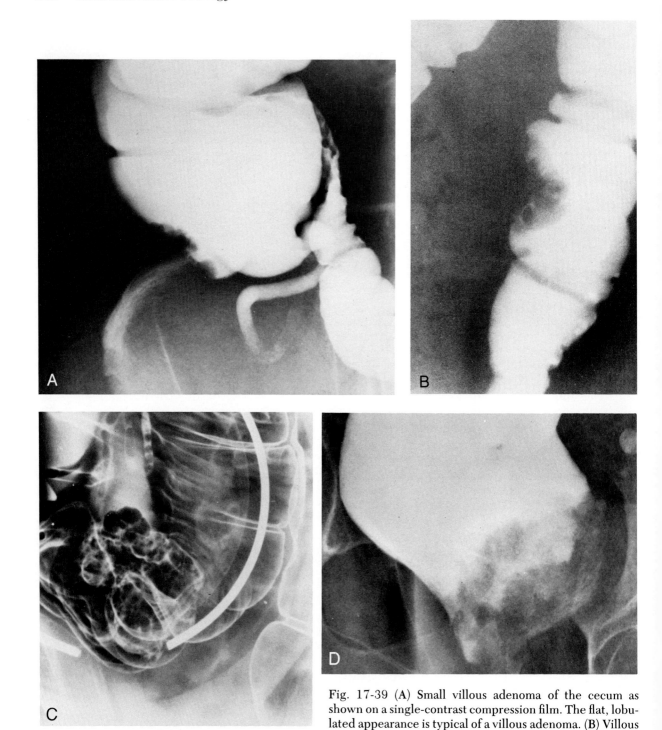

Fig. 17-39 (A) Small villous adenoma of the cecum as shown on a single-contrast compression film. The flat, lobulated appearance is typical of a villous adenoma. (B) Villous adenoma of the descending colon seen during single-contrast barium enema. The relative opacity and unclear demarcation of the peripheral portions of the lesion is due to barium mixing between the fronds of the villous adenoma. (C) Villous adenoma of the tip of the cecum, a common location for this lesion. Note the characteristic lobulation of the surface of the tumor. (D) Large, sessile villous adenoma (adenocarcinoma) of the distal rectum. The opacity and indistinct margins of the lesion are caused by barium mixing between the fronds of the tumor.

Scirrhous Carcinoma

Scirrhous carcinoma is a variant of adenocarcinoma of the colon in which the carcinoma infiltrates the colonic wall over a considerable segment. Most scirrhous carcinomas of the colon are seen in association with ulcerative colitis, and they are rather typical of colonic malignancy occurring in the later stages of that disease. The infiltrating lesion may not produce distinct margins and may approximate the appearance of a benign stricture of the colon.

Mucin-Producing Colonic Carcinomas

Mucin-producing colonic carcinomas often contain calcium that may be demonstrated roentgenologically. When these adenocarcinomas of the colon calcify, the calcifications tend to be small and flake-like. The calcification will be seen in both the primary tumor and in any metastases.

Villous Adenoma

Although a small percentage of villous adenomas detected radiologically are benign tumors, the majority are large malignant lesions. The typical lesion is a soft, bulky tumor with innumerable closely packed frond-like excrescences on its surface. There is a propensity for villous adenomas to occur in the rectum and cecum, but they are found elsewhere throughout the colon as well.

Radiologically, the typical villous adenoma is an irregular polypoid lesion, often covering a surprisingly large area of the colonic wall. The surface is usually lobulated. In addition, there is a peculiar mixing of barium into many of these lesions, the barium getting between the frond-like growths covering the surface and mixing with the tumor (Fig. 17-39).

Lymphoma

The various forms of lymphoma occur with less frequency in the colon than in the small intestine or stomach. When it occurs, lymphoma of the colon tends to have many of the malignant-appearing characteristics of carcinoma (Fig. 17-38), but over a more extensive length of colon. Often there is a large associated soft tissue mass. Lymphoma presenting as multinodular enlargement of the colonic lymphoid follicles has also been reported.

Leiomyosarcoma and Fibrosarcoma

Leiomyosarcoma and fibrosarcoma are the most frequently reported forms of colonic sarcoma other than lymphoma. Leiomyosarcomas tend to be large lesions that may outgrow their blood supply and thus become necrotic centrally, producing a large irregular ulcer within the lesion. As elsewhere in the gastrointestinal tract, any large smooth tumor measuring more than 5 cm in diameter and having a visible central ulceration should be suspected of being a leiomyosarcoma.

Carcinoid Tumors

While an occasional carcinoid tumor may occur in the colon, these lesions more often occur in the appendix or ileum. When small and localized to the appendix they are usually beyond radiologic detection. However, with increasing size, a carcinoid tumor may indent or invade the cecum. Other masses that may originate in the appendix include *mucocele, myxoglobulosis,* and *endometriosis.* These also indent the cecum when they reach sufficient size. Mucocele and its variant, myxoglobulosis, are the result of obstruction of the opening of the appendix into the cecum, and both may contain calcifications, particularly the latter.

Table 17-6. Cecal and
Ileocecal Masses

Neoplastic diseases
  Adenomatous polyp
  Lipoma
  Spindle cell tumor
  Carcinoma
  Villous adenoma
  Carcinoid tumor
  Lymphoma
Non-neoplastic diseases
  Ileocecal valve prolapse
  Appendiceal stump
  Periappendiceal abcess
  Intussusception
  Mucocele
  Duplication
  Endometriosis
  Amebiasis

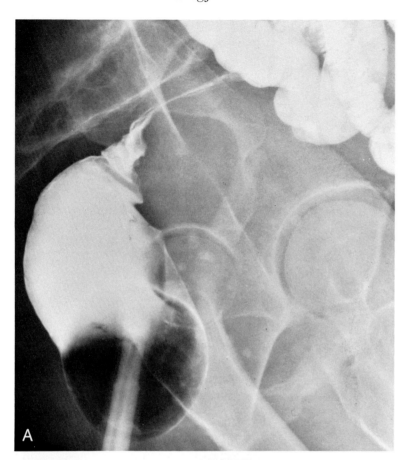

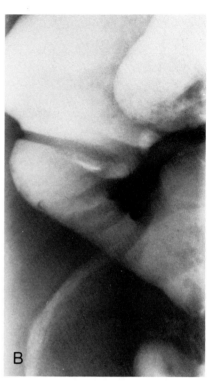

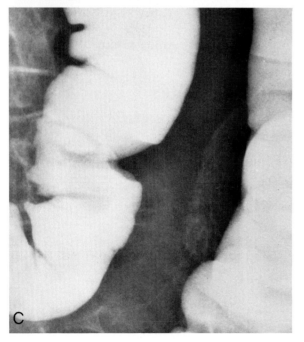

Fig. 17-40 (A) Narrowing of the rectosigmoid junction by a large tumor mass in the pouch of Douglas in a patient with carcinomatosis of the abdomen. (B) Infiltration and narrowing of the ascending colon in a patient with carcinoma of the pancreas. (C) Intramural nodule in the distal transverse colon representing a metastasis from carcinoma of the breast.

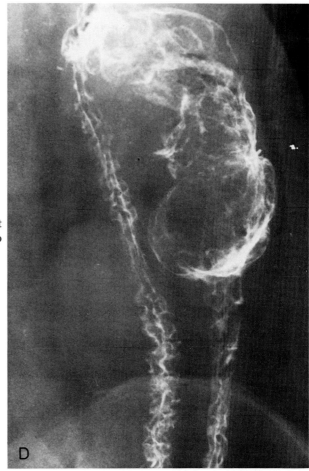

Fig. 17-40 *(continued)* (D) Large, obviously malignant polypoid lesion of the splenic flexure of the colon due to metastatic breast carcinoma.

The ileocecal region has a propensity for the development of mass lesions, and the wide variety of potential ileocecal masses is presented in Table 17-6.

Metastatic Carcinoma

Malignancies primary in other organs may metastasize to the colon by direct distension or by hematogenous seeding of the wall of the colon. Several distinct patterns of carcinoma metastatic to the colon can be recognized:

1. Carcinoma within the pouch of Douglas may involve the wall of the rectosigmoid region, pro-

ducing a bulky mass indenting the region (Fig. 17-40A).

2. Carcinomas of the stomach or pancreas may invade and indent the transverse colon along its superior aspect, or the ascending or descending colon on its medial aspect (Fig. 17-40B).

3. Hematogenous metastases manifest themselves in their earliest stages as small intramural submucosal nodules (Fig. 17-40C). They then grow rapidly and destroy the overlying mucosa, eventually becoming quite bulky and simulating a large polypoid or annular primary malignancy (Fig. 17-40D). Hematogenous metastases may also infiltrate the wall of the colon causing segmental narrowings simulating linitis plastica or granulomatous colitis. The most frequent tumors meta-

static to the colon by the hematogenous route are carcinoma of the breast and malignant melanoma.

EXTRINSIC MASSES

Over its course, the colon comes in intimate contact with most of the major organs of the abdominal cavity. Their enlargement displaces the colon, usually in a fashion characteristic for the specific organ. Hepatomegaly displaces the hepatic flexure of the colon inferiorly. Splenomegaly similarly displaces the splenic flexure inferiorly. Bulky tumors of the female reproductive organs, most commonly ovarian cysts and cystadenocarcinomas, tend to elevate the sigmoid colon up and out of the pelvis and usually displace the rectum posteriorly. Pancreatic masses often indent the superior aspect of the transverse colon and increase the distance between the transverse colon and the greater curvature of the stomach, which normally lie in close approximation. Infiltrating pancreatic disease, particularly severe pancreatitis, may cause an impression on the medial aspect of the ascending or descending colon, which lies within the same retroperitoneal space as the pancreas.

SUGGESTED READINGS

Structural Abnormalities

Bass EM: Duplication of the colon. Clin Radiol 29:205, 1978.

Beyer D, Friedmann G, Muller J: Duplication of the colon—report of two cases and review of the literature. Gastrointest Radiol 6:151, 1981.

Dick A, Green GJ: Large bowel intussusception in adults. Br J Radiol 34:769, 1961.

Dott NM: Anomalies of intestinal rotation: Their embryology and surgical aspects. Br J Surg 11:251, 1923.

Estrada RL: Anomalies of Intestinal Rotation and Fixation (Including Mentericoparietal Hernias). Springfield, IL, Charles C Thomas, 1958.

Franken EA: Gastrointestinal Radiology in Pediatrics. New York, Harper and Row, 1975, pp 172–177.

Goldberger LE, Berk RN: Cecal hernia into the lesser sac. Gastrointest Radiol 5:169, 1980.

Haskin PH, Teplick SK, Teplick JG, Haskin ME: Volvulus of the cecum and right colon. JAMA 245:2433, 1981.

Henisz A, Matesanz J, Wescott JL: Cecal herniation through the foramen of Winslow. Radiology 112:575, 1974.

Kerry RL, Lee F, Ransom HK: Roentgenologic examination in the diagnosis and treatment of colon volvulus. Am J Roentgenol 113:343, 1971.

Kim SK, Gerle RD, Rozanski R: Cathartic colitis. AJR 131:1079, 1978.

Lemaitre G, L'Herminé C, Decoulx M, et al: Radiologic aspects of chronic colitis due to laxative abuse. A study of four observations. J Belge Radiol 53:339, 1970.

Mapp E: Colonic manifestations of the connective tissue disorders. Am J Gastroenterol 75:386, 1981.

Maroy B, Ali Y, Tubiana JM, Monnier JP: Ischemic colitis and volvulus of the sigmoid colon. Ann Radiol 25:161, 1982.

Meszaros WT: The colon in systemic sclerosis (scleroderma). Am J Roentgenol 82:1000, 1959.

Pagacz AA, Vallée CA, Bovo M: Intussusception colique de l'adulte. J Can Assoc Radiol 31:107, 1980.

Sutcliffe MML: Volvulus of the sigmoid colon. Br J Surg 55:903, 1968.

teStrake L: Intussusception in adults. Diag Imaging 49:15, 1980.

Todd IP, Poster NH, Morson BC, et al: Chaga's disease of the colon and rectum. Gut 10:1009, 1969.

Young WS: Further radiological observations in caecal volvulus. Clin Radiol 31:479, 1980.

Young WS, White A, Grave GF: The radiology of ileosigmoid knot. Clin Radiol 29:211, 1978.

Inflammatory Diseases: Ulcerative Colitis and Crohn's Disease

Bartram CI: Radiology in the current assessment of ulcerative colitis. Gastrointest Radiol 1:383, 1977.

Bartram CI, Herlinger J: Bowel wall thickness as a differentiating feature betwen ulcerative colitis and Crohn's disease of the colon. Clin Radiol 30:15, 1979.

Berridge FR: Two unusual signs of Crohn's disease of the colon. Clin Radiol 32:443, 1971.

Brahme F: Granulomatous colitis. Am J Roentgenol 99:35, 1967.

Brahme F, Wenckert A: Spread of lesions in Crohn's disease of the colon. Gut 11:576, 1970.

Brunton FJ, Guyer PB: Diverticulum formation in Crohn's disease of the colon. Clin Radiol 30:39, 1979.

de Dombal FT, Geffen N, Darnborough A, et al: Radiological appearances of ulcerative colitis: An evaluation of their clinical significance. Gut 9:157, 1968.

de Dombal FT, Watts J McK, Watkinson G, Goligher JC: Local complication of ulcerative colitis: Stricture, pseudopolyps, and carcinoma of the colon and rectum. Br Med J 1:1442, 1966.

Farthing MJF, Lennard-Jones JE: Rectosacral distance and rectal size in ulcerative colitis. Br Med J 2:1266, 1977.

Ferrucci JT, Ragsdale BD, Barrett PJ, et al: Double tracking of the sigmoid colon. Radiology 120:307, 1976.

Frank PH, Riddell RH, Feczko PJ, Levin B: Radiological detection of colonic dysplasia (precarcinoma) in chronic ulcerative colitis. Gastrointest Radiol 3:209, 1978.

Fraser GM, Findlay JM: The double-contrast enema in ulcerative and Crohn's colitis. Clin Radiol 27:103, 1976.

Freeman AH, Berridge FR, Dick AP, et al: Pseudopolyposis in Crohn's disease. Clin Radiol 51:782, 1978.

Gabrielsson N, Granqvist S, Sundelin P, Thorgiersson T: Extent of inflammatory lesions in ulcerative colitis assessed by radiology, colonoscopy, and endoscopic biopsies. Gastrointest Radiol 4:395, 1979.

Goldberger LE, Neely HR, Stanner JC: Large mucosal bridges: An unusual roentgenographic manifestation of ulcerative colitis. Gastrointest Radiol 3:81, 1978.

Hildell J, Lindstrom C, Wenckert A: Radiographic appearances in Crohn's disease: I. Accuracy of radiographic methods. Acta Radiol Diag 20:609, 1978.

Hildell J, Lindstrom C, Wenckert A: Radiographic appearances in Crohn's disease: III. Colonic lesions following surgery. Acta Radiol Diag 21:71, 1980.

Joffe N: Diffuse mucosal granularity in double-contrast studies of Crohn's disease of the colon. Clin Radiol 32:85, 1981.

Kelvin FM, Gedgaudas RK: Radiologic diagnosis of Crohn's disease (with emphasis on its early manifestations). CRC Crit Rev Diagn Imaging July:43, 1981.

Kelvin FM, Oddson TA, Rice RP, et al: Double-contrast enema in Crohn's disease and ulcerative colitis. AJR 131:107, 1978.

Laufer I: Air contrast studies of the colon in inflammatory bowel disease. CRC Crit Rev Diagn Imaging 9:421, 1977.

Laufer I, Hamilton J: The radiological differentiation between ulcerative and granulomatous colitis by double contrast radiology. Am J Gastroenterol 66:259, 1976.

Laufer I, Mullens JE, Hamilton J: Correlation of endoscopy and double-contrast radiography in the early stages of ulcerative and granulomatous colitis. Radiology 118:1, 1976.

Lesher DT, Phillips JC, Rabinowitz JG: Pseudopolyposis as the only manifestation of ulcerative colitis. Am J Gastroenterol 70:670, 1978.

Lingg G, Nebel G, Dihlman W: Aphthous ulcers — early radiologic sign of Crohn's disease? Fortschr Roentgenstr 133:138, 1980.

Marshak RH, Lindner AE, Maklansky D: Granulomatous colitis. Mt Sinai J Med 46:431, 1979.

Marshak RH, Lindner AE, Maklansky D: Paracolic fistulous tracts in diverticulitis and granulomatous colitis. JAMA 243:1943, 1980.

Max RJ, Kelvin FM: Nonspecificity of discrete colonic ulceration on double-contrast barium enema study. AJR 134:1265, 1980.

Meredith JE, Carlson HD: Chronic ulcerative colitis and colon cancer. AJR 130:825, 1978.

Munro TG: Spasm in ulcerative colitis masquerading as carcinoma. J Can Assoc Radiol 30:171, 1979.

Neschis M, Siegelman SS, Parker JG: Diagnosis and management of the megacolon of ulcerative colitis. Gastrointerology 55:251, 1968.

Samach M, Train J: Demonstration of mucosal briding in Crohn's colitis. Am J Gastroenterol 74:50, 1980.

Simpkins KC, Apthoid ulcers in Crohn's disease. Clin Radiol 28:601, 1977.

Simpkins KC, Stevenson GW: The modified Malmö double-contrast barium enema in colitis: An assessment of its accuracy in reflecting sigmoidoscopic findings. Br J Radiol 45:486, 1972.

Williams HJ, Stephens DH, Carlson HC: Double-contrast radiography: Colonic inflammatory disease. AJR 137:315, 1981.

Wolf BS, Marshak RH: "Toxic" segmental dilitation of the colon during the course of fulminating ulcerative colitis: Roentgen findings. Am J Roentgenol 82:985, 1959.

Other Inflammatory Diseases

Balikian JP, Uthman SM, Khouri NF: Intestinal amebiasis. Am J Roentgenol 122:245, 1974.

Brodey PA, Fertig S, Aron JM: Campylobacter enterocolitis: Radiographic features. AJR 139:1199, 1982.

Carrera GJ, Young S, Lewicki AM: Intestinal tuberculosis. Gastrointest Radiol 1:147, 1976.

Chait A: Schistosomiasis mansoni: Roentgenologic observations in a nonendemic area. Am J Roentgenol 90:688, 1963.

El-Afifi S: Intestinal bilharziasis. Dis Colon Rectum 7:1, 1964.

Farman J, Rabinowitz J, Meyers MA: Roentgenology of infectious colitis. Am J Roentgenol 119:375, 1973.

Gardiner GA, Bird CR: Nonspecific ulcers of the colon resembling annular carcinoma. Radiology 137:331, 1980.

Guegan M, Gendre JP, Tubiana JM, et al: Radiologic examination in shigellosis. Ann Radiol 24:261, 1981.

Hill MC, Goldberg HI: Roentgen diagnosis of intestinal amebiasis. Am J Roentgenol 99:77, 1967.

Klein I: Roentgen study of lymphogranuloma venereum: Report of 24 cases. Am J Roentgenol 51:70, 1944.

Kolawole TM, Lewis EA: Radiologic observations on intestinal amebiaisis. Am J Roentgenol 122:257, 1974.

Kollitz JPM, Davis GB, Berk RN: Campylobacter colitis: A common infection born of acute colitis. Gastrointest Radiol 6:227, 1981.

Lewis EA, Kolawole TM: Tuberculous ileocolitis in Ibadan: A clinico-radiological review. Gut 13:646, 1972.

Lynch JJ, Beneventano TC: Typhoid fever: An unusual radiographic presentation with appendicitis. Am J Gastroenterol 73:168, 1980.

Martinez CR, Gilman RH, Rabbani GH, Koster F: Amebic colitis: Correlation of proctoscopy before treatment and barium enema after treatment. AJR 138:1089, 1982.

Mason GR, Dietrich P, Friedland GW, Hanks GE: The radiological findings in radiation-induced enteritis and colitis: A review of 30 cases. Clin Radiol 21:232, 1970.

Medina JT, Seamen WB, Guzman-Acosta C, Diaz-Bonnet RB: The roentgen appearance of schistosomiasis mansoni involving the colon. Radiology 85:682, 1965.

Meyer J: Radiography of the distal colon and rectum after irradiation of carcinoma of the cervic. AJR 136:691, 1981.

Palmer WL, Kirsner JB, Rodaniche EC: Studies on lymphogranuloma venereum infection of the rectum. JAMA 118:517, 1942.

Reeder MM, Hamilton LC: Tropical diseases of the colon. Semin Roentgenol 3:62, 1968.

Rodgers LF, Goldstein HM: Roentgen manifestations of radiation injury to the gastrointestinal tract. Gastrointest Radiol 2:281, 1977.

Thoeni RF, Margulis AR: Gastrointestinal tuberculosis. Semin Roentgenol 14:283, 1979.

Vaidya MG, Sodhi JS: Gastrointestinal tuberculosis: A study of 102 cases including 55 hemicolectomies. Clin Radiol 29:189, 1978.

Inflammatory Diseases: Ischemic Colitis

Bartram CI: Obliteration of thumbprinting with double-contrast enemas in acute ischemic colitis. Gastrointest Radiol 4:85, 1979.

de Dombal FT, Fletcher DM, Harris RS: Early diagnosis of ischaemic colitis. Gut 10:131, 1969.

Eisenberg RL, Montgomery CK, Margulis AR: Colitis in the elderly: Ischemic colitis mimicking ulcerative and granulomatous colitis. AJR 133:1113, 1979.

Gore RM, Calenoff L, Rogers LF: Roentgenographic manifestations of ischemic colitis. JAMA 241:171, 1979.

Marshak RH, Lindner AE: Ischemia of the colon. Semin Roentgenol 3:81, 1968.

Marshak RH, Lindner AE, Maklansky D: Ischmia of the colon. Mt Sinai J Med 48:180, 1981.

Reeders JWAJ, Rosenbusch G, Tytgat GNJ: Radiological aspects of ischaemic colitis. Diagn Imaging 50:4, 1981.

Inflammatory Diseases: Diverticular Disease

Beachley MC: Intramural masses secondary to diverticular disease of the colon. Am J Roentgenol 115:368, 1972.

Berk RN: Radiographic evaluation of spastic colon disease, diverticulosis, and diverticulitis. Gastrointest Endosc 26:26-S, 1980.

Diner WC, Barnhard HJ: Acute diverticulitis. Semin Roentgenol 8:415, 1973.

Fleischner FG: Diverticular disease of the colon: New observations and revised concepts. Gastroenterology 60:316, 1971.

Fleischner FG, Ming SC, Henken EM: Revised concepts of diverticular disease. Radiology 83:859, 1964.

Marshak RH, Lindner AE, Maklansky D: Diverticulosis and diverticulitis of the colon. Mt Sinai J Med 46:261, 1979.

Marshak RH, Lindner AE, Pochaczevsky R, Maklansky D: Longitudinal sinus tracts in granulomatous colitis and diverticulitis. Semin Roentgenol 11:101, 1976.

Williams I: Changing emphasis in diverticular disease of the colon. Br J Radiol 36:393, 1963.

Benign Neoplasms

Anderson TE, Spackman TJ, Schwartz SS: Roentgen findings in intestinal ganglioneuromatosis. Radiology 101:93, 1971.

Bussey HJR: Gastrointestinal polyposis: Progress report. Gut 11:970, 1970.

Bussey HJR: Familial Polyposis Coli. Baltimore, Johns Hopkins University Press, 1973.

Cronkhite LW Jr, Canada WJ: Generalized gastrointestinal polyposis. An unusual syndrome of polyposis, pigmentation, alopecia and onychotrophia. N Engl J Med 252:1011, 1955.

Diner WC: The Cronkhite-Canada syndrome. Radiology 105:715, 1971.

Dodds WJ: Clinical and roentgen features of the intestinal polyposis syndromes. Gastrointest Radiol 1:127, 1976.

Finkelstein AK, Stein GN, Roy RH: Colonic polyps: A radiologist's viewpoint. Radiol Clin North Am 1:175, 1963.

Fork FT: Double contrast enema and colonoscopy in polyp detection. Gut 22:971, 1981.

Gardner EJ, Richards RC: Multiple cutaneous and subcutaneous lesions occurring simultaneously with hereditary polyposis and osteomatosis. Am J Hum Genet 5:139, 1953.

Gordon RL, Evers K, Kressel HY, et al: Double-contrast enema in pelvic endometriosis. AJR 138:549, 1982.

Htoo AM, Bartram CI: The radiological diagnosis of polyps in the presence of diverticular disease. Br J Radiol 52:263, 1979.

Lane N, Fenoglio CM: The adenoma-carcinoma sequence in the stomach and colon: I. Observations on the adenoma a precursor to ordinary large bowel carcinoma. Gastrointest Radiol 1:111, 1976.

Laufer I, Smith NCW, Mullens JC: The radiological demonstration of colorectal polyps undetected by endoscopy. Gastroenterology 70:167, 1976.

Lawsen JP, Myerson PJ, Myerson DA: Colonic lymphangioma. Gastrointest Radiol 1:85, 1976.

Marshak RH, Lindner AE, Maklansky D: Familial polyposis. Am J Gastroenterol 67:177, 1977.

McAllister AJ, Richards KF: Peutz-Jehgers syndrome. Experience with twenty patients in five operations. Am J Surg 134:717, 1977.

Miller RE, Lehman G: Polypoid colonic lesions undetected by endoscopy. Radiology 129:195, 1978.

Morson B: The polyp-cancer sequence in the large bowel. Proc Roy Soc Med 67:451, 1974.

Ott DJ, Gelfand DW: Colorectal tumors: Pathology and detection. AJR 131:691, 1978.

Ott DJ, Gelfand DW, Wu WC, Kerr RM: Sensitivity of double-contrast barium enema: Emphasis on polyp detection. AJR 135:327, 1980.

Rosengren J, Hildell J, Lindstrom CG, Leandoer L: Localized colitis cystica profunda. Gastrointest Radiol 7:79, 1982.

Tavernier C, Jourde L, Dhamlencourt A-M, Delafolie A: L'endometriose colique: Diagnostic radiologique. J Radiol 61:437, 1980.

Thoeni R, Pelras A: Detection of rectal and rectosigmoid lesions by double-contrast barium enema examination and sigmoidoscopy. Radiology 142:59, 1982.

Turcot J, Despres J, St Pierre F: Malignant tumors of the central nervous system associated with familial polyposis of the colon: report of two cases. Dis Colon Rectum 2:465, 1959.

van Niekerk JP deV: Barium enema diagnosis of extensive angiomatous malformation. Br J Radiol 53:1095, 1980.

Williams SM, Woltjen JA, Le Veen RF: Lymphangioma: One of the soft lesions of the colon. Am J Gastroenterol 75:70, 1981.

Wiot JF, Felson B: Solitary benign colon tumors. Semin Roentgenol 11:123, 1976.

Yatto RP: Colonic lipomatosis. Am J Gastroenterol 77:436, 1982.

Malignant Neoplasms

Balthazar EJ: Gastrointestinal leiomyosarcoma—unusual sites: Esophagus, colon and porta hepatitis. Gastrointest Radiol 6:295, 1981.

Balthazar EJ, Rosenberg HD, Davidian MM: Primary and metastatic scirrhous carcinoma of the rectum. AJR 132:711, 1979.

Bartram CI, Hale JE: Radiological diagnosis of recurrent colonic carcinoma at the anastomosis. Gut 11:770, 1970.

Burgener FA, Hamlin DJ: Histiocytic lymphoma of the abdomen: Radiographic spectrum. AJR 137:337, 1981.

Delamarre J, Descombes P, Marti R, et al: Villous tumors of the colon and rectum: Double-contrast study of 47 cases. Gastrointest Radiol 5:69, 1980.

Fischel RE, Dermer R: Multifocal carcinoma of the large intestine. Clin Radiol 26:495, 1975.

Ginaldi S, Lindell MM, Zornoza J: The striped colon: A new radiographic observation in metastatic serosal implants. AJR 134:453, 1980.

Greenbaum EI, Friedman S: Neoplasia of the colon over a long segment. Clin Radiol 24:416, 1973.

Hodgson JR, Sauer WG: The roentgenologic features of carcinoma in chronic ulcerative colitis. Am J Roentgenol 86:91, 1961.

Joffe N: Symptomatic gastrointestinal metastases secondary to bronchogenic carcinoma. Clin Radiol 29:217, 1978.

Kaye JJ, Bragg DG: Unusual roentgenologic and clinico-pathologic features of villous adenomas of the colon. Radiology 91:799, 1968.

Khilnani MT, Marshak RH, Eliasoph J, Wolf BS: Roentgen features of metastases to the colon. Am J Roentgenol 96:302, 1966.

Lammer J, Dirschmid K, Hügel H: Carcinomatous metastases to the colon simulating Crohn's disease. Gastrointest Radiol 6:89, 1981.

Libshitz HI, Lindell MM, Dodds GD: Metastases to the hollow viscera. Radiol Clin North Am 20:487, 1982.

Marshak RH, Lindner AE, Maklansky D: Lymphoreticular disorders of the gastrointestinal tract: Roentgenographic features. Gastroinest Radiol 4:130, 1979.

Maruyama M: Radiologic Diagnosis of Polyps and Carcinoma of the Large Bowel (in English). New York,

Igaku Shoin, 1978.

Phalke IM, Smallwood CJ, Wright FW: Linitis plastica of the colon. Clin Radiol 20:224, 1969.

Ruppert GB, Smith VM: Multiple lymphomatous polyposis of the gastrointestinal tract. Gastrointest Endosc 25:67, 1979.

Sacks BA, Joffe N, Antonioli DA: Metastatic melanoma presenting clinically as multiple colonic polyps. Am J Roentgenol 129:511, 1977.

Seaman WB: Unusual roentgen manifestations of large bowel cancer. Semin Roentgenol 11:89, 1976.

Skucas J, Spataro RF, Cannucciari DP: The radiographic features of small colon cancers. Radiology 143:335, 1982.

Smith HJ, Vlasak MG: Metastasis to the colon from bronchogenic carcinoma. Gastrointest Radiol 2:393, 1978.

Welin S: The radiological detection of early carcinoma and premalignant lesions of the colon and rectum. J R Coll Surg Edinb 14:278, 1969.

Welin S, Welin G: The Double Contrast Examination of the Colon: Experiences with the Welin Modification. Stuttgart, George Thieme, 1976, pp 31–36.

Weyman PJ, Koehler RE: Roentgenologic CPC: Diffuse colonic nodularity and splenomegaly. Invest Radiol 15:2, 1980.

Wolf BS: Roentgen diagnosis of villous tumors of the colon. Am J Roentgenol 84:1093, 1960.

Young JR, Reddy ER: Peritoneal mesothelioma. Clin Radiol 31:243, 1980.

Extrinsic Masses

Abcarian H, Eftaiha M, Kraft AR, Nyhus LM: Colonic complications of acute pancreatitis. Arch Surg 114:995, 1979.

Chennells PM, Simpkins KC: The barium enema diagnosis of paracolic abscess. Clin Radiol 32:73, 1981.

Eliasoph J: Metastasis versus pancreatitis affecting the transverse colon. Mt Sinai J Med 48:201, 1981.

Kidd R, Freeny PC: Radiographic manifestations of extrinsic processes involving the bowel. Gastrointest Radiol 7:21, 1982.

Kyaw MM, Koehler PR: Pseudotumors of the colon due to adhesions. Radiology 103:597, 1972.

Schulman A, Fataar S: Extrinsic stretching, narrowing and anterior indentation of the rectosigmoid junction. Clin Radiol 30:463, 1979.

Soulard JM, et al: Colonic changes in perinephritis: Value of double-contrast examinations. J Radiol 60:503, 1979.

Appendiceal and Ileocecal Abnormalities

Bachman AL, Clemett AR: Roentgen aspects of primary appendiceal intussusception. Radiology 101:531, 1971.

Berk RN, Lasser EC: Radiology of the Ileocecal Area. Philadelphia, WB Saunders, 1975.

Euphrat EJ: Roentgen features of mucocele of the appendix. Radiology 48:113, 1947.

Hatten HP, Mostowycz L, Hagihara PF: Retrograde prolapse of the ileocecal valve. Am J Roentgenol 128:755, 1977.

Schnur MJ, Seaman WB: Prolapsing neoplasms of the terminal ileum simulating enlarged ileocecal valves. AJR 134:1136, 1980.

Short WE, Smith BD, Hoy RJ: Roentgenologic evaluation of the prominent or unusual ileocecal valve. Med Radiogr Photogr 52:2, 1976.

Simmons K, Sage MR: Mucocele of the appendix. Aust Radiol 23:33, 1979.

Skaane P, Eide TJ, Westgaard T, Gauperaa T: Lipomatosis and true lipomas of the ileocecal valve. Fortschr Roentgenstr 135:663, 1981.

Index

Page numbers followed by f represent figures; page numbers followed by t represent tables.